Herbal Medicine in Andrology
An Evidence-Based Update

Herbal Medicine in Andrology
An Evidence-Based Update

Edited by

Ralf Henkel
Department of Medical Biosciences, University of the Western Cape, Bellville,
South Africa
Department of Metabolism, Digestion and Reproduction, Imperial College London,
London, United Kingdom

Ashok Agarwal
Director, American Center for Reproductive Medicine; Professor, Lerner College of Medicine,
Cleveland Clinic, Cleveland, OH, United States

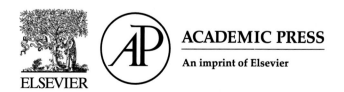

ELSEVIER

ACADEMIC PRESS
An imprint of Elsevier

Academic Press is an imprint of Elsevier
125 London Wall, London EC2Y 5AS, United Kingdom
525 B Street, Suite 1650, San Diego, CA 92101, United States
50 Hampshire Street, 5th Floor, Cambridge, MA 02139, United States
The Boulevard, Langford Lane, Kidlington, Oxford OX5 1GB, United Kingdom

Notices
Knowledge and best practice in this field are constantly changing. As new research and experience broaden our understanding, changes in research methods, professional practices, or medical treatment may become necessary.

Practitioners and researchers must always rely on their own experience and knowledge in evaluating and using any information, methods, compounds, or experiments described herein. In using such information or methods they should be mindful of their own safety and the safety of others, including parties for whom they have a professional responsibility.

To the fullest extent of the law, neither the Publisher nor the authors, contributors, or editors, assume any liability for any injury and/or damage to persons or property as a matter of products liability, negligence or otherwise, or from any use or operation of any methods, products, instructions, or ideas contained in the material herein.

Library of Congress Cataloging-in-Publication Data
A catalog record for this book is available from the Library of Congress

British Library Cataloguing-in-Publication Data
A catalogue record for this book is available from the British Library

ISBN 978-0-12-815565-3

For information on all Academic Press publications
visit our website at https://www.elsevier.com/books-and-journals

Publisher: Stacy Masucci
Editorial Project Manager: Sam Young
Production Project Manager: Maria Beranard
Cover Designer: Miles Hitchen

Typeset by SPi Global, India

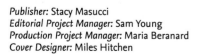

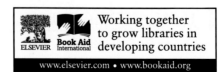

Dedication

To my late parents Waldemar and Helga Henkel for instilling the values of hard work, perseverance, and dedication. To my academic teachers, Professor Christoph Kirchner (Philipps University, Marburg, Germany) and Professor Wolf-Bernhard Schill (Justus Liebig University, Giessen, Germany) for guiding me in my academic career and continuous support. To my wife, Adv. Sharon Henkel for her unconditional love and support, without which I would not be able to do this work.

Ralf Henkel

This book is dedicated to my father Professor RC Agarwal (late) for instilling the virtues of honesty, dedication, and hard work; to my wonderful wife Meenu and sons Rishi and Neil-Yogi for their unconditional love and support; to Professor Kevin Loughlin (Harvard Medical School), Professor Anthony Thomas (late) (Cleveland Clinic), and Professor Edmund Sabanegh (Cleveland Clinic) for their friendship, guidance, and support, which left an indelible positive impression on my life; and to my associates at work, large number of researchers and students, and most importantly the patients who placed their trust in our work.

Ashok Agarwal

Contents

Contributors

Numbers in parentheses indicate the pages on which the authors' contributions begin.

Ashok Agarwal (93,129), American Center for Reproductive Medicine, Cleveland Clinic, Cleveland, OH, United States

Dulce Esperanza Alarcón-Yaquetto (47), Endocrinology and Reproduction Unit, Research and Development Laboratories (LID), Department of Biological and Physiological Sciences, Faculty of Sciences and Philosophy; High Altitude Research Institute, Universidad Peruana Cayetano Heredia, Lima, Peru

Roodabeh Bahramsoltani (67), Department of Traditional Pharmacy, School of Persian Medicine, Tehran University of Medical Sciences; PhytoPharmacology Interest Group (PPIG), Universal Scientific Education and Research Network (USERN), Tehran, Iran

Saptaparna Chakraborty (129), Department of Life Science and Bioinformatics, Assam University, Silchar, India

Rima Dada (1,9), Molecular Reproduction and Genetics, Department of Anatomy, AIIMS, New Delhi, India

Anandan Das (129), Department of Life Science and Bioinformatics, Assam University, Silchar, India

Damayanthi Durairajanayagam (93), Physiology, Faculty of Medicine, Universiti Teknologi MARA (UiTM), Sungai Buloh, Selangor, Malaysia

Elizabeth Oyebola Egieyeh (227), School of Pharmacy, University of the Western Cape, Cape Town, South Africa

Samuel Ayodele Egieyeh (227), School of Pharmacy, University of the Western Cape, Cape Town, South Africa

Lourens Johannes Christoffel Erasmus (37,123), Physiology and Environmental Health, University of Limpopo, Mankweng, Limpopo Province, South Africa

Diego Fano-Sizgorich (47), Endocrinology and Reproduction Unit, Research and Development Laboratories (LID), Department of Biological and Physiological Sciences, Faculty of Sciences and Philosophy, Universidad Peruana Cayetano Heredia, Lima, Peru

Manuel Gasco (47), Endocrinology and Reproduction Unit, Research and Development Laboratories (LID), Department of Biological and Physiological Sciences, Faculty of Sciences and Philosophy; High Altitude Research Institute, Universidad Peruana Cayetano Heredia, Lima, Peru

Annie George (215), Biotropics Malaysia Berhad, Shah Alam, Selangor Darul Ehsan, Malaysia

Gustavo F. Gonzales (47), Endocrinology and Reproduction Unit, Research and Development Laboratories (LID), Department of Biological and Physiological Sciences, Faculty of Sciences and Philosophy; High Altitude Research Institute, Universidad Peruana Cayetano Heredia, Lima, Peru

Pokhraj Guha (129), Department of Zoology, Garhbeta College, Paschim Medinipur, West Bengal, India

Ralf Henkel (9,129), Department of Medical Bioscience, University of the Western Cape, Bellville, South Africa; American Center for Reproductive Medicine, Department of Urology, Cleveland Clinic, Cleveland, OH, United States; Department of Metabolism, Digestion and Reproduction, Imperial College London, London, United Kingdom

Isadore Kanfer (175), Faculty of Pharmacy, Rhodes University, Grahamstown, South Africa; Leslie Dan Faculty of Pharmacy, University of Toronto, Canada

Kristian Leisegang (123,189), School of Natural Medicine, University of the Western Cape, Bellville, Cape Town, South Africa

Eckehard Liske (215), Departments of Life Sciences, Technical University of Braunschweig, Braunschweig, Germany

Xuesheng Ma (147), School of Natural Medicine, Faculty of Community and Health Science, University of the Western Cape, Cape Town, South Africa

Juliana Meredith (147), Red Rose Dragon Chinese Medicine and Acupuncture Centre, Riebeeck Kasteel, South Africa

Paul F. Moundipa (83), Laboratory of Pharmacology and Toxicology, Department of Biochemistry, University of Yaounde I, Yaounde, Cameroon

Chinyerum S. Opuwari (83), Department of Pre-Clinical Sciences, University of Limpopo, Polokwane, South Africa

Srinivas Patnala (189), Faculty of Pharmacy, Rhodes University, Grahamstown, South Africa

Roja Rahimi (67), Department of Traditional Pharmacy, School of Persian Medicine, Tehran University of Medical Sciences; PhytoPharmacology Interest Group (PPIG), Universal Scientific Education and Research Network (USERN), Tehran, Iran

Shubhadeep Roychoudhury (129), Department of Life Science and Bioinformatics, Assam University, Silchar, India; Department of Morphology, Physiology and Animal Genetics, Mendel University, Brno, Czech Republic

Pooja Sabharwal (1,9), Department of Rachana Sharir, CBPACS, New Delhi, India

Pallav Sengupta (93), Physiology, MAHSA University, Jenjarom, Selangor, Malaysia

Akanksha Sharma (1,9), Department of Rachana Sharir, CBPACS, New Delhi, India

Ismail Tambi (27,107), Men Wellness Clinic, Damai Service Hospital, Kuala Lumpur, Malaysia

Cinthya Vasquez-Velasquez (47), Endocrinology and Reproduction Unit, Research and Development Laboratories (LID), Department of Biological and Physiological Sciences, Faculty of Sciences and Philosophy; High Altitude Research Institute, Universidad Peruana Cayetano Heredia, Lima, Peru

About the editors

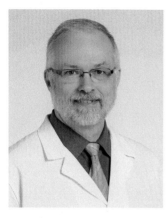

Ralf Henkel, BEd, PhD, Habil., studied Biology and Chemistry at the University of Marburg, Germany, and obtained his PhD in 1990. Ralf continued his post-doctoral training and obtained his Habilitation at the University of Giessen, School of Medicine in 1998. From 1998 to 2004, he was an Assistant, Associate and Extraordinary Professor, at the Justus-Liebig University of Giessen, Germany, before he accepted a Full Professorship at the Department of Urology at the University of Jena, Germany. From 2005 to 2020, he was Professor and Head of Department at the Department of Medical Bioscience at the University of the Western Cape, Bellville, South Africa. Currently, he is an Extraordinary Professor at that department. He is also Honorary Professor at the Universidad Peruana Cayetano Heredia, Lima, Peru, Visiting Reader in the Department of Metabolism, Digestion and Reproduction at the Imperial College London, London, United Kingdom, and Editor-in-Chief of Andrologia. Ralf has published more than 162 original and review articles as well as 47 book chapters and supervised more than 71 Hons/MSc/MD/PhD postgraduate students' theses. For his research, Ralf received 16 awards. Ralf has received 26 research grants for numerous research projects to investigate the impact of oxidative stress on sperm functions, DNA fragmentation and fertilization, as well as the effects of Herbal Medicine on male reproductive functions including prostate cancer and benign prostatic hyperplasia.

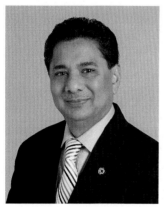

Ashok Agarwal, PhD, HCLD (ABB), ELD (ACE) is the head of Andrology Center and the director of research at the American Center for Reproductive Medicine since 1993. He holds these positions at The Cleveland Clinic Foundation, where he is the professor of surgery (urology) at the Lerner College of Medicine of Case Western Reserve University. Ashok was trained in male infertility and andrology at the Brigham and Women's Hospital and Harvard Medical School and later worked as assistant professor of urology at Harvard from 1988 to 1992. Ashok has over 28 years of experience in directing busy male infertility diagnostic facilities and fertility preservation services. He has published over 800 scientific papers and reviews in peer-reviewed scientific journals and is ranked in Scopus as the #1 author in the world in the fields of male infertility/andrology and human-assisted reproduction based on the number of peer-reviewed publications, citation scores (Scopus: 36,673; Google Scholar: 77,026), and h-index (Scopus: 103; Google Scholar: 136). He is currently the editor of more than 42 medical text books/manuals related to male infertility, ART, fertility preservation, DNA damage, and antioxidants and is active in basic and clinical research. His laboratory has trained over 1000 scientists, clinicians, graduate, and undergraduate students from the United States and more than 55 countries. Ashok is the recipient of over 100 grants totaling over 15 million dollars. His current research interests include proteomics of male infertility and the molecular markers of oxidative stress and DNA integrity in the pathophysiology of male reproduction.

Foreword

The issue of herbal medicine has gained increasing worldwide attention. Considering that about 80% of the global population have to rely on traditional remedies including herbal medicine for their primary health care, it is extremely important to investigate if and how these herbal remedies work. In the past, important medicines such as Aspirin® were initially isolated from plant extracts and then extensively investigated using modern scientific methods. This approach laid the foundation for evidence-based pharmaceutical drugs.

People in every country and region use certain specific medicinal plants. Some examples of these are St. John's wort in Europe as a mild antidepressant, coca in South America to prevent altitude sickness, or ginger in Asia as a remedy to alleviate nausea and vomiting. However, while in the western world these herbal extracts are known and clinically used for a variety of ailments, little is known about herbal remedies, their effects, usefulness, and interactions with other medicines in the field of andrology. Yet, in the past 5–10 years, in the quest of increasing the clinical repertoire to treat andrological patients, there has been an increase in the number of publications in which traditional herbal medicines were studied. In recent years, progress has been made by an increasing number of scientists who studied nontoxic plant extracts using biochemical technology to extract and evaluate defined chemical compounds and subsequently investigated their possible mechanism of action. Currently, herbal medicine for the treatment of andrological issues is mainly used in Asia, particularly in China with reference to traditional Chinese medicine, Indonesia, the Indian subcontinent, Africa, the Middle East, and South America, whereas it plays a minor role as therapeutic agents in Europe and North America.

This textbook, *"Herbal Medicine in Andrology: An Evidence-based Update,"* coedited by two highly renowned andrologists, Professor Ralf Henkel and Professor Ashok Agarwal, is the first of its kind that has gathered information about the most important plants and their extracts used all over the world to treat andrological diseases and conditions such as male infertility or prostate diseases. The editors have brought together an impressive group of international experts (biologists, clinicians, and pharmacists) to share their knowledge on the topic of herbal medicine use in andrology. The book is divided into eight sections that cover this important area of clinical andrology. The first section of the book presents an introduction to the topic with an historic overview and pharmacognosy. The second section presents an overview on the clinical presentation and indications for which herbal medicines are used, whereas the third section discusses specific herbal medicines from all regions of the world, including Chinese Medicine with reference to clinical trials in an evidence-based manner. This section is followed by sections on quality control and extraction aspects, legal regulations, herbal medicines and their interaction with other drugs, as well as its acceptance by patients and clinicians. Finally, the current status of integration of herbal medicines in clinical practice and the possible development of the market, along with the need for more research is discussed.

Hence, this book summarizes the most recent data on herbal medicine with special reference to andrology. Since medicine and pharmacy are going back to nature for the development of new drugs, this rapidly developing area of research will help in the finding of new remedies to treat patients as more information is required about the influence of herbal extracts on the hormonal profile of men in regulating spermatogenesis as well as their influence on the prostate. Herbal medicine will also open new avenues in the treatment of symptoms in the aging males.

Therefore, the aim of this book is to reach both clinicians and researchers working in the field of andrology. I believe that it will be of great value in the future progress and development of herbal medicine in andrology. I am delighted to highly recommend this first book on Herbal Medicine in Andrology as a reliable resource and important reference work for biologists and clinicians in this developing field of male reproductive health.

Wolf-Bernhard Schill

Department of Dermatology and Andrology, Justus Liebig University of Giessen, Giessen, Germany

Preface

Infertility is a global health concern affecting over 190 million couples in reproductive age of which half is due to a male factor, which contributes about 50% to infertility in general. Modern western medicines including reproductive medicine, and andrological medicine in specific, are expensive and put a strain not only on the health systems but also on couples desiring their own child, specifically in emerging economies or poor countries. About 80% of the global population relies on traditional remedies for their primary health care for traditional beliefs and because they are more affordable than western medicines. In addition, even in First World countries, many people are concerned about pharmaceutical drugs due to their known and unknown side effects and high cost. As a result, the market for herbal products is booming. On the other hand, only very few plant products such as yohimbin from the African Yohimbe tree are used in western medicine to treat andrological problems. Since herbal medicine is an under-investigated field, more light needs to be shed on the treatment options that plant products provide to treat male infertility and other kinds of andrological problems. Therefore, there is an urgent need not only to explore the opportunities that herbal medicine provides to treat andrological problems, but also to inform clinicians and scientists about the effects of herbal extracts on male reproductive functions.

This book provides a detailed description of the currently known, traditionally used herbal remedies from all over the world to treat andrological problems. Renowned experts from 10 countries have generously contributed 20 state-of-the-art chapters for this book. Our book provides detailed information on plants from different continents that can be used to treat a multitude of andrological conditions. The book also includes a brief history of herbal medicine as well as herbal pharmacognosy and aspects of quality control and legal regulations.

The combination of basic herbal science and clinical information makes our book well suited for fertility practitioners, andrologists, urologists, medical doctors, reproductive professional, and research students.

We are grateful to our contributors, who are distinguished leaders in the field with extensive experience from around the world.

This book would not have been possible without the excellent support of Elsevier. We are thankful to Tari Broderick, senior acquisition editor, and Sam Young, editorial project manager for an excellent management of this project. The editors are grateful to their families for their love and support.

We genuinely hope that this volume will support and enrich your clinical practice in clinical andrology.

Ralf Henkel
Ashok Agarwal

Introduction

Damayanthi Durairajanayagam[a], Ashok Agarwal[b], Ralf Henkel[b,c,d]

[a]Department of Physiology, Faculty of Medicine, Universiti Teknologi MARA (UiTM), Sungai Buloh, Selangor, Malaysia, [b]American Center for Reproductive Medicine, Cleveland Clinic, Cleveland, OH, United States, [c]Department of Metabolism, Digestion and Reproduction, Imperial College London, London, United Kingdom, [d]Department of Medical Bioscience, University of the Western Cape, Bellville, South Africa

Traditional medicine is practiced around the globe either as a basis for health care or as a counterpart to it, whereby it is termed as complementary medicine [1]. Both traditional and complementary medicines are a mainstay in most countries worldwide. The increasing demand for its services supports the importance of traditional and complementary medicines as part of health care. Herbal medicine is a widespread and important form of traditional and complementary medicines that has been used since ancient times. The World Health Organization (WHO) defines herbal medicines as those that include "herbs, herbal materials, herbal preparations, and finished herbal products that contain, as active ingredients, parts of plants, other plant materials, or combinations thereof" [2]. The use of herbal medicines and interest in this branch of traditional medicine continue to grow in both developing and developed countries. Herbal medicines and remedies serve as either treatment or complementary/alternative therapy for a variety of acute and chronic conditions, including infertility and other reproductive disorders.

The book *Herbal Medicine in Andrology: An Evidence-Based Update* is a unique collection of articles that highlight the current knowledge and significant aspects regarding the use of herbal medicines in dealing with issues of the male reproductive tract. This first edition of the book provides a comprehensive overview of herbal-based approaches in andrology, which are well described within 20 chapters. The contributing authors of these chapters are clinicians, pharmacists, and scientists from 20 different institutions located in 10 countries across the globe who were carefully selected based on their expertise in the field. This book is divided into three main sections: the first section defines herbal medicine and describes its development as a therapeutic modality; the second section takes a closer look at some of the commonly used herbal medicines from various regions around the world; and the third section deals with issues regarding the regulatory and procedural processes involved in developing medicinal plants into a product of standardized quality for mass consumption.

In Chapter 1 of the first section, readers are introduced to the historical background of herbal medicine use [3]. In Chapter 2, Dada and colleagues delve into the utility of herbal medicines as a treatment option as either primary or supplementary therapy [4]. They emphasize the need for conventionally trained physicians to also familiarize themselves with common herbal remedies to bolster a more open and forthcoming doctor-patient relationship. Physicians may find it informative to read scientific articles on these common herbs and secondary plant metabolites to broaden their understanding of herbal medicines and how they work. Chapter 3 explores the increased scientific focus on herbal pharmacognosy in the search for novel therapeutic molecules that have the potential to be developed into medicines for use in clinical practice [5]. Chapters 4 and 5 in the first section give an overview of clinical presentations and indications of male reproductive disorders and how these may potentially be managed using herbal medicines [6, 7].

The second section of the book probes deeper into the use of herbal medicines from various parts of the globe, such as Asia and the Indian subcontinent, China, Europe, America, Middle East, and Africa in the treatment of andrology-related issues. The 10 chapters in this section provide readers with evidence-based updates on the plant-based herbal remedies normally used to treat male reproductive disorders and offers insights into the possible mechanisms through which these herbs may be acting. Asia is a continent blessed with a cornucopia of herbs. Among the selected herbs from Asia and the Indian subcontinent that are discussed in this book are *Eleutherococcus senticosus* and *Astragalus membranaceus* [8], *Withania somnifera*, *Panax ginseng*, and *Centella asiatica* [9], *Eurycoma longifolia* jack [10], *Zingiber officinale*, and *Epimedium grandiflorum* [11], as well as *Ginkgo biloba*, *Curcuma longa*, and *Camellia sinensis* [12]. The practice of herbal therapy is deeply rooted in traditional Chinese medicine. With regards to this, Ma and Meredith have described several tonic herbs that are traditionally used in treating ailments of the reproductive tract, namely *Herba Epimedii*, *Lycium barbarum*, *Herba Cistanches*, *Semen Cuscutae*, *Radix Morindae Officinalis*, and *Fructus Psoraleae* [13]. Europe also shares a vibrant history with respect to the use of herbal medicines. For example, *Pinus pinaster* extracts serve as a source of procyanidins to combat oxidative stress, while a combination of *Urtica dioica* and *Serenoa repens (an older synonym for the species is Sabal serrulata)* are clinically used in managing benign prostatic hyperplasia-induced lower urinary tract symptoms in European practice [14]. The Americas too are immensely rich in native medicinal plants. Among the species of herbs from the geographical subregions of North America, Central America and the Caribbean, and South America that are discussed include *Lepidium meyenii* (Maca), *Serenoa repens*, and *Cucurbita pepo* [15]. The wide array of medicinal herbs traditionally used in treating andrological conditions in countries of the Middle East [16] and Africa [17] are also described.

The final section of the book deals with issues concerning the development of herbal medicines and medicinal plants that have long been utilized in traditional medicine practices into quality-controlled products for clinical use. This section highlights the multiple legal and procedural processes involved in product development before it can become a marketable product. Emphasis is placed on the need for appropriate regulatory measures to facilitate strict quality control of raw plant materials along with standardized extraction, formulation, and manufacturing procedures [18, 19]. Implementation of qualified reference standards, good manufacturing practices, and regulatory requirements contribute greatly in producing herbal medicines of standardized quality. The clinical implications of drug interactions due to coadministration of conventional and herbal medicines in andrology are also described [20]. Evidence from clinical trials performed using traditional herbs, namely *E. longifolia*, *L. meyenii*, *W. somnifera*, and *Trigonella foenum-graecum* are reviewed along with regulatory issues associated with the acceptance of herbal medicines in andrology [21]. The final chapter of this book illustrates the factors affecting the integration of traditional herbal medicine into contemporary clinical practice and propose several strategies for its improvement [22].

With limited publications available on the clinical use of herbal medicines in treating andrological patients, the chapters included in this book provide immense value to both clinicians and scientists working in the evolving field of male reproductive health. It serves as a comprehensive and valuable evidence-based resource for a wide readership that include urologists, gynecologists, reproductive endocrinologists, andrologists, and basic scientists. We hope that you, as our readers, will appreciate the tremendous value of this book and share our enthusiasm for integrating herbal medicines into evidence-based clinical management of male sexual and reproductive health disorders.

References

[1] World Health Organization. WHO traditional medicine strategy: 2014–2023. Geneva: World Health Organization; Dec 2013, ISBN:978-92-4-150609-0. Cited 23 May 2020. Available from: http://apps.who.int/iris/bitstream/10665/92455/1/9789241506090_eng.pdf.

[2] World Health Organization. WHO global report on traditional and complementary medicine 2019. Geneva: World Health Organization; 2019, ISBN:978-92-4-151543-6. Cited 23 May 2020. Available from: https://www.who.int/publications-detail/who-global-report-on-traditional-and-complementary-medicine-2019.

[3] Sharma A, Sabharwal P, Dada R. Herbal medicine—an introduction to its history. In: Henkel R, Agarwal A, editors. Herbal medicine in andrology: An evidence-based update. 1st ed. Academic Press; 2020, ISBN:978-0-1281-5565-3 [chapter 1].

[4] Dada R, Sabharwal P, Sharma A, Henkel R. Use of herbal medicine as primary or supplementary treatments. In: Henkel R, Agarwal A, editors. Herbal medicine in andrology: An evidence-based update. 1st ed. Academic Press; 2020, ISBN:978-0-1281-5565-3 [chapter 2].

[5] Leisegang K. Herbal pharmacognosy: an introduction. In: Henkel R, Agarwal A, editors. Herbal medicine in andrology: An evidence-based update. 1st ed. Academic Press; 2020, ISBN:978-0-1281-5565-3 [chapter 3].

[6] Tambi I. Overview on the clinical presentation and indications (Part A). In: Henkel R, Agarwal A, editors. Herbal medicine in andrology: An evidence-based update. 1st ed. Academic Press; 2020, ISBN:978-0-1281-5565-3 [chapter 4].

[7] Erasmus L. Overview on the clinical presentation and indications (Part B). In: Henkel R, Agarwal A, editors. Herbal medicine in andrology: An evidence-based update. 1st ed. Academic Press; 2020, ISBN:978-0-1281-5565-3 [chapter 5].

[8] Opuwari CS. Herbal medicine use to treat andrological problems: Asia and Indian sub-continent—*Eleutherococcus senticosus, Astragalus membranaceus*. In: Henkel R, Agarwal A, editors. Herbal medicine in andrology: An evidence-based update. 1st ed. Academic Press; 2020, ISBN:978-0-1281-5565-3 [chapter 6].

[9] Sengupta P, Durairajanayagam D, Agarwal A. Herbal medicine use to treat andrological problems: Asia and Indian sub-continent: *Withania somnifera, Panax ginseng, Centella asiatica*. In: Henkel R, Agarwal A, editors. Herbal medicine in andrology: An evidence-based update. 1st ed. Academic Press; 2020, ISBN:978-0-1281-5565-3 [chapter 10].

[10] Tambi I. Herbal medicine use to treat andrological problems: Asia and Indian sub-continent: *Tongkat Ali (Eurycoma longifolia* jack). In: Henkel R, Agarwal A, editors. Herbal medicine in andrology: An evidence-based update. 1st ed. Academic Press; 2020, ISBN:978-0-1281-5565-3 [chapter 11].

[11] Erasmus L. Herbal medicine use to treat andrological problems: Asia and Indian sub-continent: *Zingiber officinale, Epimedium grandiflorum*. In: Henkel R, Agarwal A, editors. Herbal medicine in andrology: An evidence-based update. 1st ed. Academic Press; 2020, ISBN:978-0-1281-5565-3 [chapter 12].

[12] Roychoudhury S, Chakraborty S, Das A, Guha P, Agarwal A, Henkel R. Herbal medicine use to treat andrological problems: Asia and Indian sub-continent: *Ginkgo biloba, Curcuma longa, Camellia sinensis*. In: Henkel R, Agarwal A, editors. Herbal medicine in andrology: An evidence-based update. 1st ed. Academic Press; 2020, ISBN:978-0-1281-5565-3 [chapter 13].

[13] Ma X, Meredith J. Herbal medicine for the treatment of andrological diseases: Traditional Chinese Medicine. In: Henkel R, Agarwal A, editors. Herbal medicine in andrology: An evidence-based update. 1st ed. Academic Press; 2020, ISBN:978-0-1281-5565-3 [chapter 14].

[14] Leisegang K. Herbal medicine use to treat andrological problems: Europe. In: Henkel R, Agarwal A, editors. Herbal medicine in andrology: An evidence-based update. 1st ed. Academic Press; 2020, ISBN:978-0-1281-5565-3 [chapter 15].

[15] Gonzales GF, Gasco M, Vasquez-Velasquez C, Fano D, Alarcón-Yaquetto DE. Herbal medicine use to treat andrological problems: Americas. In: Henkel R, Agarwal A, editors. Herbal medicine in andrology: An evidence-based update. 1st ed. Academic Press; 2020, ISBN:978-0-1281-5565-3 [chapter 7].

[16] Bahramsoltani R, Rahimi R. Herbal medicine use to treat andrological problems: Middle East. In: Henkel R, Agarwal A, editors. Herbal medicine in andrology: An evidence-based update. 1st ed. Academic Press; 2020, ISBN:978-0-1281-5565-3 [chapter 8].

[17] Opuwari CS, Moundipa PF. Herbal medicine use to treat andrological problems: Africa. In: Henkel R, Agarwal A, editors. Herbal medicine in andrology: An evidence-based update. 1st ed. Academic Press; 2020, ISBN:978-0-1281-5565-3 [chapter 9].

[18] Patnala S, Kafner I. Quality control, extraction methods and standardization: interface between traditional use and scientific investigation. In: Henkel R, Agarwal A, editors. Herbal medicine in andrology: An evidence-based update. 1st ed. Academic Press; 2020, ISBN:978-0-1281-5565-3 [chapter 16].

[19] Kafner I, Patnala S. Regulations for the use of herbal remedies. In: Henkel R, Agarwal A, editors. Herbal medicine in andrology: An evidence-based update. 1st ed. Academic Press; 2020, ISBN:978-0-1281-5565-3 [chapter 17].

[20] Moundipa PF. Herbal medicines used for andrological problems and drug interactions. In: Henkel R, Agarwal A, editors. Herbal medicine in andrology: An evidence-based update. 1st ed. Academic Press; 2020, ISBN:978-0-1281-5565-3 [chapter 18].

[21] George A, Liske E. Acceptance of herbal medicines in andrology. In: Henkel R, Agarwal A, editors. Herbal medicine in andrology: An evidence-based update. 1st ed. Academic Press; 2020, ISBN:978-0-1281-5565-3 [chapter 19].

[22] Ayodele ES, Oyebola EE. The status of integration of herbal medicines into modern clinical practice and possible development of the market. In: Henkel R, Agarwal A, editors. Herbal medicine in andrology: An evidence-based update. 1st ed. Academic Press; 2020, ISBN:978-0-1281-5565-3 [chapter 20].

Chapter 1

Herbal medicine—An introduction to its history

Akanksha Sharma[a], Pooja Sabharwal[a], and Rima Dada[b]

[a]Department of Rachana Sharir, CBPACS, New Delhi, India, [b]Molecular Reproduction and Genetics, Department of Anatomy, AIIMS, New Delhi, India

1 Introduction

Herbal medicine is a practice that includes herbs, herbal material, and preparations that contain parts of plants or combinations thereof as active ingredients. These herbs are derived from plant parts such as leaves, bark, flowers, roots, fruits, and seeds [1].

The World Health Organization (WHO) defined traditional medicine (including herbal drugs) as therapeutic practices that have been in existence for hundreds of years, before the development and expansion of modern medicine, but are still practiced presently. Herbal drugs constitute only those traditional medicines that primarily use medicinal plant preparations for therapy. The earliest recorded evidence of their use in Indian, Chinese, Egyptian, Greek, Roman, and Syrian texts dates back about 5000 years. The classical Indian texts include *Rigveda*, *Atharvaveda*, *Charaka Samhita*, and *Sushruta Samhita* [2].

Generally, it is estimated that about 80% of the global population relies on herbal remedies for their primary health care, a figure that varies in different countries [3]. Data from the WHO reveal that the population in developing countries such as India (65%–70%), Rwanda (~75%), Tanzania (50%–60%), Uganda (55%–60%), Benin (80%), and Ethiopia (90%) widely utilize their traditional and alternative medications for healthcare services. Even in developed countries such as Australia (48%–50%), Belgium (30%), France (50%), the United States (45%), and Canada (65%–70%), a remarkable proportion of the population is utilizing traditional cures occasionally for human health services [4–6].

It is hard to obtain exact figures for the aggregate number of medicinal plants on earth; in one estimation, around 35,000–70,000 plant species are being used worldwide in human healthcare services, and Indian Pharmacopeia alone incorporates more than 3000 drugs of natural origin [7].

According to the WHO, 80% of the population in developing countries depends almost entirely on traditional medicine practices and herbal medicines for their primary healthcare needs [8]. Furthermore, at the beginning of the 21st century, the worldwide annual market for herbal medicinal products approached US$60 billion [9] and the long tradition of herbal medicine continues to the present day in China, Indian, and many countries in Africa and South America.

2 Historical perspective of herbal medicine

Worldwide, people have been using herbal medicine for the treatment, control, and management of a variety of ailments since prehistoric times. The earliest written account of herbal medicine came from China and dates back to 2800 BC, and archeological remains from early civilizations have revealed that plants were used in burials and other rituals. Physical evidence of the use of herbal remedies goes back 60,000 years to a Neanderthal man's grave uncovered in Northern Iraq in 1960. An analysis of the soil revealed extraordinary quantities of plant pollen at the grave, which were medicinal plants still in use today [10].

2.1 Vedic and Medieval era

The foundation of traditional medical knowledge on the Indian subcontinent is known as the ancient Vedic era (c.1500–500 BC), during the settlements of the first Indo-Aryan tribes in Northwest India and the Ganges plain. This period corresponds to the *Vedas* (*Rigveda*, *Yajurveda*, *Samaveda*, and *Atharvaveda*). There is an intense relation between Indian traditional medicine and the *Vedas* [11]. The *Vedic* sages adopted passages from the *Vedic* scriptures relating to Ayurveda and compiled books dealing only in Ayurveda. One of these books, called the *Aatreya Samhita*, is among the oldest medical books in the world.

Herbal Medicine in Andrology. https://doi.org/10.1016/B978-0-12-815565-3.00001-1

Ayurveda is the appurtenance of *Atharvaveda*. Worldwide, people have been using herbal medicine for the treatment, control, and management of a variety of ailments since prehistoric times. In India, herbal medicine, the *Rigveda*, a collection of Hindu sacred verses, contains most aspects of Vedic science such as yoga, meditation, mantra, and Ayurveda, which are still widely practiced today.

In the later *Vedic* period, theistic philosophies like *Sankhyam*, *Yogam*, *Nyayam*, *Vaisheshikam*, *Poorvamimaamsa*, and *Utharamimaamsa*, and atheistic philosophies, namely, *Jainadarsan*, *Buddhadarsan*, and *Charvaakadarsan*, paved the way for Ayurvedic principles. *Agnivesh Samhita*, *Bhela Samhita*, *Haritha Samhita*, *Samshrutha*, and *Kashyapa Samhita* are the other books on Ayurveda written in this period.

The documents of 500 BC indicate that this medicinal system might have even earlier origins. Even though Ayurveda knowledge is 3500 years old, there has been a continuous evolution of subjects and texts dating back to three major time periods [12–14]. This highlights the nature of Ayurveda as a living tradition.

In ancient times (Prachin Kala), dating back from c.1500 BC to the 12th century AD, major compendia (Samhitās) were created and attributed to different authors like *Charaka*, *Suśruta*, and *Kashyapa*. For instance, the *Charaka Samhita*, which relates internal medicine teachings of *Punarvasu Aatreya* to his students, was originally written by one of the students, Agniveśa (1500 BC), revised by Charaka around 200 BC, and reconstructed six centuries later by *Dridhabala*.

Another important piece of work is the Suśruta Samhita, relating to surgery knowledge. Again, several authors contributed: Nagarjuna, eight centuries later related the original works of Suśruta (c.400 BCE), later reviewed by *Chandrhata* (c.1000 CE). Samhitas are the master texts on which all the current prevailing documents are based, and were periodically edited over the centuries [15]. The knowledge included in the Samhitas relates to the tremendous advances made by physicians (e.g., Charaka) and surgeons (e.g., Suśruta) to describe and study human beings functioning as a whole, that is, mind and body.

A second period (6th–12th centuries CE) was *Sangraha Kaala*, during which compilations such as *Astānga Sangraha*, *Astānga Hrudaya* (c.600 CE), and *Harita Samhita*, mostly attributed to *Vagbhatta* I and II, were developed, which were easier to read and recite, and thus were adopted widely. The medieval times (*Madhya Kaala*) marked the development of elaborate compendia on individual herbs, their properties, and classification. This era is most commonly referred to as *Nighantu Kaala* (7th–16th centuries CE), during which compilations such as *Madhava Nidana*, *Śārngadhar Samhita* (c.1300 CE), *Bhavaprakasha*, *Chakradutta*, and *Yogatarangini* were developed. This was followed by *Ras Kaala* (8th–16th centuries CE), during which exhaustive accounts of mineral and metallic preparations, with their purification and processing before internal use, were provided. These descriptions indicate the advancement in knowledge and understanding of the chemistry during this period. The most referred to text of this time was *Rasa Ratna Samuchaya* by *Vaghbhatta* in the 13th century.

During the modern period (*Adhunika Kaala*, 18th–20th centuries), many compilations were made available, mainly with commentaries on the original texts, developed in different parts of the country. These rather suggest a demand for the system to continuously evolve in the contemporary era. Currently, more than 2000 herbs, 150 minerals, and over 97,000 formulations are documented worldwide for hundreds of diseases [16, 17]. Importantly, the therapeutic mechanisms of action have also been described along with their use in diseases.

Back in the Vedic era, medicine was in such an advanced stage that eight medical specializations were developed: *Kāyachikitsā* (internal medicine), *Kumārabhritya* (pediatrics, gynecology, and obstetrics), *Bhutavidyā* (psychotherapy), Śālākya tantra (otorhinolaryngology, including ophthalmology), Śhalya chikitsā (surgery), *Agada tantra* (toxicology), *Rasayana tantra* (geriatrics, including regenerative and promotive medicine toward positive health), and *Vājīkarana tantra* (science of virility, including reproductive system health). Even the tools used for diagnosis and therapeutic modalities, including surgeries, were elaborate and advanced with some of them quite novel considering the present knowledge of medicine. Interestingly, it transpires from the textual references that Ayurveda as a medicine was highly regulated because only those who had obtained the required training and approval from a federal structure (Rajanugya) could initiate a practice [18]. It was also stated that lethargy (Rajapramada) in enforcement of this regulatory process could lead to the thriving of quacks (Rogabhisara) in the system. There was a continuing tradition of training and practice of Ayurveda through old gurukul systems and family tradition wherein the education was imparted through verbal and practical approaches (Vaidya Paramara). Some of the present-day pharmaceutical companies like Aryavaidyashala, Zandu, and Sandu have their origins from these lineages (traditional knowledge-based medicine).

Key dates of the brief history in the development of herbal medicines are [10]:

- 2800 BC: First written record of herbal medicines, the Pen Ts'ao by Shen Nung.
- c.400 BC (400 years before common era or century): First Greek herbal written; Hippocrates develops principles of diet, exercise, and happiness as the cornerstones of health.
- c.100 BC: First illustrated herbal produced in Greece.

- c. AD 50: Roman Empire spreads herbal medicine and the commerce of plants around the Empire.
- c. AD 200: Herbal practitioner, Galen, creates a system for classifying illnesses and remedies.
- c. AD 500: Hippocrates' principles followed in Britain by Myddfai practitioners throughout Saxon times.
- AD 1100s: Arab world now a major influence on medicine and healing practices.

Physician Avicenna writes the Canon of Medicine.

- AD 1200s: Black Death spreads across Europe; "qualified" apothecaries try bleeding, purging, mercury, and arsenic to stem the epidemic with no more success than traditional herbalists.
- AD 1500s: Henry VII promotes herbal medicine in the face of the growing number of untrained apothecaries and other "medical practitioners" flourishing in London. Various Acts of Parliament passed to introduce some regulation of medical practices, including protection for "simple herbalists" to practice without fear of prosecution.
- AD 1600s: Society sees the first two-tier health system emerge—herbs for the poor and exotics (plant, animal, or mineral extracts) or "drugs" for the rich. Nicholas Culpepper writes his famous herbal The English Physician, explaining in simple terms the practice of herbal medicine.
- AD 1700s: Preacher Charles Wesley advocates a sensible diet, good hygiene, and herbal medicine as the keys to a healthy life.
- AD 1800s: Herbal medicines begin to be eclipsed by mineral drug-based treatments with powerful drugs such as calomel (mercury) and laudanum (alcoholic tincture of opium) available over the counter. Serious side effects begin to be documented. The National Association of Medical Herbalists founded to defend the practice, later to become the National Institute of Medical Herbalists (NIMH).
- AD 1900s: Medicinal herbals used extensively during World War I as drugs are in short supply. The postwar period sees enormous expansion in the international pharmaceuticals industry and the discovery of penicillin. A handful of dedicated herbalists keep the tradition alive. A Modern Herbal by Hilda Leyel is published. The Pharmacy and Medicines Act of 1941 (Hansard) is an Act of the Parliament of the United Kingdom that withdraws herbal practitioner's rights to supply patients with medicines. As a result, a public outcry ensures that the Act was never enforced. After much campaigning by the NIMH, the Medicines Act 1968 of the United Kingdom reinstates practitioners' rights and the British Herbal Medicine Association (BHMA) was founded. The BHMA produce the British Herbal Pharmacopeia, of which a revised edition was published in 1990. Public concern starts to grow over the side effects of the "wonder drugs" of the 1950s and their impact on the environment.
- AD 2000: EU legislation advocates that all herbal medicines should be subject to compulsory clinical testing comparable to that undertaken for conventional drugs. Thus all herbal medicines would be licensed. Currently, the UK government is considering the possible impact and public perception of this legislation.

2.2   Present status of herbal medicine

The WHO has launched its traditional medicine in Traditional Medicine Strategy 2014–23, which aims to support member states to develop policies and strengthen the role of traditional medicine in keeping populations healthy [19]. The widespread use of herbal medicine is not restricted to developing countries as it has been estimated that 70% of all medical doctors in France and German regularly prescribe herbal medicine [20] and the number of patients seeking herbal approaches for therapy is also growing exponentially [21]. With the US Food and Drug Administration relaxing guidelines for the sale of herbal supplements [22], the market is booming with herbal products [23]. As per the available records, the herbal medicine market in 1991 in the countries of the European Union was about $6 billion (may be over $20 billion now), with Germany accounting for $3 billion, France $1.6 billion, and Italy $0.6 billion. In 1996, the US herbal medicine market was about $4 billion, which has now doubled. The Indian herbal drug market is about $1 billion and the export of herbal crude extract is about $80 million [24].

In the last few decades, curious incidents have happened to botanical medicine and it has made a significant comeback. Despite being side-lined by medical science and the pharmaceutical chemistry, the use of plants for healing purposes predates recorded history and forms the origin of much of herbal medicine. Many conventional drugs originated from plant sources: a century ago, most of the few effective drugs were plant based. Examples include aspirin (from willow bark), digoxin (from foxglove), and quinine (from cinchona bark). Although the medicinal use of willow (*Salix* sp.) dates back 6000 years [25], it was only in 1897 that the first synthetic drug, aspirin, was created out of the salicylic acid extracted from willow barks.

Herbal medicine has benefited from the objective analysis of medical science, while fanciful and emotional claims for herbal cures have been thrown out, and effective herbal treatments and plant medicine that work have been acknowledged.

Hence, herbal medicine has been found to have some impressive credentials. Developed empirically by trial and error, many herbal treatments were nevertheless remarkably effective [26]: penicillin that replaced mercury in the treatment of syphilis and put an end to so many deadly epidemics. *Atropa belladonna* (deadly nightshade; belladonna) still provides the chemical used in ophthalmological preparations and antiseptics used to treat gastrointestinal disorders. *Rauwolfia serpentina* (Indian snake root), which has the active ingredient reserpine, was the basic constituent of a variety of tranquilizers first used in the 1950s to treat certain types of emotional and mental problems. Though reserpine is seldom used today for this purpose, its discovery was a breakthrough in the treatment of mental illness. It is also the principal ingredient in a number of modern pharmaceutical preparations for treating hypertension. However, reserpine can have serious side effects, e.g., severe depression. On the other hand, tea made of *R. serpentina* has been used in India as a sedative for thousands of years [26].

Examination of the history of medicine and pharmacy reveals a definite pattern. Humankind first utilized materials found in the environment on an empirical basis to cure various ailments. These plants, animal parts, and even microorganisms were initially employed in unmodified form, then as concentrated extract to improve their intensity and uniformity of action. Subsequently, pure chemical compounds as prototypes of synthetic chemical entities were developed that possessed even greater activity [27]. In fact, plant substances remain the basis for a very large proportion of medications used today for treating heart diseases, hypertension, depression, pain, cancer, asthma, neurological disorders, irritable bowel syndrome, liver diseases, and other ailments [21, 28, 29].

By 1994, pharmacologist Norman Farnsworth had identified over 119 plant-derived substances that are used globally as drugs. Many of the prescription drugs sold in the United States are molecules derived from or modeled after naturally occurring molecules in plants. A renewed interest in natural product research has been rekindled by discoveries of novel molecules from marine organisms (such as bryostatin) and potent new chemotherapeutic agents from plants (such as Taxol). It is possible to accomplish in a few minutes what once took months to analyze in the laboratory. Even with new technology, it appears that one of the best sources for finding plant species to test is still the healer's pouch, because such plants have often been tested by generations of indigenous people. Yet, with this crescendo of enthusiasm for herbal medicine, an increasing number of aged healers are dying with their knowledge left unrecorded. Most botanists regard this estimate by the International Union for the Conservation of Nature as conservative, because it considers only species known to science; numerous undiscovered species pass from the world unrecorded and unmorned [30].

2.3 Herbal medicine during the 19th and 20th centuries

Prior to the 19th century, plant medicines were administered in their crude form as infusions (herbal teas), tinctures (alcoholic extracts), decoctions (boiled extracts of roots or stem bark), and syrup or applied externally as ointments (poultices, balms, and essential oils) and herbal baths. However, from the late 19th century onward, scientists began to discover some of the most important drugs that are still widely used in modern medicine. For example, the development of the current and popular oral hypoglycemic agent metformin was based on the use of goat's rue (*Galega officinalis*) to treat diabetes [31]. Although the direct use of plant extracts in developed countries continued to decline in the late 19th and early 20th centuries, medicinal plants still play a key role in the healthcare system of many parts of the world. However, the use of herbal supplements has increased dramatically over the past 30 years and most commonly used medicinal plants in the United States have been reviewed. Kampo medicine, the Japanese herbal medicine, dates back over 1500 years with approximately 148 formulations, and it depends entirely on traditional and herbal medicine practices for its health needs. Medicinal herbs are sold alongside vegetables and other wares in many village marketplaces. Practitioners of herbal medicines in developing countries often undergo rigorous and extended training to learn the names, uses, and preparations of native plants.

Ayurveda is a healthcare system that has been used in India for over 5000 years. Its materia medica provides a comprehensive description of over 1500 herbs and 10,000 formulations. The Indian government has recognized Ayurveda to be a complete healthcare system in comparison to Western medicine. The principal Ayurvedic book on internal medicine, the Charaka Samhita, describes 582 herbs. The main book on surgery, the Sushruta Samhita, lists some 600 herbal remedies [32].

3 Status of herbal medicine in India

India has a rich tradition of herbal medicine as evident from Ayurveda, which could not have flourished for 2000 years without any scientific basis. Ayurveda, which literally means knowledge (Veda) of life (Ayur), had its beginning in *Atharvaveda* (c.1500–1000 BC). *Charaka Samhita* and *Sushruta Samhita* are the two most famous treatises of Ayurveda; several others were compiled over the centuries such as *Bhela Samhita*, *Kashyap Samhita*, *Agnivesh tantra*, *Vagbhata's Ashtang Hridaya* (AD 500), and *Madhava Nidan* (AD 700) [33]. Vegetable products dominated *Indian Materia Medica*, which made extensive use of bark, leaves, flowers, fruits, roots, tubers, and juices. The theory of *rasa*, *vipaka*, *virya*, and *prabhava* formed the basis of Ayurveda pharmacology, which made no clear distinction between diet and drug, as both were vital components of treatment [34]. *Charaka*, *Sushruta*, and *Vagbhata* described 700 herbal drugs with their properties and clinical effects. Based on clinical effects, 50 categories of drugs have been described, such as appetizers, digestive stimulants, laxatives, and antidiarrheal, antihemorrhoid, antiemetic, antipyretic, antiinflammatory, antipruritic, antiasthmatic, antiepileptic, antihelminthic, hemopoietic, hemostatic, analgesic, sedative, promoter of life (Rasayana), promoter of strength, complexion, voice, semen and sperm, breast milk secretion, fracture and wound healing, destroyer of kidney stones drugs, etc. [33].

The advent of Western medicine in the 18th century was a setback to the practice of Ayurveda, which suffered considerable neglect at the hands of the colonial administration. After the first success of reserpine, an enormous amount of characterization of medicinal plants was done in many laboratories and university departments, but the outcome was discouraging because the effort was disorganized, thinly spread, and unfocused [34]. Molecular pharmacology now provides a new interface between Ayurveda and modern medicine. Using modern techniques, various categories of Ayurvedic drug could provide novel molecular probes. Therefore it is now possible to explore the mechanism of action of Ayurvedic drugs in terms of the current concept of molecular pharmacology. Some striking examples of Ayurvedic drugs, which are understood in terms of today's molecular pharmacology, are:

- Sarpagangha (*R. serpentina*): reserpine uniquely prevents presynaptic neuronal vesicular uptake of biogenic amines (dopamine, serotonin, and norepinephrine).
- Mainmool (*Coleus forskohlii* Briq.): forskolin directly stimulates adenylate cyclase and cyclic AMP, with inotropic and lusitropic effects on heart muscle.
- Sallaki (*Boswellia serrata*): boswellic acid inhibits 5-lipo-oxygenase and leukotriene B4 resulting in antiinflammatory and anticomplement effects.
- Shirish (*Albizia lebbeck*): prevents mast cell degranulation, similar to sodium cromoglycate.
- Aturagupta (*Mucuna pruriens*): contains L-DOPA.
- Ashwagandha (*Withania somnifera*): contains a GABA-A receptor agonist.
- Katuka (*Picrorhiza kurroa*): has antioxidant action equal to αtocopherol and an effect on glutathione metabolism in the liver and brain [33].

Sukh Dev [35] listed 15 crude Ayurvedic drugs, which have received support for their therapeutic claims. Some of *Rasayana Dravyas* have been shown to increase phagocytosis, activate macrophages, and enhance resistance to microbial invasion. Drugs like *Asparagus racemosus*, *Tinospora cordifolia*, and *Ocimum sanctum* antagonize the effect of stress. *Emblica officinalis* L., *Curcuma longa* L., *Mangifera indica* L., *Momordica charantia* L., *Santalum album* L., *Swertia chirata* Buch.-Ham., and *W. somnifera* (L.) have well-defined antioxidant properties and justify their use in traditional medicine in the past as well as the present [36].

Use of herbal medicine in jaundice, presumably viral hepatitis, has been known in India since the Vedic times. About 170 phytoconstituents isolated from 110 plants belonging to 55 families have been reported so far to possess liver protective activities. It is estimated that about 6000 commercial herbal formulations are sold worldwide as hepatoprotective drugs, of which about 40 are patent polyherbal formulations representing a variety of combinations of 93 Indian herbs from 44 families available in the Indian market [37]. In the past, a glycyrrhizin preparation was used for peptic ulcer as well as liver diseases with mixed results. However, a new Japanese preparation from glycyrrhizin, stronger neomenophagen C, appears to be very promising in the treatment of virus-related chronic liver diseases [38]. Liv 52, an extract of several plants prepared for Ayurvedic medicine was reported to improve serum biochemistry values in rats with toxic liver damage, and uncontrolled observations in patients with liver disease seemingly gave similar results [39]. Double-blind and well-designed clinical trials have also been conducted with *Argyowardhani* in viral hepatitis, *M. pruriens* in Parkinson's disease, *Phyllanthus amarus* in hepatitis, and *T. cordifolia* in obstructive jaundice [40].

India is one of the 12 mega biodiversity centers having over 45,000 plant species. About 1500 plants with medicinal uses are mentioned in ancient texts and around 800 plants have been used in traditional medicine [24]. Conversely, India has failed to make an impact in the global market with drugs derived from plants and the gap between India and other countries is widening rapidly in the herbal field [34]. The export of herbal medicine from India is negligible despite the fact that the country has a rich traditional knowledge and heritage of herbal medicine [24]. The circumstances, which tend to frustrate a major developmental initiative for herbal products, are many sided in the country:

- There is no clear definition of the target to be achieved or a time frame within which the target, if any, should be achieved.
- There is no coordination among the national laboratories that are investigating medicinal plants.

- A serious dialog between publicly funded institutions and the industry is conspicuous by its absence.
- A mechanism for regular interaction between the expert in Ayurveda and research and development groups on medicinal plants does not exist. At the political level, Ayurveda is constantly extolled, but no effort is made to unify the scattered and thinly spread effort into a powerful course of action with specified goals in the development of herbal drugs [24].

4 Problems to be solved before herbal medicine can become mainstream

To reach a stage where herbal products of assured quality and effectiveness become integrated into mainline medicinal treatment, several obstacles must be overcome, e.g., the prejudice of current practicing healthcare professionals who did not learn about phytomedicines during their academic programs and, consequently, believe all of them to be ineffective forms a barrier [41]. Hence, orthodox medical practitioners are to be convinced of the efficacy of plant extracts [42]. Equally obstinate is the opinion of some traditional herbalists who believe that unprocessed natural products have an innate superiority and that the mystical aura surrounding herbs will somehow be destroyed by extraction and standardization [41]. The use of folk beliefs and knowledge of traditional healers is a shortcut to the discovery and isolation of pharmacologically active compounds [43]. However, intellectual property rights should protect tribal and traditional knowledge, so that it can help end the "piracy" by some drug companies [44].

Major challenges that must be overcome before herbs can join mainstream medicine are the quality of the literature in the field, e.g., books, pamphlets, journals, and especially these days the internet, which is filled with misinformation, much of it written to sell products and some of it written to express a point of view based on hope, not fact, or on misinformation [41]. Most sites merely list herbs and their uses, while only few mention regulation, safety, or efficacy. Even an herb with well-recognized toxicities, such as ephedra, may have no cautionary statement [45].

Another problem is that clinicians workings with herbal products are still relatively unfamiliar with them and often do not realize the necessity of adequate dosage. Many erroneous and unreproducible results have appeared in the medical literature because the clinicians accept at face value the quality of an herb that was adulterated or misidentified. In addition, they often fail to identify specifically, that is by scientific name, the botanicals in the product tested, as well as the precise dosage administered [46].

Some countries have a rich tradition of herbal medicine as evident from Ayurveda. Ayurveda, which literally means knowledge (Veda) of life (Ayur), had its beginning in *Atharvaveda* (c.1500–1000 BC). *Charaka* Samhita and Sushruta Samhita are the two most famous treatises of Ayurveda; several others were compiled over the centuries such as *Bhela Samhita, Kashyap Samhita, Agnivesh tantra, Vagbhata's Ashtang Hridaya, Madhava Nidan Charak, Sushruta,* and *Vagbhata* that described many herbal drugs with their properties and clinical effects. Based on clinical effects, 50 categories of drug have been described, such as appetizers, digestive stimulants, laxatives, and antidiarrheal, antihemorrhoid, antiemetic, antipyretic, antiinflammatory, antipruritic, antiasthmatic, antiepileptic, antihelminthic, hemoptietic, hemostatic, analgesic, sedative, promoter of life (Rasayana), promoter of strength, complexion, voice, semen and sperm, breast milk secretion, fracture and wound healing, destroyer of kidney stones drugs, etc. [33].

Advancement of Ayurveda and plant-based solutions for medicinal services through everyday experiences is a part of the social legacy of India. In all the conventional frameworks of medication, medicinal plants assume to play a noteworthy influence and constitute the backbone. Herbs played an important role in Ayurvedic medicine. According to the *Puranas,* the Ayurveda tradition was transferred from Brahma to Prajapathi and Ashwini Kumaras and through them to Lord Indra, the King of Gods. Sage Bharadwaja is reported to have acquired the knowledge from Indra and imparted the same to Sage Aathreya.

The manufacture of Ayurvedic medicine in its modern incarnation is over a century old in India. All the major manufacturers were established between 1890 and 1920. Major players in the Indian Ayurveda sector include, among others, Kottakal Arya Vaidya Sala, Dabur, Himalaya, Zandu, and Baidyanath. All these companies started due to the needs of the time. The Ayurveda industry in India is, by exigencies of growth, largely in the small-scale sector.

5 Aim

The aim of the present review was to document herbal medicines used by traditional healers to treat and manage human diseases and ailments by some communities, and provide a platform for scientists and researchers in herbal medicine and Ayurveda fields all over the world to present their new ideas, discuss new strategies, and promote developments in all areas of herbal medicine.

6 Uses

Although herbal preparations are widely used as self-medication for acute conditions, practitioners of herbal medicine tend to concentrate on treating chronic conditions. A typical caseload might include patients with asthma, eczema, premenstrual syndrome, rheumatoid arthritis, migraine, menopausal symptoms, chronic fatigue syndrome, and irritable bowel syndrome. Herbalists do not tend to treat acute mental or musculoskeletal disorders.

References

[1] Herbal medicine: open access. http://herbal-medicine.imedpub.com/.

[2] Goswami S, Mishra KN, Singh RP, Singh P, Singh P. Sesbaniasesban, a plant with diverse therapeutic benefits: an overview. SGVU J Pharm Res Educ 2016;1:111–21.

[3] Introduction and Importance of Medicinal Plants and Herbs, National Health Portal of India. [cited 2019Nov26]. Available from: https://www.nhp.gov.in/introduction-and-importance-of-medicinal-plants-and-herbs_mtl.

[4] Katz L, Baltz RH. Natural product discovery: past, present, and future. J Ind Microbiol Biotechnol 2016;43:155–76.

[5] Fabricant DS, Farnsworth NR. The value of plants used in traditional medicine for drug discovery. Environ Health Perspect 2001;109:69–75.

[6] Bell IR, Lewis 2nd DA, Brooks AJ, Schwartz GE, Lewis SE, Walsh BT, et al. Improved clinical status in fibromyalgia patients treated with individualized homeopathic remedies versus placebo. Rheumatology (Oxford) 2004;43:577–82.

[7] Adhikari PP, Paul SB. History of Indian traditional medicine: a medical inheritance. Asian J Pharm Clin Res 2018;11(1):421.

[8] WHO. Legal status of traditional medicines and complimentary/alternative medicine: Worldwide review. WHO Publications; 2001. p. 10–4.

[9] Tilburt JC, Kaptchuk TJ. Herbal medicine research and global health: an ethical analysis. Bull World Health Organ 2008;86:594–9.

[10] https://shodhganga.inflibnet.ac.in/bitstream/10603/89648/9/09_chapter1.pdf.

[11] Lemonnier N, Zhou G-B, Prasher B, Mukerji M, Chen Z, Brahmachari S, Noble D, Auffray C, Sagner M. Traditional knowledge based medicine: a review of history, principles and relevance in this present context of P4 system medicine. Prog Prev Med 2017. http://www.progprevmed.com.

[12] Rao MS. The history of medicine in India and Burma. Med Hist 1968;12:5261.

[13] Sharma PV. Ayurveda Ka Vaijnanika Itihasa [in Hindi]. 1st ed. Varanasi: Chaukhamba Orientalia; 1975.

[14] Subbarayappa BV. The roots of ancient medicine: an historical outline. J Biosci 2001;26:135143.

[15] Patwardhan K. The history of the discovery of blood circulation: unrecognized contributions of Ayurveda masters. Adv Physiol Educ 2012;36:7782.

[16] Sen N. TKDL—a safeguard for Indian traditional knowledge. Curr Sci 2002;82(9):1070–1.

[17] Traditional Knowledge Digital Library. CSIR, Ministry of AYUSH, http://www.tkdl.res.in; 2001. [Date Accessed: 1/19/17].

[18] Sharma PV. Suśruta. Suśruta Samhita. [in Sanskrit]. Translated by Varanasi: Chaukhamba Vishwa Bharati; 2000.

[19] WHA62. 13. Traditional medicine. In: Sixty-second World Health Assembly, Geneva, 18–22 May 2009. Resolution and decision, annexes. Geneva: World Health Organisation; 2009. p. 19–21 [WHA62/2009/REC/1, accessed 3 September 2013].

[20] Murray MT, Pizzorno Jr JE. Botanical medicine—a modern perspective. In: Pizzorno Jr JE, Murray MT, editors. Text book of natural medicine, vol. 1. Churchill Livingstone; 2000. p. 267–79.

[21] Alschuler L, Benjamin SA, Duke JA. Herbal medicine—what works, what is safe. Patient Care 1997;31:48–103.

[22] Gottlieb S. US relaxes its guidelines on herbal supplements. BMJ 2000;320:207.

[23] Brevoort P. The booming US botanical market. A new overview. Herbal Gram 1998;44:33–44.

[24] Kamboj VP. Herbal medicine. Curr Sci 2000;78:35–9.

[25] DerMarderosian A, Beutler JA. Willow bark. In: DerMarderosian A, Beutler JA, editors. The review of natural products. St. Louis, MO: Facts and Comparisons Publishing Group; 2011.

[26] Dwyer J, Rattray D. Plant, people and medicine. In: Magic and medicine of plant. Reader's Digest general book; 1993. p. 48–73.

[27] Robbers JE, Speedie M, Tyler VE. Pharmacognosy and pharmacobiotechnology. Baltimore, MD: Williams and Wilkins; 1996. p. 1–14.

[28] Vickers A, Zollman C. ABC of complementary medicine: herbal medicine. BMJ 1999;319:1050–3.

[29] Carter AJ. Dwale: an anesthetic from old England. BMJ 1999;319:1623–6.

[30] Cox PA. Will tribal knowledge survive the millennium? Science 2000;287:44–5.

[31] Bailey CJ. Metformin: historical overview. Diabetologia 2017;60:1566–76.

[32] History of Herbalmedicine. [chapter1]. http://shodhganga.inflibnet.ac.in/bitstream/10603/89930/9/09chapter%201.pdf.

[33] Lele RD. Ayurveda (ancient Indian system of medicine) and modern molecular medicine. J Assoc Physicians India 1999;47:625–8.

[34] Valiathan MS. Healing plants. Curr Sci 1998;75:1122–7.

[35] Dev S. Ethnotherapeutics and modern drug development: the potential of ayurveda. Curr Sci 1997;73:909–28.

[36] Scartezzini P, Speroni E. Review on some plant of Indian traditional medicine with antioxidant activity. J Ethnopharmacol 2000;71:23–43.

[37] Bhatt AD, Bhatt NS. Indigenous drugs and liver disease. Indian J Gastroenterol 1996;15:63–7.

[38] Tandon RK. Herbal medicine in the treatment of viral hepatitis. J Gastroenterol Hepatol 1999;14(Suppl):A291–2.

[39] Jain SK, DeFilipps RA. Medicinal plants of India. Reference Publication, Inc. 1991.

[40] Pal SK, Shukla Y. Herbal medicine: current status and the future. Asian Pac J Cancer Prev 2003;4:285.

[41] Tyler VE. Phytomedicine: back to the future. J Nat Prod 1999;62:1589–92.

[42] Tattam A. Herbal medicine heads for the mainstream. Lancet 1999;353:2222.

[43] Holland BK. Prospecting for drugs in ancient text. Nature 1994;369:702.

[44] Jayaraman KS. "Indian ginseng" brings royalties for tribe. Nature 1996;381:182.

[45] Winslow LC, Kroll DJ. Herbs as medicine. Arch Intern Med 1998;158:2192–9.

[46] Schuppan D, Jia JD, Brinkhaus B, et al. Herbal product for liver diseases: a therapeutic challenge for the new millennium. Hepatology 1999;30:1099–104.

Chapter 2

Use of herbal medicine as primary or supplementary treatments

Rima Dada[a], Pooja Sabharwal[b], Akanksha Sharma[c], and Ralf Henkel[d,e,f]

[a]Molecular Reproduction and Genetics, Department of Anatomy, AIIMS, New Delhi, India, [b]PG Department of Rachna Sharir, CBPACS, New Delhi, India, [c]Department of Rachana Sharir, CBPACS, New Delhi, India, [d]Department of Medical Bioscience, University of the Western Cape, Bellville, South Africa, [e]American Center for Reproductive Medicine, Department of Urology, Cleveland Clinic, Cleveland, OH, United States, [f]Department of Metabolism, Digestion and Reproduction, Imperial College London, London, United Kingdom

1 Introduction

Herbs hold beneficial healing properties for the treatment of chronic and acute conditions, including major health concerns like cardiovascular disease, prostate problems, depression, joint inflammation, and weakened immune system. Therefore about 25% of the medicine prescribed worldwide is derived from plants, and according to the World Health Organization's essential medicine list, 11% of 252 drugs are solely of plant origin [1]. The first pharmacological compound, morphine, was produced 200 years ago from the controlled substance opium extracted from the seedpods of the poppy flower [2]. Later, scientists were using plants to make the pharmaceutical products we all know today.

1.1 What is herbal medicine?

Herbal medicines are plant-based medicines made from different combinations of plant parts, e.g., leaves, flowers, fruits, and roots. Each part of the plant has different uses and many types of chemical constituents that need different extraction strategies. The National Institute of Medical Herbalists is the leading professional body of herbal practitioners in the United Kingdom. It promotes the safe use of herbal medicine and members are aware of the importance of medicines that are being sourced from reputable manufacturers, who maintain consistent quality standards through traceability (right back to the initial batch of herbs) and certificates of genuineness to ensure the highest degree of safety, effectiveness, and sustainability.

Medicinal plants have always been used as natural remedies such as rubbing dock leaves onto nettle stings or applying lavender oil to treat burns. Herbs are used to treat a vast array of acute conditions, in both emergency and nonemergency situations, from insect bites to headaches to serious wounds. While a lot of this tradition has been lost in time, there is a resurgence of public interest in the use of local plants for minor ailments. Ayurveda clinicians are qualified in advanced first aid, and some nurses and paramedics are even practicing Ayurvedic medicine. Many herbalists run beginners' courses where one may learn a range of skills from plant identification to making remedies.

1.2 Supplement therapy

The main alternative healthcare providers use vitamin and mineral supplements to prevent diseases. Such supplements improve the survival or prognosis of patients with cancer (e.g., cervical, colon, lung, bladder, breast), allergies, Alzheimer's disease, cardiovascular disease, osteoporosis, and many other conditions.

The currently available antipyretic drugs in the allopathic system of medicine are not so effective in combating a wide variety of complications. Medicinal plants like Neem, Arjuna, Tulsi Giloye, etc. are traditionally used as antipyretics for treating fever. Since these herbal remedies are less expensive and a safer means of treatment than conventional medications, many people are choosing to revisit the traditional Indian system of medicine.

The most common reasons for the use of traditional medicine are its affordability and accessibility. Furthermore, traditional medicine is often more accepted by patients as it is believed that traditional medicine is more "natural," nontoxic, and therefore safer. Consequently, patients are of the opinion that these remedies have fewer adverse effects than chemical (synthetic) medicines. However, this assumption cannot be accepted as true, particularly when herbal remedies are taken together with prescription drugs, other herbs, or other nonprescription drugs [3–6]. Herbal remedies also satisfy the human

Herbal Medicine in Andrology. https://doi.org/10.1016/B978-0-12-815565-3.00002-3

desire for more personalized health care. Therapeutically, herbal medicines are mainly used to promote general health and treat chronic conditions rather than life-threatening conditions. Even in Europe and the United States the usage of herbal remedies increases when Western medicine is ineffective such as in patients with advanced cancer or new infectious diseases.

One reason why herbal medicine is becoming more popular is because people simply cannot afford to pay for their allopathic medication on a continuous basis. Herbal products such as herbal extracts, herbal teas, and essential oils are available in most health food markets, thus they are easier to obtain. Furthermore, since herbs are often classified as dietary supplements, they can be produced, sold, and marketed without going through the Food and Drug Administration or any other medicine regulatory council, which makes it easier to purchase and use them for medication.

1.2.1 How herbal medicines approach health problems

Anyone can be a herbalist—doctors or even laypersons use herbal products for the treatment of various diseases such as heart diseases, cancer, joint disorders, reproductive health dysfunction, diabetes, and cardiovascular diseases. Herbs can help the body to deal with the side effects of allopathic medicines or indeed help avoid higher doses of these medicines. Finally, doctors should monitor the benefits and adverse effects of self-prescribed herbal treatments consumed by their patients.

1.2.2 Herbal medicines for some common diseases

- Joints and bone disorders

Herbs have long been used in the treatment of arthritis, rheumatic disease, and musculoskeletal complaints to relieve swelling, muscle spasm and tightness, damaged tendons, and tight or lax ligaments. Often, herbs are applied outwardly to bring relief from pain and inflammation, which help the various connective tissues of the musculoskeletal system (bones, muscles, tendons, and ligaments) cooperate to give motion to the body. Apart from containing active compounds such as [6]-gingerol, which has antiinflammatory, antioxidative, and antitumorigenic properties [7], ginger is also claimed to decrease swelling and pain [8] as [6]-gingerol interacts as a heat- and pain-sensitive receptor [9].

Curcumin is a polyphenol phytochemical found in the spice turmeric, derived from the root of *Curcuma longa*. Curcumin has been shown to have potent antioxidant, antiinflammatory, and anticancer properties. It has been used as an antiinflammatory treatment in Ayurvedic medicine [10].

- Rheumatoid arthritis

Natural treatments for rheumatoid arthritis (RA) range from hot and cold compresses, magnets, massage therapy, herbs, natural supplements, and water relaxation remedies. Herbal remedies used for RA include *Boswellia serrata*, *Equisetum arvense* (horsetail), curcumin, borage seed oil, and many others [11].

Boswellia is a herb that comes from a tree native to India and its extract has been shown to significantly improve body weight and decrease ankle diameter and arthritic index [12]. The bioactive compound acetyl-11-keto-β-boswellic acid appears to attenuate not only oxidative stress and inflammation and complement activation in various cells [13, 14], but has also antiangiogenic and cytotoxic effects and could therefore be effective as adjuvant cancer therapy [15]. Similarly, *Equisetum* has also been found to exhibit significant antiinflammatory effects by modulating the functions of immunocompetent cells [16].

Many patients try to treat their RA with dietary approaches, such as fasting, vegan diets, or eliminating specific foods. A survey revealed that such approaches improved the symptoms in 15% of the patients, while 19% of patients reported worsening of the conditions [17]. Hence, there is little scientific evidence to support these approaches.

- Cardiovascular diseases

Herbal medications have also become more widely accepted and used in cardiovascular medicine. Therefore the most effective compounds of herbal extracts have undergone systematic scientific evaluations. Some of these compounds have even become historic cornerstones in the treatment of cardiovascular diseases. Garlic is one of these examples, which is thought to exert antiatherosclerotic effects by interfering with inflammatory and oxidative pathways. In addition, it is suggested that its bioactive compounds also prevent lipid deposition in blood vessels, thereby decreasing peripheral vascular resistance and vasodilatation. Garlic could also be directly involved in the relaxation of smooth muscle cells, e.g., in the pathogenesis of hypertension. These mechanisms seem to include oxidative stress and endothelial nitric oxide and hydrogen sulfide production [18, 19]. Moreover, there is evidence that garlic can reduce the endogenous synthesis and intestinal absorption of cholesterol [20, 21].

Although numerous observational and experimental clinical studies have investigated the potential efficacy of garlic for the treatment of hypertension in humans, results provided in a Cochrane study indicate that the evidence is insufficient [22].

- Skin disorders

Skin is the most extensive organ of the body and the use of herbal products in the treatment of inflammatory skin diseases results from their stages of inflammation [23]. For example, allergic eczema will require a totally different approach as this is caused by an immunologic reaction, which plays an important role in the pathogenesis of dermatitis and other skin diseases of inflammatory origin and involves the activation of T-lymphocytes.

Matricaria recutita (German chamomile) is the most commonly used medicinal plant. Its extract has antiinflammatory properties as it inhibits the synthesis of leukotrienes and prostaglandins. The bioactive compounds α-bisabolol and apigenin inhibit cyclooxygenase and 5-lipooxygenase activity, while chamazulene inhibits only 5-lipooxygenase [24, 25]. Another often-used plant for skin disorders is the *Calendula* flower (*Calendulae flos*; *Calendula officinalis*; marigold), which is used for poorly healing wounds, bruises, rashes, boils, and dermatitis. The bioactive compounds in the marigold flowers are triterpene saponins (oleanolic acid glycosides), triterpene alcohols (α-, β-amyrins, faradiol), and flavonoids (quercetin and isorhamnetin) [26], compounds that are particularly known for their antiinflammatory and antiedematous effects [27].

Hamamelis decoctions and infusions of *Hamamelis* bark (*Hamamelis virginiana*; witch hazel) and leaf are used for compresses or washes in the treatment of local inflammation of the skin [23].

- Nutritional disorders

Hippocrates, the father of modern medicine, advised to let food be our medicine and medicine be our food. He also distinguished between herbs as medicine and herbs as food on the basis of taste. Herbs as food would be bland and herbs as medicine would often have strong specific tastes to be effective as a medication, which is what herbalists several thousand years later still accept as the truth.

Some herbs like garlic, ginger, curcumin, and green tea are used as healthy foods and work well to maintain health, while others have no food use but act as powerful medicines.

- Infertility

Globally, infertility is regarded as a major public health problem. This condition is even more problematic since in many emerging economies, such as in Africa, having many children is part of the culture and childlessness has devastating consequences on both marital partners as it has not only negative psychological effects but also leads to social stigma, ridicule, isolation, and mental problems [28–30]. Since in Africa the reproductive and psychosocial burden is carried by the women [31, 32], many women turn to herbal medicine to achieve parenthood [33]. Herbal medicine may enhance fertility by supporting the natural function of the ovulation and fertility process. In general, herbal medicine is appropriate to treat any type of infertility condition. For men, clinically proven herbs are available to help improve sperm parameters such as sperm count and motility, e.g., *Ferula hermonis* root, *Phlomis brachyodon* leaves, and *Phoenix dactylifera* pollen grain. For women, herbal remedies that were used in the treatment of infertility are pollen grains from *Ceratonia siliqua*, *Anastatica hierochuntica* fruit, *Parietaria judaica* leaves, red clover, and the herbs that are traditionally used to help restore hormonal balance.

- Fertility, pregnancy, and childbirth
  Pregnant women

Reportedly, the global incidence of the use of herbal remedy usage among pregnant women ranges between 70% and 96% [34–37]. However, in developed countries such as the United States, Australia, or Italy, the usage of herbal medicines is much lower at 10%–56% [34, 38, 39]. In Ghana, for instance, despite the popular move toward Westernized prenatal medicine, herbal medicine is often used as a cure for many pregnant women in rural areas [40]. Many pregnant women most commonly used ginger, peppermint, thyme, chamomile, aniseed, green tea, tea leaf, raspberry, and echinacea leaf regularly throughout the whole duration of the pregnancy. Cultural norms, as well as personal beliefs and the need to manage personal health and illness perceptions, are reflecting a holistic approach toward health resulting in the widespread use of herbs.

Among pregnant women in Ghanaian rural areas, the most frequently used medicinal plants were ginger (*Zingiber officinale*), peppermint (*Mentha×piperita*), thyme (*Thymus* (Lamiaceae)), sage (*Salvia officinalis*), aniseed (*Pimpinella anisum*), fenugreek (*Trigonella foenum-graecum*), green tea (*Camellia sinensis*), garlic (*Allium sativum*), tea leaf (*Camellia sinensis*), raspberry (*Rubus idaeus*), and echinacea leaf (*Echinacea purpurea*) [40].

- Emotional disorders

Overall body constitution, the health of hormonal systems, neurotransmitters, and the heart may all reflect one's emotional health. There are herbs, such as St. John's Wort, that are well known and well researched and are as effective as any antidepressant drug [41]. Although other bioactive compounds such as flavonoids and tannins are also present, its most active compounds are hyperforin and hypericin [42]. Reserpine, an indole alkaloid derived from *Rauwolfia serpentina*, is a potent hypertensive [43] and poorly tolerated antipsychotic drug [44].

- Lung cancer

The aim of a treatment is to manage carcinoma, prevent or reduce its spread to other parts of the body, and improve overall survival. Medicines that act specifically on lung tissue are used for this condition. Herbal medicines helpful in this condition are: *Coptis chinensis* (Chinese goldthread), *Scutellaria barbata* (barbed skullcap), *Wedelia chinensis* (Chinese: Peng qi ju), or *Alpinia galangal* (Lengkuas) [45].

Compared to other cancers, lung cancer has a very poor prognosis, despite the latest available modern treatment [46]. The synchronic use of herbal medicines thus assumes a great deal of importance to manage tumors, improve quality of life, and improve the survival rate in patients with chronic obstructive pulmonary disease [47]. All such patients should be under the regular care and supervision of an oncology medical team.

- Hangover

A hangover is classified as a group of unpleasant signs and symptoms that can develop after drinking too much alcohol. Typical symptoms of a hangover might embrace headache, drowsiness, concentration problems, dry mouth, dizziness, fatigue, gastrointestinal distress, absence of hunger, sweating, nausea, hyperexcitability, and anxiety [48–50]. In traditional Chinese medicine, the KSS formula is offered to alleviate the symptoms of a hangover. This formula contains Kitsuraku (pith of *Citrus tangerine* Hort. et Tanaka), Shokyo (rhizome of *Z. officinale*), and brown sugar, and significantly reduces the severity of nausea, vomiting, and diarrhea if the herbal remedy was taken before the excessive alcohol intake [51]. Other remedies include:

- Bananas as they contain a natural antacid to help with nausea, and are high in magnesium, which helps relax the hammering blood vessels causing the hangover headache.
- Barley grass: Barley grass juice 24:1 extract powder can substantially mitigate hangover effects experienced by people suffering from acute alcohol toxicity.
- Cabbage: Eating raw cabbage has been used throughout history for preventing and curing hangovers.
- Chili peppers: A bowl full of hot and spicy chili is effective because chili peppers help the body fight the free radicals produced from drinking.

- Diabetes mellitus

Diabetes mellitus is a most common endocrine disorder, affecting millions of people worldwide. Diabetes consists of a group of metabolic diseases that are characterized by hyperglycemia as a result of too low insulin levels, defects in insulin action, or both. Several herbal remedies are recommended to alleviate the disease.

A. sativum is locally know as garlic and belongs to the Liliaceae family. Ethanolic extract of garlic (10 mL/kg/day) frequently shows hypoglycemic activity. Extract of garlic was a lot more economical than the antidiabetic drug glibenclamide. Ethyl acetate, ethanol, and petroleum ether extract were reported to have antidiabetic activity in streptozotocin-induced rats. Garlic shows antiplatelet and antibacterial therapeutic effects, and lowers blood pressure and cholesterol levels in the body.

For *Aloe barbadensis*, also known as Ghikanvar, a plant belonging to the Liliaceae family, it has been shown that in a rat model, oral administration of an aqueous extract of *Aloe vera* in a dose of 150 mg/kg body weight was able to significantly lower the blood glucose level [52]. On the other hand, a systematic review and metaanalysis revealed that *A. vera* may improve glycemic control in type 2 diabetic patients. However, more high-quality, randomized, controlled studies are necessary to verify the beneficial effects of this plant for diabetes [53].

- Surgical procedures

Adusumilli and coworkers [54] reported that in a large survey study including more than 3300 patients who underwent elective surgery, 65% of the patients responded, of whom 57% used herbal medicine at some point in their life. About 16.7% of the respondents continued to use herbal remedies when they had their surgical treatment. The percentage of women undergoing gynecological surgery and patients perceiving themselves as healthy had significantly higher usage of herbal medicines than patients with pulmonary symptoms, African-Americans, or patients with diabetes. Echinacea (48%), *A. vera* (30%), ginseng (28%), garlic (27%), and *Gingko biloba* (22%) were most commonly used [54]. Another study indicates that the usage of herbal products is increasing from 38.9% before treatment to 54.1% during chemotherapy [55]. This study also reports that before surgery 94.35 of patients and during chemotherapy 81.7% of patients had not been questioned about the use of herbal medicine. This indicates not only that the awareness of the use of herbal remedies among patients is increasing, but also that healthcare professionals should obtain all relevant information before the start of treatments to advise patients of the benefits and disadvantages of herbal products.

Generally, it appears that for certain medical conditions, adjunct treatment of surgery with herbal medicine has significant benefits for patients [56, 57]. However, the size and number of studies are still small, particularly for rare conditions. Therefore there is still not enough evidence available to conclude that herbal remedies have a general benefit for patients [58].

How to choose and use herbal supplements

1. Before using any herbal supplement it is always recommended to consult an Ayurvedic specialist or herbalist.
2. Do not take any irrelevant supplement, such as thyroid support supplement, when you have a healthy thyroid.
3. There are some Ayurvedic herbal supplements like Chywanprash that can be taken by almost everyone, but still, it is recommended to consult an expert before opting for any supplement.
4. There is a misconception that herbal supplements purchased from other than native countries are not reliable. However, if the quality control measures and latest herbal technologies employed to ensure the safety and efficacy of the herbal medicines are adhered to, then such an herbal product from any part of the world can be trusted.
5. Do not take any medicines without a proper label describing the list of contents and method of use.

The aim of herbal treatment is sometimes to produce sustained improvements in well-being. Practitioners usually speak in terms of attempting to treat the "underlying cause" of unwellness and should prescribe herbs aimed at correcting patterns of dysfunction rather than targeting the presenting symptoms [59].

2   Conclusion

Herbs are used around the world to treat a variety of conditions and diseases, and many studies prove their efficacy. When patients use home remedies for acute, often self-limiting conditions, such as colds, sore throats, or bee stings, it is often because professional care is not immediately available, too inconvenient, costly, or time consuming. It would be healthier than factory made medication.

Although herbal medicines are widely used all over the world, there is still a huge gap between "best scientific evidence" and what people actually use to treat a disease. In addition, despite the obvious health benefits that herbal remedies provide, there is also still a lack of acceptance of herbal medicines by healthcare professionals, especially in the Western world. Hence, it is not only important that healthcare professionals learn more about herbal medicine, but also that more high-quality scientific studies are conducted in pursuit of "evidence-based herbal medicine." Maybe then we will see "health for all" as a reality.

References

[1] Rates SM. Plants as source of drugs. Toxicon 2001;39:603–13.
[2] Wachtel-Galor S, Benzie IFF. Herbal medicine: an introduction to its history, usage, regulation, current trends, and research needs. In: Benzie IFF, Wachtel-Galor S, editors. Herbal medicine: Biomolecular and clinical aspects. 2nd ed. Boca Raton, FL: CRC Press/Taylor & Francis; 2011 [chapter 1].
[3] Canter PH, Ernst E. Herbal supplement use by persons aged over 50 years in Britain: frequently used herbs, concomitant use of herbs, nutritional supplements and prescription drugs, rate of informing doctors and potential for negative interactions. Drugs Aging 2004;21:597–605.
[4] Cohen PA, Ernst E. Safety of herbal supplements: a guide for cardiologists. Cardiovasc Ther 2010;28:246–53.
[5] Loya AM, Gonzalez-Stuart A, Rivera JO. Prevalence of polypharmacy, polyherbacy, nutritional supplement use and potential product interactions among older adults living on the United States-Mexico border: a descriptive, questionnaire-based study. Drugs Aging 2009;26:423–36.
[6] Qato DM, Alexander GC, Conti RM, Johnson M, Schumm P, Lindau ST. Use of prescription and over-the-counter medications and dietary supplements among older adults in the United States. JAMA 2008;300:2867–78.
[7] de Lima RMT, Dos Reis AC, de Menezes APM, Santos JVO, Filho JWGO, Ferreira JRO, de Alencar MVOB, da Mata AMOF, Khan IN, Islam A, Uddin SJ, Ali ES, Islam MT, Tripathi S, Mishra SK, Mubarak MS, Melo-Cavalcante AAC. Protective and therapeutic potential of ginger (*Zingiber officinale*) extract and [6]-gingerol in cancer: a comprehensive review. Phytother Res 2018;32:1885–907.
[8] Bode AM, Dong Z. The amazing and mighty ginger. In: Benzie IFF, Wachtel-Galor S, editors. Herbal medicine: Biomolecular and clinical aspects. 2nd ed. Boca Raton, FL: CRC Press/Taylor & Francis; 2011 [chapter 7].
[9] Dedov VN, Tran VH, Duke CC, Connor M, Christie MJ, Mandadi S, Roufogalis BD. Gingerols: a novel class of vanilloid receptor (VR1) agonists. Br J Pharmacol 2002;137:793–8.
[10] Kocaadam B, Sanlier N. Curcumin, an active component of turmeric (*Curcuma longa*), and its effects on health. Crit Rev Food Sci Nutr 2017;57:2889–95.
[11] Dragos D, Gilca M, Gaman L, Vlad A, Iosif L, Stoian I, Lupescu O. Phytomedicine in joint disorders. Nutrients 2017;9. pii: E70.
[12] Kumar R, Singh S, Saksena AK, Pal R, Jaiswal R, Kumar R. Effect of *Boswellia serrata* extract on acute inflammatory parameters and tumor necrosis factor-α in complete Freund's adjuvant-induced animal model of rheumatoid arthritis. Int J Appl Basic Med Res 2019;9:100–6.
[13] Ahmad S, Khan SA, Kindelin A, Mohseni T, Bhatia K, Hoda MN, Ducruet AF. Acetyl-11-keto-β-boswellic acid (AKBA) attenuates oxidative stress, inflammation, complement activation and cell death in brain endothelial cells following OGD/reperfusion. Neuromolecular Med 2019;21:505–16.
[14] Soni KK, Meshram D, Lawal TO, Patel U, Mahady GB. Fractions of *Boswellia serrata* suppress LTA4, LTC4, Cyclooxygenase-2 activities and mRNA in HL-60 cells and reduce lung inflammation in BALB/c mice. Curr Drug Discov Technol 2020. https://doi.org/10.2174/1570163817666620 0127112928 [Epub ahead of print].

[15] Pathania AS, Wani ZA, Guru SK, Kumar S, Bhushan S, Korkaya H, Seals DF, Kumar A, Mondhe DM, Ahmed Z, Chandan BK, Malik F. The anti-angiogenic and cytotoxic effects of the boswellic acid analog BA145 are potentiated by autophagy inhibitors. Mol Cancer 2015;14:6.

[16] Gründemann C, Lengen K, Sauer B, Garcia-Käufer M, Zehl M, Huber R. *Equisetum arvense* (common horsetail) modulates the function of inflammatory immunocompetent cells. BMC Complement Altern Med 2014;14:283.

[17] Tedeschi SK, Frits M, Cui J, Zhang ZZ, Mahmoud T, Iannaccone C, Lin TC, Yoshida K, Weinblatt ME, Shadick NA, Solomon DH. Diet and rheumatoid arthritis symptoms: survey results from a rheumatoid arthritis registry. Arthritis Care Res (Hoboken) 2017;69:1920–5.

[18] Ried K, Fakler P. Potential of garlic (*Allium sativum*) in lowering high blood pressure: mechanisms of action and clinical relevance. Integr Blood Press Control 2014;7:71–82.

[19] Varshney R, Budoff MJ. Garlic and heart disease. J Nutr 2016;146:416S–21S.

[20] Gebhardt R, Beck H. Differential inhibitory effects of garlic-derived organosulfur compounds on cholesterol biosynthesis in primary rat hepatocyte cultures. Lipids 1996;31:1269–76.

[21] Shouk R, Abdou A, Shetty K, Sarkar D, Eid AH. Mechanisms underlying the antihypertensive effects of garlic bioactives. Nutr Res 2014;34:106–15.

[22] Stabler SN, Tejani AM, Huynh F, Fowkes C. Garlic for the prevention of cardiovascular morbidity and mortality in hypertensive patients. Cochrane Database Syst Rev 2012;8:CD007653.

[23] Dawid-Pac R. Medicinal plants used in treatment of inflammatory skin diseases. Postepy Dermatol Alergol 2013;30:170–7.

[24] Kim S, Jung E, Kim JH, Park YH, Lee J, Park D. Inhibitory effects of (-)-α-bisabolol on LPS-induced inflammatory response in RAW264.7 macrophages. Food Chem Toxicol 2011;49:2580–5.

[25] Kiraly AJ, Soliman E, Jenkins A, Van Dross RT. Apigenin inhibits COX-2, PGE2, and EP1 and also initiates terminal differentiation in the epidermis of tumor bearing mice. Prostaglandins Leukot Essent Fatty Acids 2016;104:44–53.

[26] Muley BP, Khadabadi SS, Banarase NB. Phytochemical constituents and pharmacological activities of *Calendula officinalis* Linn (Asteraceae): a review. Trop J Pharm Res 2009;8:455–65.

[27] Leach MJ. *Calendula officinalis* and wound healing: a systematic review. Wounds 2008;20:236–43.

[28] Wischmann T, Stammer H, Scherg H, Gerhard I, Verres R. Psychosocial characteristics of infertile couples: a study by the 'Heidelberg Fertility Consultation Service'. Hum Reprod 2001;16:1753–61.

[29] Ombelet W, Cooke I, Dyer S, Serour G, Devroey P. Infertility and the provision of infertility medical services in developing countries. Hum Reprod Update 2008;14:605–21.

[30] Mumtaz Z, Shahid U, Levay A. Understanding the impact of gendered roles on the experiences of infertility amongst men and women in Punjab. Reprod Health 2013;10:3.

[31] Inhorn MC. "The worms are weak". Male infertility and patriarchal paradoxes in Egypt. Men Masculinities 2003;5:236–56.

[32] Olooto WE, Amballi AA, Banjo TA. A review of female infertility; important etiological factors and management. J Microbiol Biotechnol Res 2012;2:379–85.

[33] Kaadaaga HF, Ajeani J, Ononge S, Alele PE, Nakasujja N, Manabe YC, Kakaire O. Prevalence and factors associated with use of herbal medicine among women attending an infertility clinic in Uganda. BMC Complement Altern Med 2014;14:27.

[34] Forster DA, Denning A, Wills G, Bolger M, McCarthy E. Herbal medicine use during pregnancy in a group of Australian women. BMC Pregnancy Childbirth 2006;6:21.

[35] Fakeye TO, Adisa R, Musa IE. Attitude and use of herbal medicines among pregnant women in Nigeria. BMC Complement Altern Med 2009;9:53.

[36] Tamuno I, Omole-Ohonsi A, Fadare J. Use of herbal medicine among pregnant women attending a tertiary hospital in northern Nigeria. Int J Gynecol Obstet 2010;15:2.

[37] Hall HG, McKenna LG, Griffiths DL. Midwives' support for complementary and alternative medicine: a literature review. Women Birth 2012;25:4–12.

[38] Holst L, Wright D, Haavik S, Nordeng H. The use and the user of herbal remedies during pregnancy. J Altern Complement Med 2009;15:787–92.

[39] Cuzzolin L, Francini-Pesenti F, Verlato G, Joppi M, Baldelli P, Benoni G. Use of herbal products among 392 Italian pregnant women: focus on pregnancy outcome. Pharmacoepidemiol Drug Saf 2010;19:1151–8.

[40] Peprah P, Agyemang-Duah W, Arthur-Holmes F, Budu HI, Abalo EM, Okwei R, Nyonyo J. 'We are nothing without herbs': a story of herbal remedies use during pregnancy in rural Ghana. BMC Complement Altern Med 2019;19:65.

[41] Barnes J, Anderson LA, Phillipson JD. St John's wort (*Hypericum perforatum* L.): a review of its chemistry, pharmacology and clinical properties. J Pharm Pharmacol 2001;53:583–600.

[42] Nahrstedt A, Butterweck V. Biologically active and other chemical constituents of the herb of *Hypericum perforatum* L. Pharmacopsychiatry 1997;30(Suppl. 2):129–34.

[43] Panda SK, Das D, Tripathy BN, Nayak L. Phyto-pharmacognostical studies and quantitative determination of reserpine in different parts of Rauwolfia (spp.) of eastern Odisha by UV spectroscopy method. Asian J Plant Sci Res 2012;2:151–62.

[44] Hoenders HJR, Bartels-Velthuis AA, Vollbehr NK, Bruggeman R, Knegtering H, de Jong JTVM. Natural medicines for psychotic disorders: a systematic review. J Nerv Ment Dis 2018;206:81–101.

[45] Khan T, Ali M, Khan A, Nisar P, Jan SA, Afridi S, Shinwari ZK. Anticancer plants: a review of the active phytochemicals, applications in animal models, and regulatory aspects. Biomolecules 2019;10. pii: E47.

[46] Clausen MM, Langer SW. Improving the prognosis for lung cancer patients. Acta Oncol 2019;58:1077–8.

[47] Lin TH, Chen SI, Su YC, Lin MC, Lin HJ, Huang ST. Conventional Western treatment combined with Chinese herbal medicine alleviates the progressive risk of lung cancer in patients with chronic obstructive pulmonary disease: a nationwide retrospective cohort study. Front Pharmacol 2019;10:987.

[48] Streufert S, Pogash R, Braig D, Gingrich D, Kantner A, Landis R, Lonardi L, Roache J, Severs W. Alcohol hangover and managerial effectiveness. Alcohol Clin Exp Res 1995;19:1141–6.

[49] Wiese JG, Shlipak MG, Browner WS. The alcohol hangover. Ann Intern Med 2000;132:897–902.

[50] Verster JC. The alcohol hangover—a puzzling phenomenon. Alcohol Alcohol 2008;43:124–6.

[51] Takahashi M, Li W, Koike K, Sadamoto K. Clinical effectiveness of KSS formula, a traditional folk remedy for alcohol hangover symptoms. J Nat Med 2010;64:487–91.

[52] Noor A, Gunasekaran S, Soosai A, Vijayalakshmi MA. Antidiabetic activity of *Aloe vera* and histology of organs in streptozotocin induced diabetic rats. Curr Sci 2008;94:1070–6.

[53] Suksomboon N, Poolsup N, Punthanitisarn S. Effect of *Aloe vera* on glycaemic control in prediabetes and type 2 diabetes: a systematic review and meta-analysis. J Clin Pharm Ther 2016;41:180–8.

[54] Adusumilli PS, Ben-Porat L, Pereira M, Roesler D, Leitman IM. The prevalence and predictors of herbal medicine use in surgical patients. J Am Coll Surg 2004;198:583–90.

[55] Kocasli S, Demircan Z. Herbal product use by the cancer patients in both the pre and post surgery periods and during chemotherapy. Afr J Tradit Complement Altern Med 2017;14:325–33.

[56] Shin JS, Lee J, Lee YJ, Kim MR, Ahn YJ, Park KB, Shin BC, Lee MS, Ha IH. Long-term course of alternative and integrative therapy for lumbar disc herniation and risk factors for surgery: a prospective observational 5-year follow-up study. Spine (Phila Pa 1976) 2016;41:E955–63.

[57] Cheng CF, Lin YJ, Tsai FJ, Li TM, Lin TH, Liao CC, Huang SM, Liu X, Li MJ, Ban B, Liang WM, Lin JC. Effects of Chinese herbal medicines on the risk of overall mortality, readmission, and reoperation in hip fracture patients. Front Pharmacol 2019;10:629.

[58] Hong S, Park B, Noh H, Choi DJ. Herbal medicine for dumping syndrome: a systematic review and meta-analysis. Integr Cancer Ther 2019;18. https://doi.org/10.1177/1534735419873404. 1534735419873404.

[59] Vickers A, Zollman C. ABC of complementary medicine: herbal medicine. BMJ 1999;319:1050–3.

Chapter 3

Herbal pharmacognosy: An introduction

Kristian Leisegang

School of Natural Medicine, University of the Western Cape, Bellville, Cape Town, South Africa

1 Introduction

Pharmacognosy is the study and science of medicine from natural sources. Although usually associated with herbal medicine, this field includes animals, fungi, microbes, and minerals, as well as parts of/or entire organisms such as flowers, leaves, roots, etc. [1]. Natural medicines have been used for many thousands of years to enhance human health and treat diseases, and modern pharmaceutical medicine is largely dependent on drugs originally discovered in and isolated from natural sources [2]. In fact, natural sources are the basis for approximately 50% of all prescription medicines currently marketed [3]. Important examples include morphine, ephedrine, atropine, salicylic acid, colchicine, and tamoxifen [4]. Alternative medicinal sources increasingly investigated for therapeutic use include animals such as frogs, snakes (venom), and worms and marine species. Parasites (e.g., helminths) and fungi (e.g., psilocybin) are also included in the scope of pharmacognosy [1].

The roots of pharmacognosy are embedded in traditional medicine practices globally, and are recorded through traditional knowledge systems, folklore, incantations, materia medica, and pharmacopeias [2]. Pharmacopeia reflects investigation and standards for identity, purity, quality, and clinical efficacy of drugs, whereas material medica reflects traditional indications and applications [5]. Currently, the principles have been entrenched into pharmacological sciences through systematic evidence-based investigations related to purity, potency, extraction methodology, isolation of active constituents, consistency, efficacy, and safety [2].

Pharmacognosy remains a central feature in traditional medicine and pharmacology, with the former remaining the primary source of medicine in developing countries and emerging economies [1]. However, modern pharmacognosy includes increased scientific focus, particularly through the introduction of molecular, genomic, and metabolomic techniques, increasingly taken up in a variety of fields including molecular biology, biotechnology, proteomics, and bioinformatics [2, 6]. With the emergence of increasing global demand for more holistic, safe, and effective medicinal approaches, there is a significant resurgence in the field of pharmacognosy in recent years [5]. This chapter aims to provide an overview of herbal pharmacognosy, with a focus on secondary metabolite classes relevant to human biology, pathology, and clinical practice.

2 Herbal pharmacognosy

The use of medicinal plants dates back to prehistoric times and is well represented throughout recorded history in all cultures. Nowadays, plants remain an important source of medicine for most of the global population, and an important source of drug discovery in pharmacology [6]. Through the development of traditional medicine systems and modern scientific investigation, herbal pharmacognosy specifically focuses on plant-derived natural products for clinical application. This includes a significant variety of approaches to ensure safety, purity, and efficacy of complex multicompound products [7].

Herbal medicines are complex compounds that demonstrate multiple synergistic mechanisms of action to modulate (patho)physiological functions. However, the modern "pharmacology" approach to herbal medicine over the last 150 years has aimed to identify, isolate, and exploit specific plant compounds, particularly secondary metabolites, through more specific mechanisms of action for novel drug discovery and development [8].

3 Secondary metabolites

Plants produce a variety of biological molecules composed of different biochemical structures. These phytochemicals are commonly termed "secondary metabolites," as they are derived from primary metabolites such as carbohydrates, fats, and amino acids through numerous biochemical pathways [9–11]. Primary metabolites are concerned with growth,

Herbal Medicine in Andrology. https://doi.org/10.1016/B978-0-12-815565-3.00003-5

development, and survival, and are therefore more generic and critical for plant survival, whereas secondary metabolites are synthesized from modified metabolic pathways with more species-specific physiology relevant to innate immunity, defense against herbivores and pathogens, antioxidants, attraction of pollinators to flowers and for cellular communication as hormones and signaling molecules [12, 13]. The functions can be grouped as (i) antipathogenic against microbes, other plants, and insects as well as larger animals like herbivores, (ii) metal transporting, (iii) facilitation of plant symbiosis with other organisms, (iv) hormones, and (v) effectors of cellular differentiation [10, 14]. Classification related to nomenclature is based on chemical structure, composition, solvent solubility, or synthetic pathways [13]. The major groups include alkaloids, phenolic compounds, and terpenoids [15].

Secondary metabolites have been utilized by humans in a variety of forms as commodities through the ages, including pigments, condiments, nutrients, and medicines [9, 11]. Importantly, these secondary metabolites are largely responsible for the medicinal properties of plants, as these compounds have been shown to improve the health status in numerous diseases [13, 16]. Furthermore, each genus and subsequent species of plants have a characteristic mix of secondary metabolites, which are sometimes used for taxonomy purposes [13, 16].

4   Secondary plant metabolites

4.1   Terpenoids (isoprenoids)

Terpenoids (isoprenoids) are the largest class of natural organic compounds extracted from plants, and are typically present in plant essences and resins [17, 18]. These are derived from terpenes that are modified through the addition or removal of methyl groups or oxygen groups, and are therefore characterized by multiple hydrocarbon isoprene units and related oxygen derivatives (consisting of alcohols, ketones, aldehydes, esters, or carboxylic acid) [17, 18]. Each isoprene unit consists of five carbon atoms (C_5H_8), making the basis for the classification of terpenoids. The isoprene components are synthesized through the mevalonate pathway from acetate or via glycolytic intermediate molecules (Fig. 1) [13, 20].

Classification of terpenoids is based on the number of isoprene units that comprise the terpene (Fig. 2). This includes hemiterpenes (1 isoprene unit $= C_5H_8$), monoterpenes ($C_{10}H_{16}$), sesquiterpenes ($C_{15}H_{24}$), diterpenes ($C_{20}H_{32}$), sesterpenes ($C_{25}H_{40}$), triterpenes ($C_{30}H_{48}$), tetraterpenes ($C_{40}H_{64}$), and polyterpenes ($C > 40$). Monoterpenes constitute many plant essential oils, including those from vegetables, fruits, and herbs, and may prevent carcinogenesis at both the initiation and promotion stages [21, 22]. Sesquiterpenes are mostly in higher plants, and have increasing research supporting anticancer, cytotoxic, antiviral, and antibiotic properties [21]. Tetraterpenes include carotenoids, an important group of colorful pigments and pollinator attractors in flowers, fruits, and vegetables [21]. Some examples of terpenoids include isoprene (hemiterpene), geraniol (monoterpene), steroids (triterpene), carotenoids and lycopene (tetraterpene), and ubiquinones and tocopherols (polyterpenes) [13].

Well-defined activities of terpenoids in plants include maintenance of cell membrane fluidity, phytohormone activity, and immune function [18]. Furthermore, these compounds provide a communication tool for plants due to their volatility, as well as for pollinators, and provide a basis for culinary flavors and fragrances [13, 23]. Physiological benefits include expectorant activities in relieving cough and as an analgesic to relieve pain [17, 18]. They are also important nutritional sources for cancer protection (e.g., lycopene) [21]. With more than 40,000 different terpenoids isolated and identified, alongside the physiological activity in humans, these have become economically important compounds in both pharmaceutical and agricultural uses (pesticides) [24].

4.2   Glycosides

Glycosides are a heterogeneous and diverse group of secondary metabolites with significant bioactivity, which include phenol, alcohol, or sulfur-related compounds [13, 25]. They are characterized by one or more sugar components combined with a bioactive nonsugar component (a lipophilic aglycone joined with a hydrophilic glycone unit) through a glycosidic bond (Fig. 3) [13, 25]. In plant biology, these compounds are typically used to store energy in the form of sugars, which are hydrolyzed to increase their chemical availability by releasing the aglycone unit [25]. In humans, this typically occurs within the colon [13].

Glycosides are classified based on the aglycone unit, the glycone unit, or the type of glycosidic bond. Arising from the classification based on the aglycone sugar unit, clinically useful groups include alcoholic, anthraquinone, cardiac (steroidal), coumarin, cyanogenic, flavonoid, phenolic (saponins), and thioglycoside molecules [25]. Therefore, they are a very heterogeneous group based on their structure, making glycosides difficult to work with, to study, and clinically apply [13].

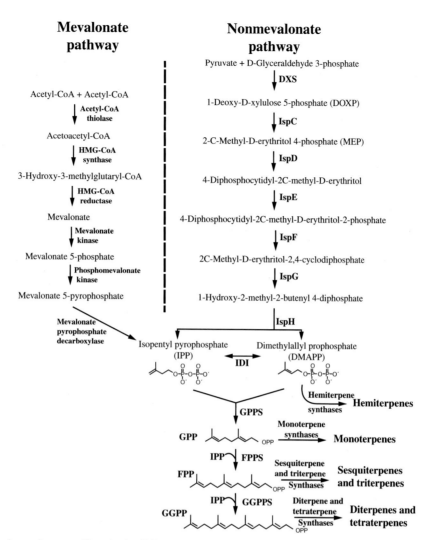

FIG. 1 Biosynthetic pathways for terpenoid production [19].

4.3 Saponins

Saponins are a diverse group of plant molecules that are characterized by one or more hydrophilic glycosides combined to a lipophilic triterpene or steroid molecule such as an aglycone unit. The aglycone unit consists of a range of polycyclic organic structures, and dietary monosaccharides such as D-glucose and D-galactose are the most abundant hydrophilic component [13, 26]. Saponins are classified based on the skeletons of the aglycon side chains that are attached to the saccharide portion, alongside the number of saccharide chains, giving rise to the chemical nomenclature system (Fig. 4) [8, 28]. They contribute significantly to pathogen resistance and food quality in crops, hence having agricultural and economic importance [29]. These molecules are further characterized by the active components forming colloidal solutions that lather to produce soap-like foam and precipitate cholesterol when shaken in water [13, 30]. Molecular properties include solubilization, emulsification, and foaming [13]. These physiochemical properties, alongside increasing evidence of biological properties, are driving an increased consumer demand and scientific interest in these molecules [26]. Therefore, saponins represent significant importance and commercial interest for the food, cosmetic, pharmacological, and clinical fields [26].

Saponins are found predominantly in terrestrial plants, including Sapindaceae (such as soapberry and horse chestnut), *Gynostemma pentaphyllum*, *Panax ginseng* (ginsenosides), and *Astragalus* spp. [8, 28]. However, they also naturally occur in starfish and sea cucumbers [29]. Saponins have been shown to have antibacterial, antitumor, anticholesterol, and immune-modulating properties [28, 30]. Other demonstrated effects include reduced lipogenesis and improvement of nonalcoholic fatty liver and hyperuricemia [31]. Significantly more research into saponins is warranted, as this diverse group with the potential for high-value drug discovery remains underexplored [29].

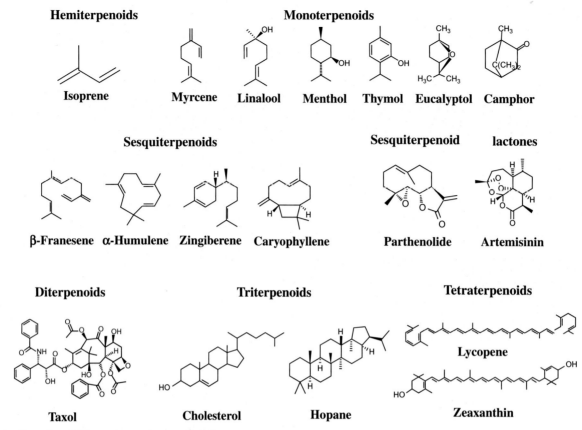

FIG. 2 Examples of different classes of terpenoids [19].

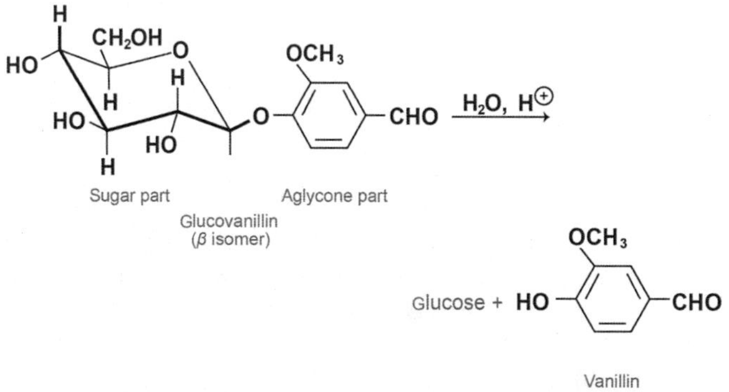

FIG. 3 Bonding of sugar component and aglycone component in glycosides, using glucovanillin as a specific example. The bonding is through oxygen to the carbonyl carbon.

4.4 Phenolic compounds

Phenols are compounds characterized by a hydroxyl functional group joined to an aromatic hydrocarbon, which are alcohols with higher acidity due to the aromatic ring. When more hydroxyl groups are present, they are termed "polyphenols" (also see tannins below) [13]. Soluble phenols are generally found in cell vacuoles, where insoluble phenols are found predominantly in cell walls [32]. Phenols, both soluble and insoluble, are considered one of the most important groups of secondary metabolites, particularly relevant to human health. They are predominantly found in fruits, vegetables, teas, and other antioxidant-rich compounds such as coffee and cocoa [13, 21]. Some foods, like apples and pears, berries, grapes,

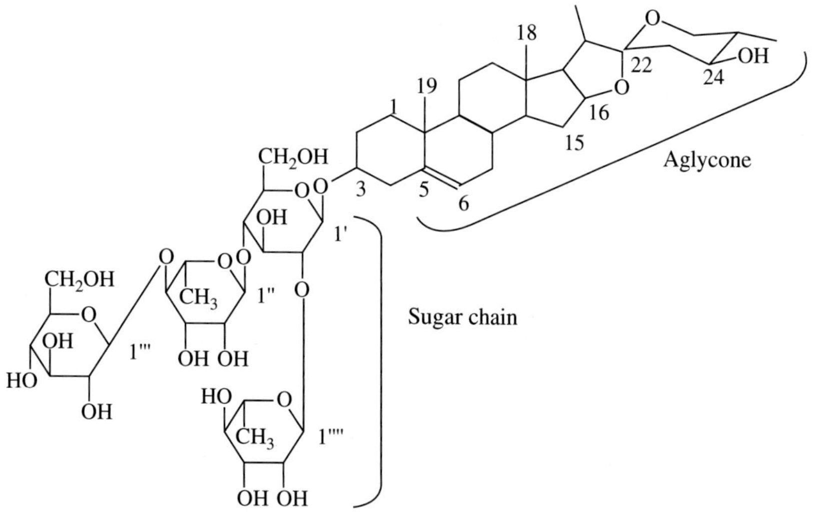

FIG. 4 Structure of a saponin [27]. *From Zhou D, Li X, Chang W, Han Y, Liu B, Chen G, Li N. Antiproliferative steroidal glycosides from rhizomes of Polygonatum sibiricum. Phytochemistry 2019;164:172–83. https://doi.org/10.1016/j.phytochem.2019.05.013.*

and cherries, have > 250 mg polyphenols per 100 g [32]. They contribute to bitterness, color, odor, and redox stability in food, and protection against pathogen aggressiveness and ultraviolet (UV) radiation [32]. The content of phenols in plants is highly dependent on environmental factors, including soil type, rainfall, sun exposure, pathogen exposure, harvesting, fruit ripening, storage methods and duration, and food preparation and cooking [32].

These compounds have significant antioxidant capacity, alongside antiinflammatory, antimicrobial, and anticancer properties, which offers protection from a broad range of chronic and oxidative stress-mediated diseases [13, 17, 33]. The total polyphenol intake in humans is generally inversely correlated to the risk of numerous chronic noncommunicable and degenerative diseases including cardiovascular and neurodegenerative diseases, diabetes, cancer, and osteoporosis [32].

To date, more than 8000 polyphenols have been identified. Yet, the terminology and classification remain unclear and even confusing. All these polyphenolic compounds arise from phenylalanine or shikimic acid as close precursors, and primarily occur as conjugated forms in which one or more sugar components are bound to hydroxyl groups (Fig. 5) [32]. Alternative structures can include direct joining of sugars (as monosaccharides or polysaccharides) to an aromatic carbon, or they may exist in close association with organic acids, carboxylic acid, amines, or lipids that link other phenols [32]. Classification systems are based on the number of hydroxyl groups, chemical composition, and substitutes in the aromatic rings, as well as the number of aromatic rings. The main subclassification groups of polyphenols include bioflavonoids, phenolic acids, stilbenes, and lignans [13].

4.4.1 Flavonoids

This is the most well-researched group of polyphenols, typically found predominantly in flowers as coloring pigments for pollinator attraction. Essentially, they comprise basic units of two aromatic rings to form an oxygenated heterocycle [32]. Further classification into major subgroups is based on the type of heterocycle involved, such as anthocyanins, flavones, flavonols, flavanones, flavonols, and isoflavones (Fig. 6) [13]. Additional variation in each group is based on the hydroxyl group arrangements and the presence of posttranslational modifications like alkylation or glycosylation. Important medicinal examples of flavonoids include compounds such as quercetin and catechins [32].

Flavonoids are hydrophilic pigments typically found in the vacuoles of plant cells [13]. They are further involved in nitrogen fixation, chemical messaging, cell cycle inhibition, and enhancement of symbiotic relationships [13, 32]. Flavonoids are reported to have broad benefits in treating chronic diseases, including obesity complications and cancer, through immunomodulation and antioxidant effects [17]. The insurgence of numerous chronic diseases, such as atherosclerosis, diabetes, cancer, and degenerative diseases, is inversely correlated with flavonoid intake [13]. However, intake for medicinal purpose requires further investigation, particularly for the identification of the most effective flavonoid and relative concentration in the prevention and management strategies of different disease models. It is postulated that increased consumption above

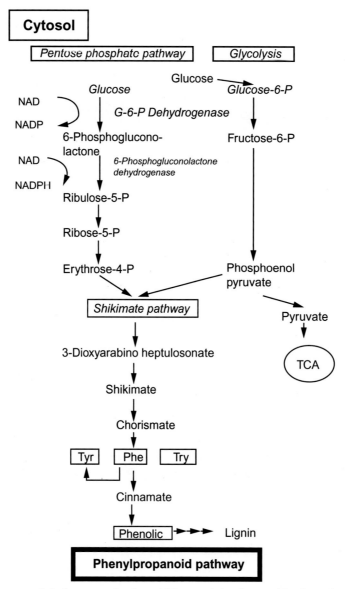

FIG. 5   Biosynthesis of phenolic compounds in the pentose phosphate, shikimate and phenylpropanoid pathways in plants [34].

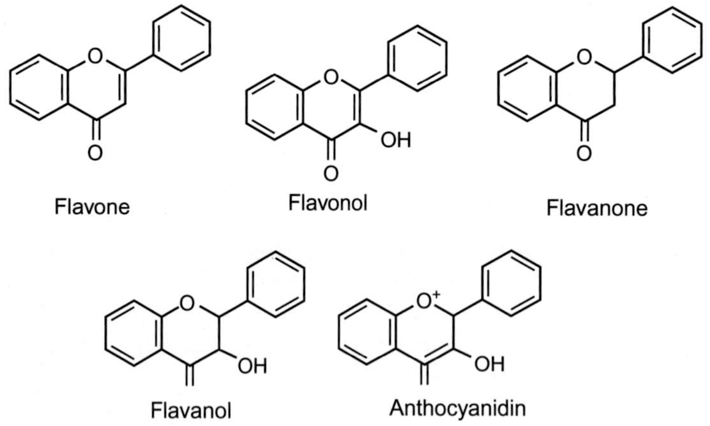

FIG. 6   Generic structures of flavonoids [35].

the recommended normal nutritional intake may be detrimental to health, probably through the establishment of reductive stress [13].

4.4.2 Phenolic acids

Phenolic acids are abundant metabolites in foods. They are divided into two subclasses: (a) derivatives of benzoic acid and (b) derivatives of cinnamic acid. The latter are significantly more common in edible plants, and mostly consist of caffeic, ferulic, and coumaric acids [32].

4.4.3 Stilbenes

Stilbenes consist of two phenyl rings that are joined by a methylene bridge. These have significant antifungal properties [32]. Resveratrol is one of the most well-studied stilbenes found in red grape seeds and skins, as well as in red wine [32].

4.4.4 Lignans

The basic structure of lignans include two phenolic molecules with a dibenzylbutane structure [32]. The latter is formed by the dimerization of two cinnamic acid residues [32]. Many lignans, such as secoisolariciresinol, have phytoestrogenic activity [32].

4.5 Tannins

Tannins are a class of polyphenolic molecules containing hydroxyl or carboxyl groups that form complexes with macromolecules such as carbohydrates [36, 37]. They make a significant proportion of total plant biomass, contributing up to 10% of the dry weight of tree leaves, although they are typically found in the bark and wood in higher abundance [21, 36–38]. Tannins are used in a range of industries, including leather tanning, wood adhesives, animal feed, fisheries, the manufacture of beverages, and potential applications being explored in wood preservation, corrosive prevention, binding in Teflon, and epoxy adhesives [39]. With characteristic astringent properties, tannins are largely responsible for dry mouth associated with consumption of tea, red wine, and unripe fruits [40]. Importantly, they are also gaining importance in reducing reliance on fossil fuels in an effort to reduce the detrimental environmental impact of increased atmospheric carbon dioxide [41, 42]. A central feature and advantage of tannins is that they have strong antioxidant properties because of their phenolic structure [13, 39]. Moreover, they play a prominent role in UV protection and other biological threats from animals and pathogenic microorganisms [43].

The synthesis of these compounds relies on the shikimic (phenylpropanoid) pathway, also responsible for isoflavones, coumarins, and aromatic amino acids [13]. They are generally hydrophobic, with some exceptions in those of high molecular weight [13]. All tannins are broadly classified into two groups, namely, hydrolysable and condensed tannins (Fig. 7) [45]. Hydrolysable tannins are simple phenols [45], particularly represented by gallotannins, formed through the esterification of gallic acid and subsequent binding to a hydroxyl group of a carbohydrate (e.g., glucose). These compounds are specifically gaining significant interest for the development of future antimicrobial drugs [39]. Moreover, hydrolysable tannins, such as ellagic acid, can be reduced by weak acids and bases to produce phenolic acid alongside carbohydrates [13]. On the other side, condensed tannins are derived from polyhydroxy-flavan-3-ol oligomers and they make most of the

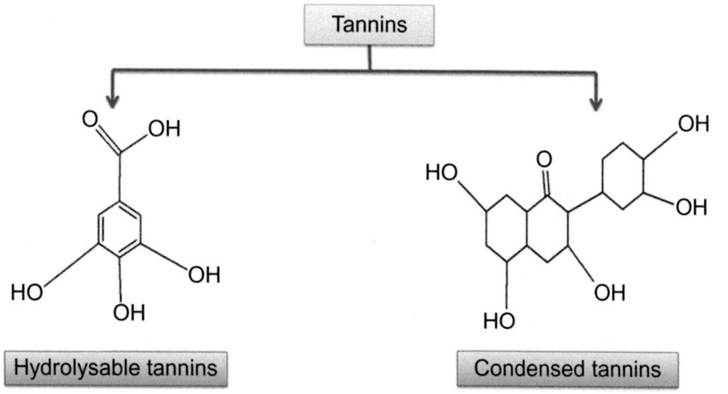

FIG. 7   Types of tannins and their basic structures [44].

total global production of tannins [46]. These consist of repeating tannins units formed by the condensation of flavans, with no sugar residues. These are also known as flavonoids or proanthocyanidins, such as biologically beneficial catechins and epicatechin [39].

4.6 Alkaloids

Alkaloids are organic nitrogenous compounds, most widely found in dicotyledonous plants [17, 47]. These are typically synthesized in bacteria, fungi, and larger animals from an amino acid base and are generally of low molecular weight, have a negative oxidation state, and are used as defense response to pathogens and predators [13]. Examples include nicotine, caffeine, morphine, atropine, ephedrine, and quinine. Alkaloids are a very large and diverse group with physiological and medicinal effects, significant structural diversity and no clear defining or classification systems [13]. Since they are derivatives of amino acids, there is no clear defining point between alkaloids and many other nitrogen-containing molecules, including polypeptides, nucleotides, and nucleic acids, that are not termed "alkaloids" [48]. Classification and nomenclature are traditionally based on the source species, particularly prior to the understanding of chemical structures. Recent classification can also be based on similarities of the carbon skeleton (such as indole, isoquinoline, and pyridine) or the precursor amino acid [49]. This can further lead to a subclassification in true alkaloids and protoalkaloids (nitrogen-based derived from amino acids), polyamine alkaloids (derivatives of true alkaloids), peptide alkaloids, and pseudoalkaloids (which do not originate from amino acids) [13]. Many of them are used in medicine, as purified extractions, or synthetically manufactured in a range of clinical disciplines and applications, including antimicrobial, antiarhythmic, antimutagenic, anticancer, analgesic, and antimalarial activities [13].

4.7 Essential oils

Essentials oils are volatile compounds that are aromatic and highly fragrant. This function of essential oils is plant protection from pathogens and predators, alongside pollination [13, 50]. These compounds are all lipophilic, but do not include nonaromatic fatty acids and other lipids in vegetable sources [13]. The effect on human biology is postulated to be primarily through the stimulation of the olfactory nerve that communicates directly with the limbic system [13, 51, 52].

5 Conclusion

Medicines derived from natural sources have been used extensively in human history, dating back tens of thousands of years. These sources include animals, plants, and minerals. In recent years, pharmacognosy has developed, broadly to study the science of these natural medicines. Herbal pharmacognosy specifically focuses on current and potential pharmacological and medicinal applications of plant compounds, with a specific focus on secondary plant metabolites. Scientific interest in these metabolites has significantly increased in recent years, relevant to human applications. In addition to traditional medicine, pharmaceutical development, and clinical practice, herbal applications include industrial uses and biofuel sources, pigments, cooking, and nutrition, among others. Mechanisms of action of secondary metabolites on human biology and pathophysiology are broad. However, a significant focus is on the antioxidant- and redox-regulating activity, associated with the prevention and potential treatment of numerous diseases, specifically noncommunicable chronic diseases. Moreover, increasing investigation about the application of secondary plant metabolites in reproductive biology and andrology shows their potential for the development of novel therapeutic strategies for both established and idiopathic reproductive dysfunction. Significant interdisciplinary research is required to establish appropriate herbs, secondary metabolites, extraction methods, standardized medicines, isolate identification and drug development within human health, disease, and reproductive dysfunction.

References

[1] Orhan IE. Pharmacognosy: science of natural products in drug discovery. Bioimpacts 2014;4(3):109–10.
[2] Dhami N. Trends in pharmacognosy: a modern science of natural medicines. J Herbal Med 2013;3:123–31.
[3] Kennedy DO, Wightman EL. Herbal extracts and phytochemicals: plant secondary metabolites and the enhancement of human brain function. Adv Nutr 2011;2(1):32–50.
[4] Ahmad I, Aqil F, Owais M. Modern phytomedicine: turning medicinal plants into drugs. In: Modern phytomedicine: Turning medicinal plants into drugs; 2006. p. 1–384.

[5] Roy Upton RH. Traditional herbal medicine, pharmacognosy, and pharmacopoeial standards: a discussion at the crossroads. In: Evidence-based validation of herbal medicine. Elsevier Inc.; 2015. p. 46–85.

[6] Heinrich M, Anagnostou S. From pharmacognosia to DNA-based medicinal plant authentication—pharmacognosy through the centuries. Planta Med 2017;83(14–15):1110–6.

[7] Pferschy-Wenzig EM, Bauer R. The relevance of pharmacognosy in pharmacological research on herbal medicinal products. Epilepsy Behav 2015;52:344–62.

[8] Li J, Wang R, Yang L, Wang Z. Structure and biological action on cardiovascular systems of saponins from *Panax notoginseng*. Zhongguo Zhong Yao Za Zhi 2015;40(17):3480–7.

[9] Staniek A, Bouwmeester H, Fraser PD, Kayser O, Martens S, Tissier A, et al. Natural products—modifying metabolite pathways in plants. Biotechnol J 2013;8(10):1159–71.

[10] Demain AL, Fang A. The natural functions of secondary metabolites. Adv Biochem Eng Biotechnol 2000;69:1–39. https://doi.org/10.1007/3-540-44964-7_1.

[11] Springob K, Kutchan T. Introduction to the different classes of natural products. In: Osbourne A, Lanzotti V, editors. Plant-derived natural products. Springer Science; 2009.

[12] Piasecka A, Jedrzejczak-Rey N, Bednarek P. Secondary metabolites in plant innate immunity: conserved function of divergent chemicals. New Phytol 2015;206(3):948–64.

[13] Kabera JN. Plant secondary metabolites: biosynthesis, classification, function and pharmacological properties. J Pharm Pharmacol 2014;2:377–92.

[14] Richard NB, Roger MW. Secondary metabolites in plant defence mechanisms. New Phytol 1994;127(4):617–33.

[15] Bohlmann J, Keeling CI. Terpenoid biomaterials. Plant J 2008;54(4):656–69.

[16] Wang Y, Li JY, Han M, Wang WL, Li YZ. Prevention and treatment effect of total flavonoids in *Stellera chamaejasme* L. on nonalcoholic fatty liver in rats. Lipids Health Dis 2015;14(1):1–9.

[17] Yao H, Qiao YJ, Zhao YL, Tao XF, Xu LN, Yin LH, et al. Herbal medicines and nonalcoholic fatty liver disease. World J Gastroenterol 2016;22(30):6890–905.

[18] Arendt P, Pollier J, Callewaert N, Goossens A. Synthetic biology for production of natural and new-to-nature terpenoids in photosynthetic organisms. Plant J 2016;87(1):16–37.

[19] Abdallah II, Quax WJ. A glimpse into the biosynthesis of terpenoids. KnE Life Sci 2017;3(5):81.

[20] Grayson DH. Monoterpenoids. Nat Prod Rep 1996;13(3):195.

[21] Jamwal K, Bhattacharya S, Puri S. Plant growth regulator mediated consequences of secondary metabolites in medicinal plants. J Appl Res Med Aromat Plants 2018;9:26–38. https://doi.org/10.1016/j.jarmap.2017.12.003.

[22] Gould MN. Cancer chemoprevention and therapy by monoterpenes. Environ Health Perspect 1997;105(Suppl. 4):977–9.

[23] Maffei ME. Sites of synthesis, biochemistry and functional role of plant volatiles. S Afr J Bot 2010;76(4):612–31.

[24] Moses T, Pollier J, Thevelein JM, Goossens A. Bioengineering of plant (tri)terpenoids: from metabolic engineering of plants to synthetic biology in vivo and in vitro. New Phytol 2013;200(1):27–43.

[25] Bartnik M, Facey PC. Glycosides. In: Pharmacognosy: Fundamentals, applications and strategy. Elsevier Inc.; 2017. p. 101–61.

[26] Guclu-Ustundag Ö, Mazza G. Saponins: properties, applications and processing. Crit Rev Food Sci Nutr 2007;47(3):231–58.

[27] Moghimipour E, Handali S. Saponin: properties, methods of evaluation and applications. Annu Res Rev Biol 2015;5(3):207–20.

[28] Dong J, Liang W, Wang T, Sui J, Wang J, Deng Z, et al. Saponins regulate intestinal inflammation in colon cancer and IBD. Pharmacol Res 2019;144:66–72.

[29] Osbourn A, Goss RJM, Field RA. The saponins-polar isoprenoids with important and diverse biological activities. Nat Prod Rep 2011;28(7):1261–8.

[30] Liu X, Yu J, Liu M, Shu J, Huang H. Research progress of bioactivity of steroidal saponins in recent ten years. Zhongguo Zhong Yao Za Zhi 2015;40(13):2518–23.

[31] Zhao YC, Xue CH, Zhang TT, Wang YM. Saponins from sea cucumber and their biological activities. J Agric Food Chem 2018;66:7222–37.

[32] Pandey K, Rizvi S. Plant polyphenols as dietary antioxidants in human health and disease, oxidative medicine and cellular longevity. Oxid Med Cell Longev 2009;2(5):270–8.

[33] Faghihzadeh F, Adibi P, Rafiei R, Hekmatdoost A. Resveratrol supplementation improves inflammatory biomarkers in patients with nonalcoholic fatty liver disease. Nutr Res 2014;34(10):837–43.

[34] Lin D, Xiao M, Zhao J, Li Z, Xing B, Li X, et al. An overview of plant phenolic compounds and their importance in human nutrition and management of type 2 diabetes. Molecules 2016;21(10):1374. https://doi.org/10.3390/molecules21101374.

[35] Balasundram N, Sundram K, Samman S. Phenolic compounds in plants and agri-industrial by-products: antioxidant activity, occurrence, and potential uses. Food Chem 2006;99(1):191–203.

[36] Arbenz A, Avérous L. Tannins: a resource to elaborate aromatic and biobased polymers. In: Biodegradable and biobased polymers for environmental and biomedical applications. Hoboken, NJ: John Wiley & Sons, Inc.; 2016. p. 97–148.

[37] Barbehenn RV, Constabel CP. Tannins in plant-herbivore interactions. Phytochemistry 2011;72(13):1551–65.

[38] Mueller-Harvey I. Analysis of hydrolysable tannins. Anim Feed Sci Technol 2001;91(1–2):3–20.

[39] Shirmohammadli Y, Efhamisisi D, Pizzi A. Tannins as a sustainable raw material for green chemistry: a review. Ind Crops Prod 2018;126:316–32.

[40] Schmid R, McGee H. On food and cooking: the science and Lore of the kitchen. Taxon 1989;38(3):446.

[41] Luckeneder P, Gavino J, Kuchernig R, Petutschnigg A, Tondi G. Sustainable phenolic fractions as basis for furfuryl alcohol-based co-polymers and their use as wood adhesives. Polymers (Basel) 2016;8(11):396.

[42] de Hoyos-Martínez PL, Merle J, Labidi J, Charrier-El Bouhtoury F. Tannins extraction: a key point for their valorization and cleaner production. J Clean Prod 2019;206:1138–55. Elsevier Ltd.

[43] Tondi G, Thevenon MF, Mies B, Standfest G, Petutschnigg A, Wieland S. Impregnation of Scots pine and beech with tannin solutions: effect of viscosity and wood anatomy in wood infiltration. Wood Sci Technol 2013,47(3):615–26.

[44] Ghosh D. Tannins from foods to combat diseases. Int J Pharma Res Rev 2015;4(5):40–4.

[45] Aroso IM, Araújo AR, Pires RA, Reis RL. Cork: current technological developments and future perspectives for this natural, renewable, and sustainable material. ACS Sustain Chem Eng 2017;5(12):11130–46.

[46] Hemingway R, Karchesy J. Chemistry and significance of condensed tannins. Newyork and London: Springer Science & Business Media, Plenum Publishing; 2012.

[47] Stegelmeier BL, Brown AW, Welch KD. Safety concerns of herbal products and traditional Chinese herbal medicines: dehydropyrrolizidine alkaloids and aristolochic acid. J Appl Toxicol 2015;35(12):1433–7.

[48] Giweli AA, Džamić AM, Soković M, Ristić MS, Janaćković P, Marin PD. The chemical composition, antimicrobial and antioxidant activities of the essential oil of *Salvia fruticosa* growing wild in Libya. Arch Biol Sci 2013;65(1):321–9.

[49] Savithramma N, Rao ML, Suhrulatha D. Screening of medicinal plants for secondary metabolites. Middle-East J Sci Res 2011;8(3):579–84.

[50] Angelucci FL, Silva VV, Dal Pizzol C, Spir LG, Praes CEO, Maibach H. Physiological effect of olfactory stimuli inhalation in humans: an overview. Int J Cosmet Sci 2014;36(2):117–23.

[51] Schnaubelt K, Beasley J. Advanced aroatherapy: The science of essential oil therapy. Vermont: Healing Arts Press Rochester; 1998.

[52] Meamarbashi A. Instant effects of peppermint essential oil on the physiological parameters and exercise performance. Avicenna J Phytomedicine 2014;4(1):72–8.

Chapter 4.1

Overview on the clinical presentation and indication

Ismail Tambi

Men Wellness Clinic, Damai Service Hospital, Kuala Lumpur, Malaysia

1 Testosterone deficiency

1.1 Testosterone

Testosterone is derived from cholesterol and, in men, 95% of the amount is synthesized primarily in the interstitial cells of Leydig in the testes, while the remaining 5% are produced by the adrenal glands [1]. During puberty, the increase in testosterone production promotes the growth of spermatogenic tissue in the testicles, male fertility, penis enlargement, increased libido, and frequency of erection [1]. The amount of testosterone synthesized is regulated by the hypothalamic-pituitary-testicular axis [2].

When testosterone levels are low, gonadotropin-releasing hormone (GnRH) is released by the hypothalamus, which in turn stimulates the pituitary gland to release FSH and LH [2]. Follicle-stimulating hormone (FSH) and luteinizing hormone (LH) stimulate the testes to synthesize testosterone, which when elevated will inhibit the release of GnRH and FSH/LH, respectively, through a negative feedback loop which acts on the hypothalamus and pituitary [2]. In normal males, approximately 98% of the testosterone circulates in the blood bound to protein, of which approximately 60% is weakly bound to albumin and other proteins and 40% is bound with higher binding affinity to sex hormone binding globulin (SHBG) [3, 4]. The remaining 2% is free or unbound. The fraction available to the tissues (also termed bioavailable testosterone) is believed to be the free plus the albumin-bound testosterone, consisting of approximately half of the total plasma testosterone [5].

Testosterone bound to albumin is biologically available due to rapid dissociation. Testosterone is important throughout life in men as it is the principal steroidal hormone that awakes manhood in a male child and maintains health and well-being [6]. Typical manly body features like increased muscle strength and mass, broad shoulders and expanded rib cage, deepening of the voice, and growth of the Adam's apple become evident as testosterone peaks [7]. Other features include enlargement of sebaceous glands, oily face and acne, and decrease in baby fat in the face as well as pubic hair extends to thighs and up toward umbilicus, development of facial hair (sideburns, beard, moustache), male pattern loss of scalp hair (androgenetic alopecia), increase in chest hair, peri-areolar hair, perianal hair, leg hair, and armpit hair [5]. Growth spurts brought about by growth hormone enhance growth of jaw, brow, chin, nose, and remodeling of facial bone contours toward manly features with completion of bone maturation initiated by testosterone [6]. A male child who is devoid of testosterone will lack all the above features and will have a female physical feature with a childlike voice [7]. Considering that testosterone is important throughout life, any deficiency of testosterone at any phase of man's life will result with testosterone deficiency [7].

1.2 Factors affecting testosterone levels

Testosterone production is enhanced in sexually active men [8] and influences sexual function, mood, and visuospatial cognition in older men [9]. Falling in love, establishing a relationship, and marriage dampen testosterone production [10]. Testosterone charged men are more prone to extramarital affairs or divorce [11]. Fatherhood subdues testosterone production in positive paternal care [11].

Herbal Medicine in Andrology. https://doi.org/10.1016/B978-0-12-815565-3.00004-7

Men flirting with women may experience a surge of testosterone [12]. Watching a sexually explicit movie can increase testosterone by 35%, peaking for 60–90 min after the end of the film [13]. Vitamin A deficiency may lead to suboptimal plasma testostcrone levels while vitamin D3 in levels of 400–1000 IU/d (10–25 µg/d) raises testosterone levels [11]. On the other hand, zinc deficiency lowers testosterone level but over-supplementation has no effect on serum testosterone [14]. Men exposed to scents of ovulating women maintained a stable testosterone level compared to men exposed to nonovulating women [15]. Resistance training exercises increase testosterone levels [16]. However, endurance training in men lowers their testosterone levels [17].

Reduction in body weight may result in an increase in testosterone levels. Fat cells synthesize the enzyme aromatase, which converts testosterone into estradiol, the female sex hormone [18]. There is no clear association between body mass index (BMI) and testosterone levels [19]. Aggressive and dominating behavior can occasionally stimulate increased testosterone release in men [20]. Sleep, especially REM sleep, on the other hand, increases nocturnal testosterone levels which contributed to nocturnal penile tumescence (NPT) [21]. Testosterone levels gradually reduce as men age, an effect referred to as "andropause" or LOH (late-onset hypogonadism) [20]. In elderly males, normal levels of testosterone decrease the risk of cardiovascular disease, decrease the visceral fat mass, total cholesterol, and glycemic control, and increase lean body mass [22].

Natural or man-made antiandrogens including spearmint tea can reduce testosterone levels [23]. However, the root extract of Tongkat Ali (Ali's walking stick in Malay language), a well-known Malaysian jungle shrub known as *Eurycoma longifolia jack,* in the standardized water-soluble form, enhances serum testosterone levels significantly [24].

1.3   Testosterone replacement therapy (TRT)

Testosterone replacement therapy is known as a hormone replacement therapy (HRT) that maintains serum testosterone levels in the normal range [8]. The natural decline in testosterone production has led to a scientific and medical interest in this therapy [8]. However, it is still unclear if the supplementation with testosterone in patients with low testosterone levels due to aging is beneficial or harmful [25]. Androgen deficiency may have serious consequences in men, and this condition requires diagnosis and appropriate treatment. When administered properly, androgens are safe. On the other hand, when administered inappropriately or abused, they may cause considerable harm [25]. Testosterone is used as a medication for the treatment of low testosterone production or hypogonadism, and gender dysphoria in transgender men [26].

2   Poor semen quality and infertility

Semen is an organic fluid that is a combination of the secretions of the testes and the accessory sexual glands, namely the seminal vesicles, the prostate, the Cowper's gland, and the epididymis that besides spermatozoa contains proteolytic and other enzymes as well as fructose, which promote the survival of spermatozoa [27]. Semen is ejected through the process of ejaculation, which is the end result of sexual stimulation through masturbation or vaginal sexual intercourse [27]. Semen quality is a measure of the ability of the male germ cells, the spermatozoa, to accomplish fertilization and pregnancy. It is also regarded as a measure of male fertility [28] and decrease in semen quality involves both sperm quantity and quality [28]. In addition, decreased semen quality is a major factor of male infertility; specifically with the sperm, fertilizing capacity being a major indicator [28]. Fecundity starts to decline when the sperm concentrations fall below $30–55 \times 10^6$/mL, yet the WHO lower reference value for normal values is currently 15×10^6/mL [28]. Over the past 15 years, multiple studies have reported median sperm concentrations of $41–55 \times 10^6$/mL in young men (mean age 18–21 years) from the general population, suggesting that many of them have suboptimal semen quality [29]. Between 19 and 29 years of age, sperm numbers remain fairly constant, provided the growth hormone and the pubertal hormonal status are functioning normally [29]. It is interesting to note that as men get older semen volume, sperm motility, and sperm morphology decline but not the sperm concentration [30].

2.1   Factors that affect quality of semen

The reasons for poor semen quality and adverse trends are not well established, however some associations suggest heavy smoking and heavy drinking are associated with worse seminal parameters than moderate smoking/drinking and nonsmoking/abstaining from alcohol [29]. Strong evidence has shown that smoking is associated with increased sperm DNA damage and male infertility [31]. Obese men have lower circulating testosterone, which affects semen quality, namely poor low sperm count [32].

Specific pharmaceutical medications affect the quality of semen in a negative manner [33]. Specifically, selective serotonin reuptake inhibitor (SSRIs) such as paroxitine causes sperm DNA fragmentation [33]. Calcium channel blockers like nifedipine affect sperm motility and structural changes in both the head and tail regions of sperm [34]. Antiepileptic medications including carbamazepine, phenytoin, and valproate have specific drug-dependent side effects, including abnormal sperm morphology, reduced motility, and lower sperm count [33]. Similarly, highly active antiretroviral therapy (HAART) like saquinavir increased rates of abnormal sperm morphology and decreased sperm motility [35]. However, semen quality is not affected by proton-pump inhibitors (PPIs), such as omeprazole, a commonly used medication to treat upper gastrointestinal disorders including gastrointestinal reflux disease and peptic ulcer disease [36].

Industrial chemical and components of polycarbonate plastic and epoxy resins, which contain endocrine disrupting compounds, xenoestrogens like bisphenol A, nonylphenol, and octylphenol have been associated with decreased sperm quality on exposure by interfering with the normal reproductive hormonal process of spermatogenesis [37]. In addition, pesticides like diphenyl trichloroethane (DDT) and hexachlorobenzene affect reproductive hormonal functions and cause disruption of spermatogenesis resulting in decreased semen quality [37].

On the other hand, a healthy dietary pattern like the higher intakes of legumes, vegetables, cereals, fruits, and olive oil are associated with good semen quality, particularly sperm concentration and progressive motility among male partner of couples planning pregnancy [38]. Low-fat dairy intake, particularly low-fat milk, was also related to higher sperm concentration and progressive motility [39]. In addition, fish consumption was positively associated with total sperm count and morphology, whereas processed meat consumption was negatively associated with sperm morphology [39]. Phytoestrogens like isoflavone supplements have little to no effect on sperm concentration, count, motility, and cause no changes in testicular or ejaculate volume [40]. *Eurycoma longifolia Jack* locally known as Tongkat Ali is a common shrub found along the slopes in hilly terrains of the Malaysian rainforest. A aqueous decoction of the root of Tongkat Ali is a well-known traditional supplement for the enhancement of sexuality and fertility. The standardized extract of the *Eurycoma longifolia Jack* significantly improves semen volume, sperm concentration, sperm motility, and the percentage of morphologically normal sperm in men with idiopathic infertility [41].

3 Aging males' symptoms (AMS)

The Aging Males' Symptoms Score Chart (Fig. 1) is an instrument to measure the severity of aging symptoms in men, and their impact on quality of life [42]. This quality of life scale for elderly males was originally developed in Germany in 1999 [41]. Like women during their menopausal transition, men also develop similar complaints like nervousness, lethargy, depression, loss of libido, increase sweating, and insomnia [42]. The AMS score scale was designed (a) to assess symptoms of aging (independent of those which are disease-related) between groups of males under different conditions, (b) to evaluate the severity of symptoms over time, and (c) to measure changes pre- and postandrogen replacement. Elderly males going through climacteric, experience impaired memory, lack of concentration, nervousness, depression, insomnia, periodic sweating or hot flushes, bone and joint complaints, and reduction in muscle mass [43]. The scale was designed as self-administered scale to assess symptoms of aging. The scale comprises 17 questions divided into three symptom blocks: psychological (five issues), somatic (seven questions), and sexual symptoms (five issues). The sum of the issues, which results in variation from one to five points, was considered as the general symptom score. The general score for somatic, psychological, and sexual symptoms was categorized, being classified as having psychological symptoms the subjects who obtain scores ≥ 12 points; with somatic symptoms, the subjects who have scores ≥ 13 points; and with sexual symptoms those subjects who have scores ≥ 8 points. The general symptom score was dichotomized so that those who submit score ≥ 27 points were classified as having aging symptoms, while those with values below that score were classified without symptoms. The AMS scale is a valuable tool for assessing health-related quality of life and symptoms in aging men and used worldwide [44].

4 Erectile dysfunction

Erectile dysfunction (ED) is defined as the inability to achieve or maintain an erection adequate enough for satisfactory sexual intercourse [45]. Normal penile erection is dependent on the overall health of the individual, the penile vascular bed, and the perineal and ischiocavernosus muscles that support the proximal penis [45, 46]. A man's ability to achieve normal penile erections depends on adequate arterial blood inflow and trapping within the corpora cavernosa (veno-occlusion) to maintain increasing pressure and volume to achieve penile rigidity [46, 47]. Erection thus involves sinusoidal relaxation, arterial dilatation, and venous compression [47]. This veno-occlusive function of the corpora cavernosa contribute to the increased blood flow into the corpora cavernosa that creates the structural rigidity necessary to prevent collapse of the

AMS Questionnaire

Which of the following symptoms apply to you at this time? Please mark the appropriate box for each symptom. For symptoms that do not apply, please mark "none."

Symptoms Score =	None 1	Mild 2	Moderate 3	Severe 4	Extremely severe 5
1. **Decline in your feeling of general well-being** (general state of health, subjective feeling)......	☐	☐	☐	☐	☐
2. **Joint pain and muscular ache** (lower back pain, joint pain, pain in a limb, general back ache)......	☐	☐	☐	☐	☐
3. **Excessive sweating** (unexpected/sudden episodes of sweating, hot flushes independent of strain)......	☐	☐	☐	☐	☐
4. **Sleep problems** (difficulty in falling asleep, difficulty in sleeping through, waking up early and feeling tired, poor sleep, sleeplessness)......	☐	☐	☐	☐	☐
5. **Increased need for sleep, often feeling tired**......	☐	☐	☐	☐	☐
6. **Irritability** (feeling aggressive, easily upset about little things, moody)......	☐	☐	☐	☐	☐
7. **Nervousness** (inner tension, restlessness, feeling fidgety)......	☐	☐	☐	☐	☐
8. **Anxiety** (feeling panicky)......	☐	☐	☐	☐	☐
9. **Physical exhaustion/lacking vitality** (general decrease in performance, reduced activity, lacking interest in leisure activities, feeling of getting less done, of achieving less, of having to force oneself to undertake activities)......	☐	☐	☐	☐	☐
10. **Decrease in muscular strength** (feeling of weakness)......	☐	☐	☐	☐	☐
11. **Depressive mood** (feeling down, sad, on the verge of tears, lack of drive, mood swings, feeling nothing is of any use)......	☐	☐	☐	☐	☐
12. **Feeling that you have passed your peak**......	☐	☐	☐	☐	☐
13. **Feeling burnt out, having hit rock-bottom**......	☐	☐	☐	☐	☐
14. **Decrease in beard growth**......	☐	☐	☐	☐	☐
15. **Decrease in ability/frequency to perform sexually**......	☐	☐	☐	☐	☐
16. **Decrease in the number of morning erections**......	☐	☐	☐	☐	☐
17. **Decrease in sexual desire/libido** (lacking pleasure in sex, lacking desire for sexual intercourse)......	☐	☐	☐	☐	☐

Have you got any other major symptoms?   Yes.......☐   No.....☐

If Yes, please describe: _____

_____

Thank you very much for your cooperation

FIG. 1 AMS questionnaire.

penile column, depends on the integrity of neural, vascular, and endocrine systems as well as the fibro-elastic properties of the corporal cavernosal tissue [46–48]. Other types of sexual dysfunction such as premature ejaculation and low libido may occur. However, the most common and disruptive problem in men is ED [45]. Although most men will experience periodic episodes of ED, these episodes tend to become more frequent with advancing age [45, 48].

ED is an international problem with prevalence and severity increasing with age [48]. Several studies have demonstrated that a wide range of causes like medical conditions and lifestyle habits contribute to erectile dysfunction [45, 48]. The most important organic causes of ED are cardiovascular disease and diabetes, neurological problems (for example, trauma from prostatectomy surgery), hormonal insufficiencies (hypogonadism), and drug side effects [45–47].

Psychological impotence is defined as a condition where an erection or penetration fails due to thoughts or feelings (psychological reasons) rather than physical impossibility and can often be helped. In psychological impotence, a strong response to placebo treatment has been reported [46]. Besides treating the underlying causes such as low testosterone, the first-line treatment of erectile dysfunction consists of a trial of phosphodiesterase-5 (PDE5 inhibitor) (such as sildenafil or tadalafil) [45]. In some cases, treatment can involve applying prostaglandin gel in the urethra, prostaglandin injections into the penis, a penile prosthesis, a penis erect aid vacuum pump, or vascular reconstructive surgery [49].

5   Hypogonadism

Male hypogonadism is characterized by a deficiency of testosterone—a critical hormone for sexual, cognitive, and body function and development [50] A large number of men with hypogonadism remain undiagnosed and untreated [50]. Clinically low testosterone levels can lead to the absence of secondary sex characteristics, infertility, muscle wasting, and other abnormalities [51]. Low testosterone levels may be due to testicular, hypothalamic, or pituitary abnormalities [52]. In individuals who also present with clinical signs and symptoms like loss of libido, erectile dysfunction, changes in mood, fatigue and lethargy, clinical guidelines recommend treatment with testosterone replacement therapy [53].

There are two basic types of hypogonadism: primary hypogonadism and secondary hypogonadism. While in primary hypogonadism, the problem originates in the testicles, known as primary testicular failure, in secondary hypogonadism, a problem in the hypothalamus or the pituitary gland—parts of the brain that signal the testicles to produce testosterone—is the cause [53]. The hypothalamus produces the gonadotropin-releasing hormone (GnRH), which signals the pituitary gland to make the follicle-stimulating hormone (FSH) and luteinizing hormone (LH) [53]. LH, in turn, then signals the Leydig cells in the testis to produce testosterone [53].

Either type of hypogonadism may be caused by an inherited (congenital) trait or something that happens later in life (acquired), such as an injury or an infection [54]. Stress, excessive physical activity, and weight loss have all been associated with hypogonadism. Some have attributed this to stress-induced hypercortisolism, which would suppress hypothalamic function [55–57].

5.1   Signs and symptoms of hypogonadism

Hypogonadism is suspected when the serum testosterone levels are less than 300 ng/dL in combination with at least one clinical sign or symptom including the absence or regression of secondary sex characteristics, anemia, muscle wasting, reduced bone mass or bone mineral density, oligozoospermia, and abdominal adiposity [54]. Symptoms of post-pubescent hypogonadism include sexual dysfunction (erectile dysfunction, reduced libido, diminished penile sensation, difficulty attaining orgasm, and reduced ejaculate), reduced energy and stamina, depressed mood, increased irritability, difficulty concentrating, changes in cholesterol levels, anemia, osteoporosis, and hot flushes [53, 58]. On the contrary, in the prepubertal male, if treatment is not initiated, signs and symptoms include sparse body hair and delayed epiphyseal closure [59].

Early diagnosis can reduce risks associated with hypogonadism, prevent problems of delayed puberty in young boys, and protect men against the development of osteoporosis and other conditions [59]. The diagnosis of hypogonadism is based on symptoms and the evaluation of blood parameters, particularly on testosterone levels [54]. Testosterone replacement therapy is the primary treatment option for hypogonadism [54]. Ideally, the therapy should provide physiological testosterone levels, typically in the range of 300–800 ng/dL (based on the guidelines from the American Association of Clinical Endocrinologists) [60].

6   The prostate

The prostate is an accessory sex organ, contributing about 20%–30% to the total seminal ejaculate volume at the time of orgasm [57, 61]. Prostatic secretions are important in optimizing conditions for fertilization by enhancing the viability of sperm in both male and female reproductive tracts [61]. In adult men, the average measurements for the prostate are 3.4 cm in length, 4.4 cm in width, and 2.6 cm in thickness; the weight of the normal gland is between 15 and 20 g. It is located in the pelvis, under the urinary bladder and in front of the rectum [61].

The prostate lies immediately below the base of the bladder surrounding the proximal portion of the urethra and consists of canals and follicles lined with columnar epithelial cells and surrounded by a fibromuscular stroma consisting of connective tissue and smooth muscle [62]. The prostate surrounds part of the urethra, the tube that carries urine from the bladder during urination and semen during ejaculation [57]. Consequently, due to its proximity, prostate diseases affect urination, ejaculation, and rarely defecation [57].

6.1 Benign prostatic hyperplasia

Benign prostatic hyperplasia (BPH), also called prostate enlargement, is a noncancerous increase in the size of the prostate [63]. BPH is a progressive disease that is commonly associated with bothersome lower urinary tract symptoms (LUTS) such as frequent urination, urgency, nocturia, decreased and intermittent force of stream, and the sensation of incomplete bladder emptying. Complications can include urinary tract infections, bladder stones, and chronic kidney problems [64]. The term BPH actually refers to a histologic condition, namely the presence of stromal glandular hyperplasia within the prostate gland [65].

In a large-scale Multinational Survey of the Aging Male, 34% of men in the United States and 29% of European men aged 50–80 years reported moderate to severe LUTS [63]. The underlying mechanism involves the prostate pressing on the urethra thereby making it difficult to pass urine out of the bladder [66]. Diagnosis is typically based on symptoms and examination after ruling out other possible causes [66]. The clinical diagnosis of BPH is based on a history of LUTS (lower urinary tract symptoms), a digital rectal exam, and exclusion of other causes of similar signs and symptoms [66]. The degree of LUTS does not necessarily correspond to the size of the prostate [66]. While an enlarged prostate gland on rectal examination that is symmetric and smooth supports a diagnosis of BPH, an asymmetrical, firm, or nodular prostate raises concern for prostate cancer [66]. Validated questionnaires such as the American Urological Association Symptom Index (AUA-SI), the International Prostate Symptom Score (I-PSS), and more recently the UWIN score (urgency, weak stream, incomplete emptying, and nocturia) are useful aids to the diagnosis of BPH and quantifying the severity of symptoms [66].

Lifestyle factors such as exercise, weight gain, and obesity appear to have an impact on LUTS [66]. Encouraging activity, regulating fluid intake (especially in the evening), and limiting bladder irritants in the diet are advisable [66]. Bladder irritants include excessive amounts of alcohol, caffeine, and highly seasoned or irritative food. Treatment options include lifestyle changes, medications, a number of procedures, and surgery [67].

For patients with more significant symptoms, medications may include α-blockers such as terazosin or 5α-reductase inhibitors such as finasteride [66, 68]. Surgical removal of part of the prostate may be carried out in those who do not improve with other measures [67]. Alternative medicine, such as saw palmetto, does not appear to help [68].

7 Prostate cancer

Prostate cancer is the development of cancer in the prostate [69]. Most prostate cancers are slow growing; however, some grow relatively quickly [70]. The cancer cells may spread from the prostate to other areas of the body, particularly the bones and lymph nodes [70]. Initially the disease may not cause symptoms, but in later stages, it can lead to difficulty in urinating, blood in the urine, or pain in the pelvis, back, or when urinating [71].

7.1 Risk factors of prostate cancer

Factors that increase the risk of prostate cancer include older age, a family history of the disease, and race [72]. About 99% of the cases occur in males over the age of 50 [72]. Having a first-degree relative with the disease increases the risk two- to threefold [72]. In the United States, it is more common in the African American population than the White American population [71]. Other factors that may be involved include a diet high in processed meat, red meat, or milk products or low in certain vegetables [72]. An association with gonorrhea has been found, but a reason for this relationship has not been identified [73]. An increased risk is associated with the breast cancer genes 1 and 2 mutation (BRCA1 and BRCA2 gene mutations) [74].

7.2 Prostate cancer screening

Prostate cancer is diagnosed by biopsy with medical imaging being done to determine if the cancer has spread to other parts of the body [71]. Prostate-specific antigen (PSA) testing increases the cancer detection, but it is controversial regarding whether it improves outcomes, that is, decrease the risk of death from prostate cancer [71]. Testing, if carried out, is more reasonable in those with a longer life expectancy [72]. While 5α-reductase inhibitors appear to decrease low-grade cancer risk, they do not affect high-grade cancer risk and thus are not recommended for prevention [72]. Supplementation with vitamins or minerals does not appear to affect the risk [72]. In the United Kingdom, the National Health Service (2018) does not mandate, nor advice for PSA test, but allows patients to decide based on their doctor's advice [75]. The American Urological Association (AUA 2013) guidelines call for weighing the benefits of preventing prostate cancer mortality in one man for every 1000 men screened over a 10-year period against the known harms associated with diagnostic tests and treatment [76]. The American Urological Association in 2018 states that men under the age of 55 and over the age of 69 should not be routinely screened. The greatest benefit of screening appears to be in men aged 55–69 years. To reduce the harms of screening, a routine screening interval of 2 years or more may be preferred over annual screening in those men who have participated in shared decision-making and decided on screening. Screening is done by measuring of PSA (blood test) [76].

8 Outline of management of prostate cancer

Many cases are managed with active surveillance or watchful waiting [71]. Other treatments may include a combination of surgery, radiation therapy, hormone therapy, or chemotherapy [71]. When the cancer only occurs inside the prostate, it may be curable. In those patients in whom the disease has spread to the bones, pain medications, bisphosphonates, and targeted therapy among others may be useful [71]. Outcomes depend on the person's age and other health problems as well as how aggressive and extensive the cancer is [71]. Most men with prostate cancer do not end up dying from the disease [71].

References

[1] Griffin JE, Wilson JD. Disorders of the testes and the male reproductive tract. In: Wilson JD, Foster DW, Kronenberg HM, Larsen PR, editors. Williams textbook of endocrinology. 9th ed. Philadelphia, PA: W.B. Saunders Co.; 1998. p. 819–75.
[2] Mooradian AD, Morley JE, Korenman SG. Biological actions of androgens. Endocr Rev 1987;8(1):1–28.
[3] Dunn JF, Nisula BC, Rodbard D. Transport of steroid hormones: binding of 21 endogenous steroids to both testosterone-binding globulin and corticosteroid-binding globulin in human plasma. J Clin Endocrinol Metab 1981;53(1):58–68.
[4] Bhasin S, Bagatell CJ, Bremner WJ, Plymate SR, Tenover JL, Korenman SG, Nieschlag E. Issues in testosterone replacement in older men. J Clin Endocrinol Metab 1998;83(10):3435–48.
[5] Griffin JE, Wilson JD. Disorders of the testes. In: Braunwald E, Fauci AS, Kasper DL, Hauser SL, Longo DL, Jameson JL, editors. Harrison's principles of internal medicine. 15th ed. New York: McGraw Hill; 2001. p. 2143–54.
[6] McClure RD. Endocrine investigation and therapy. Urol Clin N Am 1987;14:471–88.
[7] Bassil N, Alkaade S, Morley JE. The benefits and risks of testosterone replacement therapy: a review. Ther Clin Risk Manag 2009;5(3):427–48.
[8] Pinyerd B, Zipf WB. Puberty-timing is everything! J Pediatr Nurs 2005;20(2):75–82.
[9] Gray PB, Singh AB, Woodhouse LJ, Storer TW, Casaburi R, Dzekov J, Dzekov C, Sinha-Hikim I, Bhasin S. Dose-dependent effects of testosterone on sexual function, mood and visuospatial cognition in older men. J Clin Endocrinol Metab 2005;90:3838–46.
[10] Marazziti D, Canale D. Hormonal changes when falling in love. Psychoneuroendocrinology 2004;29(7):931–6.
[11] Booth A, Dabbs JM. Testosterone and Men's Marriages. Soc Forces 1993;72(2):463–77.
[12] Roney JR, Mahler SVand Maestripieri D. Behavioral and hormonal responses of men to brief interactions with women. Evol Hum Behav 2003;24(6):365–75.
[13] Pirke KM, Kockott G, Dittmar F. Psychosexual stimulation and plasma testosterone in man. Arch Sex Behav 1974;3(6):577–84.
[14] Prasad AS, Mantzoros CS, Beck FW, Hess JW, Brewer GJ. Zinc status and serum testosterone levels of healthy adults. Nutrition 1996;12(5):344–8.
[15] Miller SL, Maner JK. Scent of a woman: men's testosterone responses to olfactory ovulation cues. Psychol Sci 2010;21(2):276–83.
[16] Vingren JL, Kraemer WJ, Ratamess NA, Anderson JM, Volek JS, Maresh CM. Testosterone physiology in resistance exercise and training: the upstream regulatory elements. Sports Med 2010;40:1037–53.
[17] Craig BW, Brown R, Everhart J. Effects of progressive resistance training on growth hormone and testosterone levels in young and elderly subjects. Mech Ageing Dev 1989;49(2):159–69.
[18] Håkonsen LB, Thulstrup AM, Aggerholm AS, Olsen J, Bonde JP, Andersen CY, Bungum M, Ernst EH, Hansen ML, Ernst EH, Ramlau-Hansen CH. Does weight loss improve semen quality and reproductive hormones? Results from a cohort of severely obese men. Reprod Health 2011;8(1):24.
[19] MacDonald AA, Herbison GP, Showell M, Farquhar CM. The impact of body mass index on semen parameters and reproductive hormones in human males: a systematic review with meta-analysis. Hum Reprod Update 2010;16(3):293–311.
[20] Schultheiss OC, Campbell KL, DC MC. Implicit power motivation moderates men's testosterone responses to imagined and real dominance success. Hormones Behav 1999;36(3):234–41.
[21] Andersen ML, Tufik S. The effects of testosterone on sleep and sleep-disordered breathing in men: its bidirectional interaction with erectile function. Sleep Med Rev 2008;12(5):365–79.
[22] Stanworth RD, Jones TH. Testosterone for the aging male; current evidence and recommended practice. Clin Interv Aging 2008;3(1):25–34.

[23] Kumar V, Kural MR, Pereira BM, Roy P. Spearmint induced hypothalamic oxidative stress and testicular anti-androgenicity in male rats—altered levels of gene expression, enzymes and hormones. Food Chem Toxicol 2008;46(12):3563–70.

[24] Tambi MI, Imran MK, Henkel RR. Standardised water-soluble extract of *Eurycoma longifolia*, Tongkat Ali, as testosterone booster for managing men with late-onset hypogonadism. Andrologia 2012;44(1):226–30.

[25] Bagatell CJ, Bremner WJ. Androgens in men: uses and abuses. N Engl J Med 1996;334(11):707–14.

[26] Myers JB, Meacham RB. Androgen replacement therapy in the aging male. Rev Urol 2003;5(4):216–26.

[27] Kimball JW. Sexual reproduction in humans. In: Kimball's Biology. The Saylor Foundation; 2006 [online textbook].

[28] Irtanen HE, Jørgensen N, Toppari J. Semen quality in the 21st century. Nat Rev Urol 2017;14:120–30.

[29] Levine H, Jørgensen N, Martino-Andrade A, Mendiola J, Weksler-Derri D, Mindlis I, Pinotti R, Swan and Shanna H. Temporal trends in sperm count: a systematic review and meta-regression analysis. Hum Reprod Update 2017;23(6):646–59.

[30] Kidd SA, Eskenazi B, Wyrobek AJ. Effects of male age on semen quality and fertility: a review of the literature. Fertil Steril 2001;75(2):237–48.

[31] Boeri L, Capogrosso P, Ventimiglia E, Pederzoli F, Cazzaniga W, Chierigo F, Dehò F, Montanari E, Montorsi F, Salonia A. Heavy cigarette smoking and alcohol consumption are associated with impaired sperm parameters in primary infertile men. Asian J Androl 2019;21(5):478–85.

[32] Stokes VJ, Anderson RA, George JT. How does obesity affect fertility in men—and what are the treatment options? Clin Endocrinol 2015;82(5):633–8.

[33] Brezina PR, Yunus FN, Zhao Y. Effects of pharmaceutical medications on male fertility. J Reprod Infertil 2012;13(1):3–11.

[34] Kanwar U, Anand RJ, Sanyal SN. The effect of nifedipine, a calcium channel blocker, on human spermatozoal functions. Contraception 1993;48(5):453–70.

[35] Kehl S, Weigel M, Müller D, Gentili M, Horne-mann A, Sütterlin M. HIV-infection and modern antiretroviral therapy impair sperm quality. Arch Gynecol Obstet 2011;284(1):229–33.

[36] Keihani S, Craig JR, Zhang C, Presson AP, Myers JB, Brant WO, Aston KI, Emery BR, Jenkins TG, Carrell DT, Hotaling JM. Proton-pump inhibitor use does not affect semen quality in sub fertile men. Asian J Androl 2018;20(3):290–3.

[37] Mortimer D, Barratt CLR, Bjorndahl L, De Jager C, Jequier AM, Muller CH. What should it take to describe a substance or product as 'sperm-safe. Hum Reprod Update 2013;19:11–45.

[38] Oostingh EC, Steegers-Theunissen RPM, de Vries JHM, Laven JSE, Koster MPH. Strong adherence to a healthy dietary pattern is associated with better semen quality, especially in men with poor semen quality. Fertil Steril 2017;107:916–23.

[39] Afeiche M, Bridges N, Williams P, Gaskins A, Tanrikut C, Petrozza J, Hauser R, Chavarro J. Dairy intake and semen quality among men attending a fertility clinic. Fertil Steril 2014;101:1280–7.

[40] Mitchell JH, Cawood E, Kinniburgh D, Provan A, Collins AR, Irvine DS. Effect of a phytoestrogen food supplement on reproductive health in normal males. Clin Sci 2001;100(6):613–8.

[41] Tambi MI, Imran MK. *Eurycoma longifolia* Jack in managing idiopathic male infertility. Asian J Androl 2010;12(3):376–80.

[42] Heinemann LAJ, Zimmermann T, Vermeulen A, Thiel C. A new 'aging male's symptoms' (AMS) rating scale. Aging Male 1999;2:105–14.

[43] Heinemann LAJ, Thiel C, Assmann A, Zimmermann T, Hummel W, Vermeulen A. Sex differences of "climacteric symptoms" with increasing age? A pooled analysis of cross-sectional population-based surveys. Aging Male 2003;3:124–31.

[44] Nieschlag E, Swerdloff R, Behre HM, Gooren LJ, Kaufman JM, Legros JJ, Lunenfeld B, Morley JE, Schulman C, Wang C, Weidner W, Wu FC. Investigation, treatment and monitoring oflate-onset hypogonadism in males. ISA, ISSAM, and EAU recommendations. Eur Urol 2005;48:1–4.

[45] Heinemann LAJ, Saad F. Measurement of quality of life specific for aging males. In: HPG S, editor. Hormone replacement therapy and quality of life. London, New York, Washington: Parthenon Publishing Group; 2002. p. 63–83.

[46] Cunningham GR, Rosen RC. In: Martin KA, editor. Overview of male sexual dysfunction [UpToDate, Waltham, MA]; 2018.

[47] Nehra A, Goldstein I, Pabby A, Nugent M, Huang YH, de las Morenas A, Krane RJ, Udelson D, Saenz de Tejada I, Moreland RB. Mechanisms of venous leakage: a prospective clinicopathological correlation of corporeal function and structure. J Urol 1996;156:1320–9.

[48] Nicolosi A, Moreira ED, Shirai M, Bin Mohd Tambi MI, Glasser DB. Epidemiology of erectile dysfunction in four countries: cross-national study of the prevalence and correlates of erectile dysfunction. Urology 2003;61:201–6.

[49] Yaman O, Yilmaz E, Bozlu M, Anafarta K. Alterations of intracorporeal structures in patients with erectile dysfunction. Urol Int 2003;71:87–90.

[50] Yassin AA, Saad F. Testosterone and erectile dysfunction. J Androl 2008;29:593–604.

[51] Trinick TR, Feneley MR, Welford H, Carruthers M. International web survey shows high prevalence of symptomatic testosterone deficiency in men. Aging Male 2011;14:10–5.

[52] Wu FC, Tajar A, Beynon JM, et al, EMAS Group. Identification of late-onset hypogonadism in middle-aged and elderly men. N Engl J Med 2010;363:123–35.

[53] Lejeune H, Huyghe E, Droupy S. Hypoactive sexual desire and testosterone deficiency in men. Prog Urol 2013;23:621–8.

[54] Dohle GR, Arver S, Bettocchi C, et al. EAU 2014 guideline on male hypogonadism; 2014, ISBN:978-90-79754-83-0.

[55] Cumming DC, Quigley ME, Yen SS. Acute suppression of circulating testosterone levels by cortisol in men. J Clin Endocrinol Metab 1983;57:671–3.

[56] Brownlee KK, Moore AW, Hackney AC. Relationship between circulating cortisol and testosterone: influence of physical exercise. J Sports Sci Med 2005;4(1):76–83.

[57] Carli G, Bonifazi M, Lodi L, Lupo C, Martelli G, Viti A. Changes in the exercise-induced hormone response to branched chain amino acid administration. Eur J Appl Physiol Occup Physiol 1992;64(3):272–7.

[58] Lunenfeld B, Arver S, Moncada I, et al. How to help the aging male? Current approaches to hypogonadism in primary care. Aging Male 2012;15:187–97.

[59] Silveira, Latronico A. Approach to the patient with hypogonadotropic hypogonadism. J Clin Endocrinol Metab 2013;98(5):1781–8.

[60] Hypogonadism Task Force AACE. Medical guidelines for clinical practice for the evaluation and treatment of hypogonadism in adult male patients—2002 updated. Endocr Pract 2002;8:434–56.

[61] Lang EK. Radiology of the Lower Urinary Tract. Berlin Heidelberg: Springer-Verlag; 1994. p. 167–8.

[62] Huggins C, Scott WW, Heinen JH. Chemical composition of human semen and of the secretions of the prostate and seminal vehicles. Am J Phys 1942;136(3):467–73.

[63] Lee C, Kozlowski J, Grayhack J. Intrinsic and extrinsic factors controlling benign prostatic growth. Prostate 1997;31:131–8.

[64] Alan C, Kırılmaz B, Koçoğlu H, Ersay AR, Ertung Y, Eren AE. Comparison of effects of alpha receptor blockers on endothelial functions and coagulation parameters in patients with benign prostatic hyperplasia. Prostatic diseases and male voiding dysfunction. Urology 2011;77:1439–43.

[65] Nordling J. Efficacy and safety of two doses (10 and 15 mg) of alfuzosin or tamsulosin (0.4 mg) once daily for treating symptomatic benign prostatic hyperplasia. BJU Int 2005;95:1006–12.

[66] Kim EH, Larson JA, Andriole GL. Management of benign prostatic hyperplasia. Ann Rev Medi (Rev) 2016;67:137–51.

[67] Abrams P, Chapple C, Khoury S, Roehrborn C, de la Rosette J. International Scientific Committee. Evaluation and treatment of lower urinary tract symptoms in older men. J Urol 2009;181(4):1779–87.

[68] Silva J, Silva CM, Cruz F. Current medical treatment of lower urinary tract symptoms/BPH: do we have a standard? Curr Opin Urol January 2014;24(1):21–8.

[69] National Cancer Institute. Prostate Cancer; 1980. Archived from the original on 12 October 2014.

[70] National Cancer Institute. Prostate Cancer Treatment (PDQ) – Health Professional Version. National Cancer Institute; 2014.

[71] Catalona WJ. Prostate Cancer Screening. Med Clin N Am 2018;102(2):199–214.

[72] Stewart BW, Wild CP. World Health Organization. In: World cancer report 2014; 2014. p. 11, ISBN:978-9283204299. Chapter 5.

[73] Caini S, Gandini S, Dudas M, Bremer V, Severi E, Gherasim A. Sexually transmitted infections and prostate cancer risk: a systematic review and meta-analysis. Cancer Epidemiol 2014;38(4):329–38.

[74] Lee MV, Katabathina VS, Bowerson ML, Mityul MI, Shetty AS, Elsayes KM. BRCA-associated cancers: role of imaging in screening, diagnosis, and management. Radiographics 2016;37(4):1005–23.

[75] Wayback Machine, NHS Choices. Should I have a PSA test?; 2018. Archived 28 January 2018.

[76] Carter HB, Albertsen PC, Barry MJ, Etzioni R, Freedland SJ, Greene KL, Holmberg L, Kantoff P, Konety BR, Murad MH, Penson DF, Zietman AL. Early detection of prostate cancer guideline. American Urological Association; 2018.

Chapter 4.2

Overview on the clinical presentation and indications: Part B

Lourens Johannes Christoffel Erasmus

Physiology and Environmental Health, University of Limpopo, Mankweng, Limpopo Province, South Africa

1 Clinical indications

1.1 Introduction

Human sexuality is complex and multidimensional, and can include aspects ranging from diseased states to impaired reproductive capabilities and more. Among these diseased states, prostatitis syndrome as a primary male sexual health concern has been recognized as a commonly encountered clinical scenario [1]. However, despite numerous advances it remains difficult to manage [2]. Furthermore, other male reproductive issues such as infertility, decreased libido, and effective male contraception can cause sexual dissatisfaction. Of particular interest in male infertility is the presence of antisperm antibodies. These antibodies can adversely affect pre- and postfertilization events [3] resulting in decreased sperm motility, gamete interaction, and impaired fetal development. In addition, a decreased libido can contribute toward infertility and compromise sexual quality of life. There are tremendous inter- and intrapersonal variations in the intensity of libido [4], which frequently challenges the clinical management thereof. In contrast to these infertility concerns, there is also the desire to effectively manage fertile couples through contraception [5]. However, while much progress has been made in the field of female contraception, an effective and reversible male contraceptive remains somewhat elusive.

1.2 Prostatitis

Prostatitis relates to a series of disorders, ranging from acute bacterial infection to chronic pain syndromes with a prevalence of approximately 8.2% [6]. Furthermore, it accounts for almost 8% of visits to urologists, and up to 1% of visits to primary-care physicians [7]. However, the condition is poorly understood, underdiagnosed, and is difficult to treat [8]. Based on the National Institutes of Health classification, diagnosis comprises four clinical entities [9]: acute bacterial prostatitis (type I), chronic bacterial prostatitis (type II) chronic prostatitis/pelvic pain syndrome (type III), and asymptomatic prostatitis (type IV) [10].

1.2.1 Type I: Acute bacterial prostatitis

Acute bacterial prostatitis comprises approximately 10% of all prostatitis diagnoses, with a peak incidence in men of 20–40 years of age and in those older than 70 years [11]. This results from retrograde infection of bacteria, such as *Escherichia coli* and *Enterococcus* spp. [12], from the urinary tract into the prostate [13]. Clinical presentations include dysuria, urinary frequency and urgency, urinary obstruction (hesitancy, weak urinary stream, and incomplete voiding), pelvic pain [14], and systemic symptoms such as fever and chills [10]. This is easily diagnosed clinically [10]. In addition, urinary symptoms may be irritative (e.g., dysuria, urinary frequency, urinary urgency) or obstructive (e.g., hesitancy, poor/interrupted stream, straining to void, incomplete emptying/urinary retention) [10, 15]. Pain may be experienced in the suprapubic, rectal, or perineal regions, or in the external genitalia [16–18]. The presence of painful ejaculation, hematospermia, decreased libido, and painful defecation have been reported [15, 19]. Prostate-specific antigen (PSA) in the serum is not indicated to be assessed, but is raised in 70% of cases and remains elevated for up to 2 months after the infection [19]. Diagnosis is based on a microscopic analysis of a midstream urine sample. This urine sample analysis is subject to evidence of leukocytes and confirmation via a microbiological culture [20]. Initial therapy with antimicrobials is empiric and experience based [21]. It is recommended that either a broad-spectrum penicillin derivative with a beta-lactamase inhibitor, third-generation cephalosporin, or fluoroquinolone possibly in association with aminoglycoside be used to treat bacterial infections [22, 23].

Herbal Medicine in Andrology. https://doi.org/10.1016/B978-0-12-815565-3.00011-4

In the diagnosis of acute bacterial prostatitis, helpful clues include rapid onset of symptoms, systemic manifestations, and prostatic tenderness [15]. In general, digital rectal examination reveals warm, tender, diffusely enlarged, and possibly indurated prostate [15].

1.2.2 Type II: Chronic bacterial prostatitis

Chronic bacterial prostatitis is a persistent bacterial infection of the prostate lasting more than 3 months [10]. Even though chronic bacterial prostatitis may develop from acute bacterial prostatitis, some men have no clinical history of the latter [15]. Unlike acute bacterial prostatitis, those affected do not appear to be symptomatically ill. Clinical presentation is indistinguishable from CP/CPPC, and may include irritative voiding symptoms, pain in the epididymis, testes, back or penis, low-grade fever, arthralgia, and myalgia [10, 15]. Signs may also include urethral discharge, hematospermia, and evidence of secondary cpididymo-orchitis [15]. Many patients are asymptomatic between episodes, although detectable pathogens persist on localization tests [10]. On physical examination, patients are generally afebrile [10]. On digital rectal examination the prostate mostly appears to be normal, but in some cases it may be swollen, firm, or tender [10, 15]. As a bacterial infection, management of chronic bacterial prostatitis depends on the use of antibiotics with good tissue penetration into the prostate. As a recommended first-line agent fluoroquinolones have demonstrated the best tissue concentrations [24, 25]. Other antimicrobials, such as trimethoprim and sulfamethoxazole, may be considered. However, tissue penetration is not on par with fluoroquinolones and there is evidence of uropathogenic resistance [25].

1.2.3 Type III: Chronic abacterial prostatitis (chronic pelvic pain syndrome)

The hallmark symptom of CP/CPPS is pain ascribed to the prostate with no obvious indication of infection [10]. Although poorly understood, symptoms may originate from the prostate, other structures within the pelvis, or by neuropathic mechanisms within the sensory nervous system [8]. The use of the term CCPS emphasizes that the prostate may only be partially responsible for the pain experienced and that the symptomatic management thereof would unequivocally require a more holistic approach.

Symptoms are generally grouped into four complexes: pain symptoms, voiding symptoms, sexual dysfunction, and psychosocial symptoms [26]. Pain can be felt in the perineum, lower abdomen, groin, lower back, testes, or tip of the penis [15]. Voiding symptoms include hesitancy and weak stream, urinary urgency and frequency, and occasionally dysuria or urethral burning independent of micturition [15]. Sexual dysfunction may include premature ejaculation [27], impotence, ejaculatory pain [28, 29], and loss of libido [15], mediated through vascular, endocrine, psychogenic, and neuromuscular mechanisms [30]. The psychosocial impact emphasizes the role of depression and anxiety on these men as well as cognitive and behavioral consequences [8]. Its diagnosis is frequently based on exclusion of other urologic conditions such as voiding dysfunction and bladder cancer, in association with its presentation. Commonly used medications include antimicrobials, α-blockers, and antiinflammatory agents [10].

1.2.4 Type IV: Asymptomatic inflammatory prostatitis

Asymptomatic inflammatory prostatitis (AIP) has been recognized as a distinct subtype since 1995, where symptoms are typically absent, but it can cause an elevated PSA or pyuria. The National Institutes of Health created a new category for asymptomatic inflammatory prostatitis (type IV). This category includes cases that lack clinical symptoms and exhibit either histopathological findings of inflammation and/or presence of leukocytes in prostatic secretions or semen tested for other diseases [31]. Morphologically, the diagnosis can be confirmed through transrectal ultrasound scan or prostatic biopsy [32]. While the diagnosis is normally incidental, during urologic evaluation for others [10], treatment is predominantly based on the primary reason for the urologic assessment [32]. There is general consensus that this condition does not require additional diagnosis or therapy [20]. However, while evidence-based data is lacking, antimicrobial therapy can be suggested to patients with raised PSA [33]. However, when the indication for biopsy is an elevated PSA level, it is essential to remember that normalization of the PSA value following antibiotic or 5α-reductase inhibitor therapy does not rule out the diagnosis of prostate cancer, and continued urologic evaluation is justified [10].

1.3 Male accessory gland infection

Male urogenital tract infection, also known as male accessory gland infection (MAGI), is a clinical diagnostic term used to define infectious diseases of the male reproductive tract [34]. These infections can occur as prostatitis, prostatic-vesiculitis, or prostate-vesiculo-epididymitis [35], resulting from the canalicular spreading of microorganisms via the male reproductive tract [36]. The frequency of MAGI among infertile men varies significantly from 2% to 18% [37]. Various microorganisms such as *E. coli, Neisseria gonorrhoeae, Chlamydia trachomatis, Ureaplasma urealyticum, Mycoplasma hominis, Candida albicans,* and *Trichomonas vaginalis,* when present in the male urogenital tract, are associated with abnormal sperm parameters, especially motility and mitochondrial sperm function, and chromatin and DNA integrity [35]. The range of microorganisms implicated hint on sexual as well as nonsexual causality.

MAGI often presents as urethral infection with a chronic course, capable of affecting more than one accessory gland [35], including but not limited to the prostate. In effect, this means that there can be a clinical overlap between MAGI and infectious prostatitis [34]. In symptomatic cases, clinical presentation can vary significantly and can comprise suprapubic/perineal pain, dysuria, frequency, urgency, and hematuria [38]. However, it is often either asymptomatic or pauci-symptomatic which complicates the diagnosis [37]. Laboratory confirmation of MAGI is linked to elevated concentration of cytokines and reactive oxygen species (ROS), as well as leukocytospermia [39].

MAGI is a common and potentially curable cause of male infertility [34]. MAGI can deteriorate the quality of spermatozoa and can impair the function of male accessory glands. Therefore, it is considered a potentially correctable cause of male infertility. These infections are associated with decreased semen volume as well as reduced levels of α-glucosidase, fructose, and zinc in seminal plasma, which implies impaired accessory gland function [40]. Three possible mechanisms have been proposed: (i) accessory gland dysfunction [40], (ii) favoring an inflammatory microenvironment, with specific emphasis on oxidative stress and cytokine production especially TNF-α, IL-6, and IL-10 [41–43], and (iii) in rare instances obstruction of seminal routes [35, 39]. The most frequent spermatozoa alterations attributable to bacterial infections include a decreased sperm concentration, loss of motility, alterations to sperm morphology, and impaired acrosome reactions [44]. Furthermore, in urogenital infections sperm concentration, seminal plasma α-glucosidase, fructose, and zinc concentrations are significantly decreased. Such decreases are associated with reduced seminal volume and an increased pH [45]. Treatment of MAGI is usually directed at relieving symptoms, such as reduction/eradication of microorganisms, normalization of inflammation, and improvement of sperm parameters [36]. In addition, when assisted reproductive technologies are considered for infertile couples, sperm preparation methods used generally focus on reducing the bacterial load in semen samples used for insemination purposes [46].

1.4 Antisperm antibodies

Antisperm antibodies (ASA) are immunoglobulins IgG, IgA, and/or IgM that impair sperm functions [3], such as sperm penetration into the cervical mucous, sperm capacitation, acrosome reaction, and sperm-ovum binding [47]. This affects approximately 8%–21% of infertile men, demonstrated with significant titres of ASA in their ejaculate. Importantly, ASA are demonstrated in 1.2%–19% of fertile men, suggesting ASA do not necessarily equate to infertility [48–50]. ASA have been detected in men and women [51], isolated from seminal plasma, blood serum, cervical mucous, and oviductal fluid/follicular fluid [52, 53]. IgA and IgG ASA have been identified in the ejaculates of men with demonstrated antisperm autoimmunity; however, IgM is rarely detected and does not appear to have any clinical significance [54]. IgA and IgG can have an immobilizing, agglutinating, or cytotoxic impact on the mobility of spermatozoa, and may disrupt many of the steps required in normal fertilization [55]. However, some evidence suggests that spermatogenesis is not affected by ASA [56].

The blood-testis barrier (BTB) provides protection against autoimmunity. It is formed by the Sertoli cells that isolate the tubular content from the vasculature and limited lymphatic drainage in the testis [57]. In addition, various other immunoregulatory mechanisms are involved in the prevention of antisperm immunity, such as seminal plasma immunosuppressive factors, as well as systemic nonspecific and specific factors [58]. Autoimmunization against sperm may be initiated when the BTB is compromised via testicular trauma/torsion, undescended testicles, vasectomy reversal, tubal obstruction, testicular cancer, or inflammation/infection [55, 59, 60]. Recently, proteomic analysis revealed that certain sperm proteins are capable of inducing ASA [61]. However, controversy still remains regarding the association between ASA and various inflammatory/infectious conditions, such as chronic urethritis, CP, and chronic epididymitis. Furthermore, evidence suggest that inflammation- and infection-related obstructions of the male reproductive tract do not seem as significant as generally considered [62, 63]. Not surprisingly, there seems to be disagreement whether inflammatory and infectious diseases should be considered significant risks in male infertility. However, the exact mechanisms involved in the pathogenesis of ASA remain poorly understood [34, 64].

Antisperm antibodies are found in both fertile and infertile men; therefore, its mere presence is not indicative of infertility per se. Nevertheless, there is scientific support of its impact on the inhibition of sperm motility and viability [65], acrosome reaction [53], and interference with the process of fertilization [66], causing low sperm binding to the oocyte [67]. Infertility can result only if the circulating antibodies are present within the reproductive tract and on the surface of the living sperm [68], and when the level of ASA binding is high enough (> 50%) [69, 70].

In identifying the relevant antigens of ASA an appropriate causal treatment can be established; it can further contribute to the development of tools for immunocontraception [71]. Direct assessment of sperm antibodies on the sperm surface, using methods such as direct immune bead tests and mixed agglutination reaction [3], is the preferred method as capacitation of sperm can assist in defining antibody reactivity [72]. Indirect measurements that are designed to follow ASA in the seminal fluid, sperm extracts, cervical mucous, and sera include tests such as sperm immobilization test (SIT), tray agglutination test (TAT), gel agglutination test (GAT), and flow cytometry [61].

Antisperm antibodies can impair the fertilizing capacity of human spermatozoa. In the treatment of infertility resulting from sperm surface antibodies, both intrauterine insemination (IUI) and in vitro fertilization (IVF) revealed high pregnancy rates. Furthermore, ovarian hyperstimulation followed by IUI is a less invasive procedure than IVF [73]. However, in severe cases where the sperm head is involved, intracytoplasmic sperm injection (ICSI) is considered the primary choice of treatment [74].

1.5 Male contraception

Current estimates exceed seven billion, and it is anticipated that the world population would double in less than four decades [75]. Numerous challenges exist in male contraceptive development [76]. Considering the target of action, male contraceptives can be classified into three categories: those that (i) impede sperm transport in the female reproductive system, (ii) suppress spermatogenesis [77], and (iii) methods that disrupt maturation [78].

1.5.1 Affecting sperm transport/movement

Condoms provide a physical barrier preventing sperm from entering the vagina; they are produced from either latex or polyurethane. It is used by approximately 11.6% of men in the United States and by 2.4% of men in sub-Saharan Africa [79]. They are relatively free from any side effects, offers protection against many sexually transmitted diseases, and their main drawback is their marginal contraceptive efficacy [80]. As a sole means of contraception it would offer an efficacy of 15%–20% *per annum*; however, in younger couples with high spontaneous fertility the failure rates might be higher [81].

Vasectomy is a surgical procedure most appropriate for men who desire no further fertility. This procedure is performed under local anesthesia and the vas deferens is interrupted bilaterally through a small incision in the scrotum [82]. The widely adopted and very popular "no-scalpel" technique [83] relies on a single midline puncture in the scrotal raphe [84]. This highly effective method, with a failure rate of < 1%, has few complications [85]. The primary reproductive drawback being the delayed onset of azoospermia, which can take up to 4 months, during which time additional contraception is recommended. Furthermore, bleeding and hematomas may develop [86], while in rare cases wound infection necessitates the use of antibiotics.

Numerous procedures for vaso-occlusion have been undertaken as an alternative to vasectomy. These devices either block the flow of sperm or render the sperm dysfunctional in the vas deferens. During Reversal Inhibition of Sperm Guidance (RISUG), a solution of 60 mg of styrene maleic anhydride (SMA), a crystal clear polymer dissolved in 120 μL of dimethyl sulfoxide (DMSO) (1:2), is injected bilaterally [5] into the vas deferens and induces infertility within 10 days [87, 88].

1.5.2 Hormonal methods affecting spermatogenesis

The quest for an improved male contraceptive method prompted investigations into a hormonally derived contraceptive equivalent to the estrogen-progesterone birth control pill used by women. The arguments to support the development of androgen monotherapy stems from basic reproductive physiology. Even though the use of monotherapy for contraception is not without merit, the desire for greater rates of azoospermia stimulated studies on combination therapy. Among the first combinations to be investigated was the combination of testosterone with a progestin (synthetic progestogen) [89]. Reports on the combination of testosterone with medroxyprogesterone acetate (DMPA) indicated poor contraceptive outcomes [90]. However, more recently it was reported that combining the injectable DMPA form with either testosterone implants or TU resulted in significant oligozoospermia (< 1 million/mL) [89, 91]. Furthermore, substituting DMPA with the potent progestin levonorgestrel (LNG) induced much higher levels of azoospermia [92]. Similarly, azoospermia may result when a long-acting LNG implant is used in conjunction with TU [93]. Etonogestrel combined with either testosterone decanoate [94] or TU [95] suppressed spermatogenesis, in 80%–90% of men, to such an extent that sperm counts were < 1 million/mL. Other progestins of note are cyproterone, which exhibits antiandrogenic properties [96, 97], and nesterone a 19-norprogesterone-derived progestin that can be applied as a transdermal gel [98, 99].

Further advances in male hormonal contraception incorporated the use of a gonadotropin-releasing hormone (GnRH) agonist. The sustained use of GnRH analogs will suppress the synthesis and release of gonadotropins, resulting in the depletion of testicular testosterone [100]. The combination of GnRH agonist with testosterone could not achieve adequate suppression of spermatogenesis. This most probably be due to the lack of follicle-stimulating hormone (FSH) suppression [101]. However, when including a progestin into this combination the result was severe oligozoospermia [102].

1.5.3 Nonhormonal methods affecting spermatogenesis

The intent to disrupt spermatogenesis through nonhormonal mechanisms initiated the investigations into adjudin, an antisperm compound that interrupts the adhesion of spermatids to the Sertoli cells, causing untimely spermiation and subsequent infertility [103]. In adult rats, adjudin induced complete infertility following 5 weeks of treatment, which was accompanied by unaltered serum testosterone and gonadotropin levels [104]. Conjugating adjudin to an FSH-b mutant specifically targeting the Sertoli cells was necessitated by reports of liver inflammation in a 29-day study [103], which also succeeded in significantly reducing the dose required for contraception [104]. However, due to the fact that the testis is an immune-privileged area, some concerns exist regarding the development of anti-FSH autoantibodies [105]. In addition, H2-gamendazole, an antisperm compound, rapidly acts via the Sertoli cells through a transient increase in interleukin 1A which disrupts the spermatid-Sertoli cell junction. This impairment in apical ectoplasmic specialization [106] results in the premature release of spermatids. An attractive target for the discovery of male contraceptive drugs is the human testis-specific and bromodomain-containing protein (hBRDT). This protein is essential for chromatin remodeling during spermatogenesis [107], and if inhibited would suppress spermatogenesis. Rodent models, using the BRDT-inhibitor JQ1, illustrated reversible suppression of spermatogenesis [108] without affecting the endocrine signaling pathways [109].

A further area of interest is the epididymis, where specific molecular targets are an emerging field of research. The epididymal protease inhibitor (Eppin) is one such target as it promotes normal semen function [110, 111]. In primates immunized with Eppin, seven out of nine were unable to father pregnancies this effect was reversible in five of the seven primates when the immunizations were stopped [112]. To date, only animal models exist in exploiting Eppin as a potential contraceptive mechanism [113]. In the epididymis, N-acetyl-β-D-hexosaminidase enzyme (NAH) enters the sperms. This enzyme, which has two variant forms, A and B, promotes fertilization. However, sperm cells only contain the latter type [114]. Inhibiting the B (HEX-B) variant will result in a decreased ability to bind to and cleave the ZO glycoproteins [115]. In vivo rodent efficiency rates, when using a ZP-glycoprotein analog to block HEX-B, were approximately 90% without overt adverse effects and restoration of fertility within 1 week after the treatment was discontinued [116].

A molecular mechanism of interest is the manipulation of calcium channels, which is important in optimal sperm physiology [117, 118]. Of particular interest is the role of Catsper ion channel, which is a sperm-specific, Ca^{2+}-permeable, pH-dependent, and low-voltage-dependent channel that is essential for the hyperactivity of sperm flagellum, chemotaxis toward the egg, capacitation, and acrosome reaction [119]. Nifedipine, a hypertensive drug, induces antispermatogenic activity by targeting the Catsper channel and preventing Ca^{2+}-influx [120], rendering the sperm incapable of fertilization. Other Ca^{2+}-channel blockers are compounds such as HC-056456, NNC55-0396, nimodipine, quinindium, clofilium, theophylline, and ketamine [119], all potentially viable as therapeutic agents in male contraception.

1.5.4 Herbal extracts and contraception

The use of herbal extracts in fertility treatment is as old as the human race itself. From the use of crude extracts, as mostly practiced in traditional medicine, to the more advanced isolation of fractions and compounds, herbal medicine has provided a potential source of male contraception discovery. One of the most known phenolic compounds isolated from cottonseeds, gossypol, acts as an inhibitor for numerous dehydrogenase enzymes. Furthermore, it exhibits proapoptotic properties that affects spermatogenesis as well as sperm motility. However, an earlier systematic review of gossypol and triptolide concluded that neither was effective or safe to use [121]. The concerns regarding triptolide, isolated from *Tripterygium wilfordii*, were its immunosuppressive effects and irreversible infertility [122].

The contraceptive capabilities of papaya seed extracts have been disseminated since the late 1970s [123, 124]. Recently, a compound identified as 1,2,3,4-tetrahydropyridin-3-yl octanoate was isolated from *Carica papaya* seeds [125]. This compound at a concentration of 12.5 ng/μL significantly decreased sperm motility and viability and increased sperm abnormalities [125]. Furthermore, its contraceptive capabilities are widely recognized, but there seems to be concerns regarding the noted weight loss, which might be associated with toxicity [126, 127]. Of interest is that the use of a chloroform extract in Langur monkeys for a period of 1 year found a steady decrease in sperm production without any evidence of toxicity [128].

1.6 Libido

Human sexuality is invariably complex. It integrates multifactorial dimensions dealing with biological, psychological, interpersonal, and behavioral concepts [129]. Similarly, libido demarcates a person's overall sexual drive or desire for sexual activity, and it is affected by biological [130], psychological, and social factors [131]. Therefore, a decreased libido is associated with a lack or absence of desire for sexual activity or even the absence of sexual fantasies itself [132]. While a decreased libido is widely accepted as the most prominent presentation of low testosterone levels in men [133–135], it is challenging to measure comprehensively. However, there is a consensus that correcting low testosterone levels could prove invaluable in the treatment of androgen deficiency (AD) symptoms such as a reduced libido [136].

Many drugs, prescribed or otherwise, are known to affect male sexual functions. These effects can be undesirable and distressing, and a concerted effort should be made to minimize their negative impacts. Drugs such as antihypertensives and antidepressants are some of the most prominent drugs that can affect libido. Antihypertensives that may reduce libido include enalapril [137], lisinopril [138], spironolactone [139, 140], amiloride hydrochloride [141], hydrochlorothiazide, and chlorthalidone [142, 143]. Antidepressants include selective serotonin reuptake inhibitors (SSRI) [144, 145] and antipsychotics [146, 147]. Further prescription drugs reducing libido include statins [148–150], cardiac glycosides [151], gonadotropin-releasing hormone agonists [152], and enzyme-inducing AEDs, such as carbamazepine, phenytoin, phenobarbital, and primidone [153].

2 Conclusion

Advances in the clinical management of CP/CPPS is at least partially attributed to the increased appreciation of the role of psychosocial factors and pelvic floor pain. Acknowledgment of these domains corresponds with the increased use of their respective therapies. The significance of male genital infections in infertility appears to be uncertain in countless respects. Furthermore, it remains important to distinguish between the different forms of asymptomatic infections and remember that the diagnosis of MAGI can no longer rely on the classical parameters only. Unexplained infertility, in the presence of a normal semen analysis, is often ascribed to ASA as a causality. While clinicians are encouraged to pay close attention to ASA, there is also recognition of the cost involved in detecting these antibodies. Access to more affordable tests to identify ASA can play a significant role in the management of infertility. Despite beliefs regarding male participation in family planning, male hormonal contraception among others is a realistic prospect. However, progress in reproductive technology will require commitment and resources directed toward the research and development of these hormonal contraceptives. Therefore, until such a reliable and safe contraceptive method is developed, women will, unfortunately, still have to endure most of the burden of contraception. In theory, various hormones can alter sexual behavior such as libido. Epidemiological as well as intervention studies emphasize the role of testosterone. However, the involvement of other hormones is less clearly understood. At present, research findings are disappointing either due to lack of consistency or side effects.

References

[1] Roberts RO, Lieber MM, Bostwick DG, Jacobsen SJ. A review of clinical and pathological prostatitis syndromes. Urology 1997;49:809–21.
[2] Doiron RC, Tripp D, Tolls V, Nickel JC. The evolving clinical picture of chronic prostatitis/chronic pelvic pain syndrome (CP/CPPS): a look at 1310 patients over 16 years. Can Urol Assoc J 2018;12:196–202.
[3] Ashrafizadeh M, Ahmadi Z. The relationship between the anti-sperm antibodies and immunologic infertility. Int J Biochem Physiol 2018;3:000134.
[4] Alidu H, Amidu N, Owiredu WKBA, Gyasi-Sarpong CK, Bawah AT, Dapare PPM, Agyemang Prempeh EB. Testosterone and its bioactive components are associated with libido and the metabolic syndrome in men. Adv Sex Med 2017;7:105–19.
[5] Amory JK. Male contraception. Fertil Steril 2016;106:1303–9.
[6] Krieger JN, Lee SW, Jeon J, Cheah PY, Liong ML, Riley DE. Epidemiology of prostatitis. Int J Antimicrob Agents 2008;31:S85–90.
[7] Collins MM, Stafford RS, O'Leary MP, Barry MJ. How common is prostatitis? A national survey of physician visits. J Urol 1998;159:1224–8.
[8] Rees J, Abrahams M, Doble A, Cooper A. Prostatitis Expert Reference Group (PERG). Diagnosis and treatment of chronic bacterial prostatitis and chronic prostatitis/chronic pelvic pain syndrome: a consensus guideline. BJU Int 2015;116:509–25.
[9] Anon. Executive summary: NIH workshop on chronic prostatitis; 1995. Bethesda, Maryland.
[10] Sharp VJ, Takacs EB, Powell CR. Prostatitis: diagnosis and treatment. Am Fam Physician 2010;82:397–406.
[11] Roberts RO, Lieber MM, Rhodes T, Girman CJ, Bostwick DG, Jacobsen SJ. Prevalence of a physician-assigned diagnosis of prostatitis: the Olmsted County study of urinary symptoms and health status among men. Urology 1998;51:578–84.
[12] Brede CM, Shoskes DA. The aetiology and management of acute prostatitis. Nat Rev Urol 2011;8:207–12.
[13] Deguchi T. Diagnosis and treatment of prostatitis. J Japan Med Assoc 2004;130:251–5.
[14] Krieger JN, Nyberg Jr L, Nickel JC. NIH consensus definition and classification of prostatitis. JAMA 1999;282:236–7.
[15] Attar KH, Hamid R, Peters J. Diagnosis and management of prostatitis: a urological challenge. Trends Urol Gynaecol Sex Health 2007;12:26–30.

[16] Millán-Rodríguez F, Palou J, Bujons-Tur A, Musquera-Felip M, Sevilla-Cecilia C, Serrallach-Orejas M, Baez-Angles C, Villavicencio-Mavrich H. Acute bacterial prostatitis: two different sub-categories according to a previous manipulation of the lower urinary tract. World J Urol 2006;24:45–50.

[17] Lipsky BA, Byren I, Hoey CT. Treatment of bacterial prostatitis. Clin Infect Dis 2010;50:1641–52.

[18] Ramakrishnan K, Salinas RC. Prostatitis: acute and chronic. Prim Care 2010;37:547–63.

[19] Ludwig M. Diagnosis and therapy of acute prostatitis, epididymitis and orchitis. Andrologia 2008;40:76–80.

[20] Benelli A, Hossain H, Pilatz A, Weidner W. Prostatitis and its management. Eur Urol Suppl 2017;16:132–7.

[21] Naber KG. Antimicrobial treatment of bacterial prostatitis. Eur Urol Suppl 2003;2:23–6.

[22] Wagenlehner FM, Pilatz A, Bschlwipfer T, Diemer T, Linn T, Meinhardt A, Schagdarsurengin U, Dansranjavin T, Schuppe HC, Weidner W. Bacterial prostatitis. World J Urol 2013;31:711–6.

[23] Grabe M, Bartoletti R, Bjerklund Johansen TE, Cai T, Çek M, Köves B, Naber KG, Pickard RS, Tenke P, Wagenlehner F, Wullt B. EAU guidelines on urological infections. European Association of Urology Guidelines; 2015.

[24] Charalabopoulos K, Karachalios G, Baltogiannis D, Charalabopoulos A, Giannakopoulos X, Sofikitis N. Penetration of antimicrobial agents into the prostate. Chemotherapy 2003;49:269–79.

[25] Nickel JC, Moon T. Chronic bacterial prostatitis: an evolving clinical enigma. Urology 2005;66:2–8.

[26] Weidner W, Schiefer HG. In: Garraway M, editor. Inflammatory disease of the prostate: Frequency and pathogenesis. New York: Springer; 1998. p. 85–93.

[27] Sadeghi-Nejad H, Wassermann M, Weidner W, Richardson D, Goldmeier D. Sexually transmitted diseases and sexual function. J Sex Med 2010;7:389–413.

[28] Shoskes DA, Landis R, Wang Y, Nickel C, Zeitlin SI, Nadler R, the Chronic Prostatitis Collaborative Research Network Study Group. Impact of post-ejaculatory pain in men with category III chronic prostatitis/chronic pelvic pain syndrome. J Urol 2004;172:542–7.

[29] Illie CP, Mischianu DL, Pemberton RJ. Painful ejaculation. BJU Int 2007;99:1335–9.

[30] Tran CN, Shoskes DA. Sexual dysfunction in chronic prostatitis/chronic pelvic pain syndrome. World J Urol 2013;31:741–6.

[31] Gurunadha Rao Tunuguntla HS, Evans CP. Management of prostatitis. Prostate Cancer Prostatic Dis 2002;5:172–9.

[32] Nickel JC. Prostatitis. Can Urol Assoc J 2011;5:306–15.

[33] Wagenlehner F, Naber KG, Bschleipfer T, Brähler E, Weidner W. Prostatitis and male pelvic pain syndrome. Dtsch Arztebl Int 2009;106:175–83.

[34] Weidner W, Krause W, Ludwig M. Relevance of male accessory gland infection for subsequent fertility with special focus on prostatitis. Hum Reprod Update 1999;5:421–32.

[35] La Vignera S, Vicari E, Condorelli RA, D'Agata R, Calogero AE. Male accessory gland infection and sperm parameters. Int J Androl 2011;34:E330–47.

[36] La Vignera S, Vicari E, Condorelli RA, Franchina C, Scalia G, Morgia G, Perino A, Schillaci R, Calogero AE. Prevalence of human papilloma virus infection in patients with male accessory gland infection. Reprod Biomed Online 2015;30:385–91.

[37] La Vignera S, Condorelli R, Vicari E, D'Agata R, Calogero AE. High frequency of sexual dysfunction in patients with male accessory gland infections. Andrologia 2012;44:438–46.

[38] Raynor MC, Carson CC. Urinary infections in men. Med Clin N Am 2011;95:43–54.

[39] Krause W. Male accessory gland infection. Andrologia 2008;40:113–6.

[40] Marconi M, Pilatz A, Wagenlehner F, Diemer T, Weidner W. Impact of infection on the secretory capacity of the male accessory glands. Int Braz J Urol 2009;35:299–308.

[41] Vicari E. Seminal leukocyte concentration and related specific reactive oxygen species production in patients with male accessory gland infections. Hum Reprod 1999;14:2025–30.

[42] Lotti F, Maggi M. Interleukin 8 and the male genital tract. J Reprod Immunol 2013;100:54–65.

[43] Castiglione R, Salemi M, Vicari LO, Vicari E. Relationship of semen hyperviscosity with IL-6, TNF-α, IL-10 and ROS production in seminal plasma of infertile patients with prostatitis and prostato-vesiculitis. Andrologia 2014;46:1148–55.

[44] Fraczek M, Kurpisz M. Mechanisms of the harmful effects of bacterial semen infection on ejaculated human spermatozoa: potential inflammatory markers in semen. Folia Histochem Cytobiol 2015;53:201–17.

[45] La Vignera S, Condorelli RA, Vicari E, Salmeri M, Morgia G, Favilla V, Cimino S, Calogero AE. Microbiological investigation in male infertility: a practical overview. J Med Microbiol 2014;63:1–14.

[46] Keck C, Gerber-Schäfer C, Clad A, Wilhelm C, Breckwoldt M. Seminal tract infections: impact on male fertility and treatment options. Hum Reprod Update 1998;4:891–903.

[47] Sinisi AA, Di Finizio B, Pasquali D, Scurini C, D'Apuzzo A, Bellastella A. Prevalence of antisperm antibodies by Sperm MAR test in subjects undergoing a routine sperm analysis for infertility. Int J Androl 1993;16:311–4.

[48] Pattinson HA, Mortimer D. Prevalence of sperm surface antibodies in male partners of infertile couples as determined by the immunobead screening. Fertil Steril 1987;48:466–9.

[49] Vazquez-Levin MH, Marín-Briggiler CI, Veaute C. Antisperm antibodies: invaluable tools toward the identification of sperm proteins involved in fertilization. Am J Reprod Immunol 2014;72:206–18.

[50] Francavilla F, Barbonetti A. Male autoimmune infertility. In: Krause W, Naz R, editors. Immune infertility. Cham: Springer; 2017. p. 187–96.

[51] Husted S, Hjort T. Comparison of the occurrence of spermatozoal antibodies in male and female blood donors. Clin Exp Immunol 1974;17:61–9.

[52] Al-Dujaily SS, Chakir WK, Hantoosh SF. Direct antisperm antibody examination of infertile men. Glob J Med Res 2012;12:37–41.

[53] Bozhedomov VA, Nikolaeva MA, Ushakova IV, Lipatova NA, Bozhedomova GE, Sukhikh GT. Functional deficit of sperm and fertility impairment in men with antisperm antibodies. J Reprod Immunol 2015;112:95–101.

[54] Hjort T. Antisperm antibodies: antisperm antibodies and infertility: an unsolvable question? Hum Reprod 1999;14:2423–9.

[55] Lheureux H, Randriamahazo RT, Mons J, Gabriele M. Effects of sperm treatment on the antisperm antibodies IgG and IgA. Int J Immunol 2017;5:49–52.

[56] Meinertz H, Linnet L, Fogh-Andersen P, Hjort T. Antisperm antibodies and fertility after vasovasostomy: a follow-up study of 216 men. Fertil Steril 1990;54:315–21.

[57] Setchell BP, Voglmayer JK, Waites GM. A blood-testis barrier restricting passage from blood rete testis fluid but not into lymph. J Physiol 1969;200:73–85.

[58] Sainio-Pollanen S, Saari T, Simell O, Pollanen P. CD28-CD80/CD86 interactions in testicular immunoregulation. J Reprod Immunol 1996;31:145–63.

[59] Khatoon M, Chaudhari AR, Singh R. Effect of gender on antisperm antibodies in infertile couples in central India. Indian J Physiol Pharmacol 2012;56:262–6.

[60] Menge AC, Christman GM, Ohl DA, Naz RK. Fertilization antigen-1 removes antisperm autoantibodies from spermatozoa of infertile men and results in increased rates of acrosome reaction. Fertil Steril 1999;71:256–60.

[61] Nowicka-Bauer K, Kamieniczna M, Cibulka J, Ulcova-Gallova Z, Kurpisz M. Proteomic identification of sperm antigens using serum samples from individuals with and without antisperm antibodies. Andrologia 2016;48:693–701.

[62] Dohle GR. Inflammatory-associated obstructions of the male reproductive tract. Andrologia 2003;35:321–4.

[63] Engeler DS, Hauri D, John H. Impact of prostatitis NIH IIIB (prostatodynia) on ejaculate parameters. Eur Urol 2003;44:546–8.

[64] Imtiaz F, Alam N, Khatoon F, Mahmood A. Antisperms antibodies in infertile males attending a Tertiary Care Hospital in Karachi. Pak J Med Sci 2012;28:171–4.

[65] Marey MA, Yousef MS, Kowsar R, Hambruch N, Shimizu T, Pfarrer C, Miyamoto A. Local immune system in oviduct physiology and pathophysiology: attack or tolerance? Domest Anim Endocrinol 2016;56:S204–11.

[66] Taneichi A, Shibahara H, Takahashi K, Sasaki S, Kikuchi K, Sato I, Yoshizawa M. Effects of sera from infertile women with sperm immobilizing antibodies on fertilization and embryo development in vitro in mice. Am J Reprod Immunol 2003;50:146–51.

[67] Ferrer MS, Klabnik-Bradford J, Anderson DE, Bullington AC, Palomates RA, Miller LMJ, Stawicki R, Miesner M. Sperm-bound antisperm antibodies prevent capacitation of bovine spermatozoa. Theriogenology 2017;89:58–67.

[68] Bronson R, Cooper G, Rosenfeld D. Sperm antibodies: their role in infertility. Fertil Steril 1984;42:171–83.

[69] Barratt CLR, Dunphy BC, McLeod I, Cooke ID. The poor prognostic value of low to moderate levels of sperm surface-bound antibodies. Hum Reprod 1992;7:95–8.

[70] Fallick ML, Lin WW, Lipshultz LI. Leydig cell tumours presenting as azoospermia. J Urol 1999;161:1571–2.

[71] Haidl G. Characterization of fertility related antisperm antibodies—a step towards causal treatment of immunological infertility and immunocontraception. Asian J Androl 2010;12:793–4.

[72] Esteves S, Schneider D, Verza S. Influence of antisperm antibodies in the semen on intracytoplasmic sperm injection outcome. Int Braz J Urol 2007;33:795–802.

[73] Felemban A, Hassonah SM, Felimban N, Alkhelb H, Hassan S, Alsalman F. Sperm surface antibodies: IUI vs. IVF treatment. J Obstet Gynaecol Res 2018;1:80–4.

[74] Lombardo F, Gandini L, Dondero F, Lenzi A. Antisperm immunity in natural and assisted reproduction. Hum Reprod Update 2001;7:450–6.

[75] Tulsiani DRP. New approaches to male contraception. Gynaecol Obstet (Sunnyvale) 2016;6:e114. https://doi.org/10.4172/2161-0932.1000e114.

[76] Dorman E, Bishai D. Demand for male contraception. Expert Rev Pharmacoecon Outcomes Res 2012;12:605–13.

[77] Abou-Haila A, Tulsiani DRP. Mammalian sperm acrosome: formation, contents and function. Arch Biochem Biophys 2000;379:173–82.

[78] Young CH, Barfield JP, Cooper TG. Physiological volume regulation by spermatozoa. Mol Cell Endocrinol 2006;250:98–105.

[79] United Nations. Trends in contraceptive use worldwide 2015. United Nations, Department of Economic and Social Affairs, Population Division; 2015.

[80] D'Anna LH, Korosteleva O, Warner L, Douglas J, Paul S, Metcalf C, McIlvaine E, Malotte CK, RESPECTS-2 Study Group. Factors associated with condom use problems during vaginal sex with main and non-main partners. Sex Transm Dis 2012;39:687–9.

[81] Martinez GM, Chandra A, Abma JC, Jones J, Mosher WD. Fertility, contraception, and fatherhood: data on men and women from cycle 6 (2002) of the 2002 National Survey of Family Growth. Vital Health Stat 2006;23:1–142.

[82] Schmidt SS. Vasectomy by section, luminal fulguration and fascial interposition: results from 6248 cases. Br J Urol 1995;76:373–4.

[83] Li SQ, Goldstein M, Zhu J, Huber D. The no-scalpel vasectomy. J Urol 1991;145:341–4.

[84] Nirapathpongporn A, Huber DJ, Krieger JN. No scalpel vasectomy at the King's birthday vasectomy festival. Lancet 1990;335:894–5.

[85] Philp T, Guillebaud J, Budd D. Complications of vasectomy: review of 16,000 patients. Br J Urol 1984;56:745–8.

[86] Schwingl PJ, Guess HA. Safety and effectiveness of vasectomy. Fertil Steril 2000;73:923–36.

[87] Dey D, Chatterjee A, Banji D, Bhowmik BB. Current status of male contraception. Am J Phytomedicine Clin Ther 2013;1:282–90.

[88] Lohiya NK, Alam I, Hussain M, Khan SR, Ansari AS. RISUG: an intra-vasal injectable male contraceptive. Indian J Med Res 2014;140:S63–72.

[89] Turner L, Conway AJ, Jimenez M, Liu PY, Forbes EA, Mclachlan RI, Handelsman DJ. Contraceptive efficacy of a depot progestin and androgen combination in men. J Clin Endocrinol Metabol 2003;88:4659–67.

[90] Barfield A, Melo J, Coutinho E, Alvarez-Sanchez F, Faundes A, Brache V, Leon P, Frick J, Bartsch G, Weiske WH, Brenner P, Mishell Jr D, Bernstein G, Ortiz A. Pregnancies associated with sperm concentrations below 10 million/mL in clinical studies of a potential male contraceptive method, monthly depot medroxyprogesterone acetate and testosterone esters. Contraception 1979;20:121–7.

[91] Gu YQ, Tong JS, Ma DZ, Wang XH, Yuan D, Tang WH, Bremner WJ. Male hormonal contraception: effects of injections of testosterone undecanoate and depot medroxyprogesterone acetate at eight-week intervals in Chinese men. J Clin Endocrinol Metabol 2004;89:2254–62.

[92] Bebb RA, Anawalt BD, Christensen RB, Paulsen CA, Bremner WJ, Matsumoto AM. Combined administration of levonorgestrel and testosterone induces more rapid and effective suppression of spermatogenesis than testosterone alone: a promising male contraceptive approach. J Clin Endocrinol Metabol 1996;81:757–62.

[93] Gui YL, He CH, Amory JK, Bremner WJ, Zheng EX, Yang J, Yang PJ, Gao ES. Male hormonal contraception: suppression of spermatogenesis by injectable testosterone undecanoate alone or with levonorgestrel implants in Chinese men. J Androl 2004;25:720–7.

[94] Brady BM, Amory JK, Perheentupa A, Zitzmann M, Hay CJ, Apter D, Anderson RA, Bremner WJ, Pollanen P, Nieschlag E, Wu FC, Kersemaekers WM. A multicentre study investigating subcutaneous etonogestrel implants with injectable testosterone decanoate as a potential long-acting male contraceptive. Hum Reprod 2006;21:285–94.

[95] Mommers E, Kersemaekers WM, Elliesen J, Kepers M, Apter D, Behre HM, Beynon J, Bouloux PM, Costantino A, Gerbershagen HP, Grønlund L, Heger-Mahn D, Huhtaniemi I, Koldewijn EL, Lange C, Lindenberg S, Meriggiola MC, Meuleman E, Mulders PF, Nieschlag E, Perheentupa A, Solomon A, Väisälä L, Wu FC, Zitzmann M. Male hormonal contraception: a double-blind, placebo-controlled study. J Clin Endocrinol Metabol 2008;93:2572–80.

[96] Meriggiola MC, Bremner WJ, Paulsen CA, Valdiserri A, Incorvaia L, Motta R, Pavani A, Capelli M, Flamigni C. A combined regimen of cyproterone acetate and testosterone enanthate as a potentially highly effective male contraceptive. J Clin Endocrinol Metabol 1996;81:3018–23.

[97] Meriggiola MC, Bremner WJ, Costantino A, Di Cintio G, Flamigni C. Low dose of cyproterone acetate and testosterone enanthate for contraception in men. Hum Reprod 1998;13:1225–9.

[98] Kumar N, Koide SS, Tsong Y, Sundaram K. Nestorone: a progestin with a unique pharmacological profile. Steroids 2000;65:629–36.

[99] Ilani N, Roth MY, Amory JK, Swerdloff RS, Dart C, Page ST, Bremner WJ, Sitruk-Ware R, Kumar N, Blithe DL, Wang C. A new combination of testosterone and nestorone transdermal gels for male hormonal contraception. J Clin Endocrinol Metabol 2012;97:3476–86.

[100] Hori J, Koga D, Kakizaki H, Watanabe T. Differential effects of depot formulations of GnRH agonist leuprorelin and antagonist degarelix on the seminiferous epithelium of the rat testis. Biomed Res (Tokyo) 2018;39:197–214.

[101] Behre HM, Nashan D, Hubert W, Nieschlag E. Depot gonadotropin-releasing hormone agonist blunts the androgen-induced suppression of spermatogenesis in a clinical trial of male contraception. J Clin Endocrinol Metabol 1992;74:84–90.

[102] Wang C, Festin MPR, Swerdloff RS. Male hormonal contraception: where are we now? Curr Obstet Gynaecol Rep 2016;5:38–47.

[103] Mok KW, Mruk DD, Lie PP, Lui WY, Cheng CY. Adjudin, a potential male contraceptive, exerts its effects locally in the seminiferous epithelium of mammalian testes. Reproduction 2011;141:571–80.

[104] Mruk DD, Cheng CY. Testin and actin are key molecular targets of adjudin, an antispermatogenic agent, in the testes. Spermatogenesis 2011;1:137–46.

[105] Aliyu B, Onwuchekwa C. Birth control: contraceptive drugs/pills and methods in the last decades. Trop J Obstet Gynaecol 2018;35:233–40.

[106] Tash JS, Attardi B, Hild SA, Chakrasali R, Jakkaraj SR, Georg GI. A novel potent indazole carboxylic acid derivative blocks spermatogenesis and is contraceptive in rats after a single oral dose. Biol Reprod 2008;78:1127–38.

[107] Gao N, Ren J, Hou L, Zhou Y, Xin L, Wang J, Yu H, Xie Y, Wang H. Identification of novel potent human testis-specific and bromodomain-containing protein (BRDT) inhibitors using crystal structure-based virtual screening. Int J Mol Med 2016;38:39–44.

[108] Matzuk MM, McKeown MR, Filippakopoulos P, Li Q, Ma L, Agno JE, Lemieux ME, Picaud S, Yu RN, Qi J, Knapp S, Bradner JE. Small molecule inhibition of BRDT for male contraception. Cell 2012;150:673–84.

[109] Zdrojewicz Z, Konieczny R, Papier P, Szten F. Brdt bromodomains inhibitors and other modern means of male contraception. Adv Clin Exp Med 2015;24:705–14.

[110] Chen Z, He W, Liang Z, Yan P, He H, Tang Y, Zhang J, Shen Z, Ni B, Wu Y, Li J. Protein prime-peptide boost as a new strategy induced and Eppin dominant B-cell epitope specific immune response and suppressed fertility. Vaccine 2009;27:733–40.

[111] Silva EJ, Hamil KG, Richardson RT, O'Rand MG. Characterization of EPPIN's semenogelin I binding site: a contraceptive drug target. Biol Reprod 2012;87:1–8.

[112] O'Rand MG, Widgren EE, Sivashanmugam P, Richardson RT, Hall SH, French FS, VandeVoort CA, Ramachandra SG, Ramesh V, Rao AJ. Reversible immunocontraception in male monkeys immunized with Eppin. Science 2004;306:1189–90.

[113] Khourdaji I, Zillioux J, Eisenfrats K, Foley D, Smith R. The future of male contraception: a fertile ground. Transl Androl Urol 2018;7:S220–35.

[114] Averal HI, Stanley A, Marugaian P, Palanisami A, Akbarsha MA. Specific effect of vincristine on epididymis. Indian J Exp Biol 1996;34:53–6.

[115] Hall JC, Perez FM, Kochins JG, Pettersen CA, Li Y, Tubbs CE, LaMarche MD. Quantification and localization of N-acetyl-beta-D-hexosaminidase in the adult rat testis and epididymis. Biol Reprod 1996;54:914–29.

[116] Tassi C, Angelini A, Beccari T, Capodicasa E. Fluorimetric determination of activity and isoenzyme composition of N-acetyl-beta-D-hexosaminidase in seminal plasma of fertile men and infertile patients with secretory azoospermia. Clin Chem Lab Med 2006;44:843–7.

[117] Marquez B, Ignotz G, Suarez SS. Contributions of extracellular and intracellular Ca2 + to regulation of sperm motility: release of intracellular stores can hyperactivate Catsper1 and Catsper2 null sperm. Dev Biol 2007;303:214–21.

[118] Chung JJ, Shim SH, Everley RA, Gygi SP, Zhuang X, Clapham DE. Structurally distinct Ca(2+) signaling domains of sperm flagella orchestrate tyrosine phosphorylation and motility. Cell 2014;157:808–22.

[119] Sun X-H, Zhu Y-Y, Wang L, Liu H-L, Ling Y, Li Z-L, Sun L-B. The Catsper channel and its roles in male fertility: a systematic review. Reprod Biol Endocrinol 2017;15:65. https://doi.org/10.1186/s12958-017-0281-2.

[120] Babcock DF. Wrath of the wraiths of Catsper3 and Catsper4. Proc Natl Acad Sci U S A 2007;104:1107–8.

[121] Lopez LM, Grimes DA, Schulz KF. Non-hormonal drugs for contraception in men: a systematic review. Obstet Gynaecol Surv 2005;60:746–52.

[122] Qian SZ. *Tripterygium wilfordii*, a Chinese herb effective in male fertility regulation. Contraception 1987;36:335–45.

[123] Dhar SK, Gupta S, Chanduke NA. Antifertility studies of some indigenous plants. In: Proceedings of the XIth Annual Conference of the Indian Pharmacological Society, New Delhi; 1978.

[124] Gopalakrishnan M, Rajasekbarasetty MR. Effect of papaya (*Carica papaya* Linn.) on pregnancy and oestrus cycle in albino rats of Wistar strain. Indian J Physiol Pharmacol 1978;22:66–70.

[125] Julaehaa E, Permatasaria Y, Mayantia T, Diantinib A. Antifertility compound from the seeds of *Carica papaya*. Proc Chem 2015;17:66–9. 3rd International Seminar on Chemistry 2014.

[126] Lohiya NK, Mishra PK, Pathak N, Manivannan B, Bhande SS, Panneerdoss S, Sriram S. Efficacy trial on the purified compounds of the seeds of *Carica papaya* for male contraception in albino rat. Reprod Toxicol 2005;20:135–48.

[127] Rajasekaran M, Bapna JS, Lakshmanan S, Ramachandran Nair AG, Veliath AJ, Panchanadam M. Antifertility effect in male rats of oleanolic acid, a triterpene from *Eugenia jambolana* flowers. J Ethnopharmacol 1988;24:115–21.

[128] Lohiya NK, Manivannan B, Mishra PK, Pathak N, Sriram S, Bhande SS, Panneerdoss S. Chloroform extract from *Carica papaya* seeds induces long-term reversible azoospermia in Langur monkey. Asian J Androl 2002;4:17–26.

[129] World Health Organization. Defining sexual health. Retrieved from http://www.who.int/reproductivehealth/topics/sexual_health/sh_definitions/en; 2006.

[130] Nagarajah AK, Pai NB, Rao S, Rao TS, Goyal N. Biology of sexual dysfunction. Online J Health Allied Sci 2009;8:1–7.

[131] Brotto L, Atallah S, Johnson-Agbakwu C, Rosenbaum T, Abdo C, Byers ES, Graham C, Nobre P, Wylie K. Psychological and interpersonal dimensions of sexual function and dysfunction. J Sex Med 2016;13:538–71.

[132] Coretti G, Baldi I. The relationship between anxiety disorders and sexual dysfunction. Psychiatr Times 2007;24:16–21.

[133] Wang C, Nieschlag E, Swerdloff RS, Behre H, Hellstrom WJ, Gooren LJ, Kaufman JM, Legros JJ, Lunenfeld B, Morales A, Morley JE, Schulman C, Thompson IM, Weidner W, Wu FC. ISA, ISSAM, EAU, EAA and ASA recommendations: investigation, treatment and monitoring of late onset hypogonadism in males. Int J Impot Res 2009;21:1–8.

[134] Matsumoto AM. Andropause: clinical implications of the decline in serum testosterone levels with aging in men. J Gerontol A Biol Sci Med Sci 2002;57:M76–99.

[135] Morley JE. Testosterone and behaviour. Clin Geriatr Med 2003;19:605–16.

[136] Travison TG, Morley JE, Araujo AB, O'Donnell AB, Mckinlay JB. The relationship between libido and testosterone levels in aging men. J Clin Endocrinol Metabol 2006;91:2509–13.

[137] Grimm Jr RH, Grandits GA, Prineas RJ, McDonald RH, Lewis CE, Flack JM, Yunis C, Svendsen K, Liebson PR, Elmer PJ. Long-term effects on sexual function of five antihypertensive drugs and nutritional hygienic treatment in hypertensive men and women. Treatment of Mild Hypertension Study (TOMHS). Hypertension 1997;29:8–14.

[138] Ma R, Yu J, Xu D, Yang L, Lin X, Zhao F, Bai F. Effect of felodipine with irbesartan or metoprolol on sexual function and oxidative stress in women with essential hypertension. J Hypertens 2012;30:210–6.

[139] Conaglen M, Conaglen V. Drug-induced sexual dysfunction in men and women. Aust Prescr 2013;36:42–5.

[140] Jansen PM, Frenkel WJ, Van den Born BJ, De Bruijne EL, Deinum J, Kerstens MN, Arnoldus JH, Woittiez AJ, Wijbenga JA, Zietse R, Danser AH, Van den Meiracker AH. Determinants of blood pressure reduction by eplerenone in uncontrolled hypertension. J Hypertens 2013;31:404–13.

[141] Anon. Midamor product monograph, www.aapharma.ca/downloads/en/PIL/midamor_pm.pdf; 2010.

[142] Bulpitt CJ, Dollery CT. Side effects of hypotensive agents evaluated by a self-administered questionnaire. Br Med J 1973;3:485–90.

[143] Chang SW, Fine R, Siegel D, Chesney M, Black D, Hulley SB. The impact of diuretic therapy on reported sexual function. Arch Intern Med 1991;151:2402–8.

[144] Mir S, Taylor D. Sexual adverse effects with new antidepressants. Psychiatr Bull 1998;22:438–41.

[145] Stahl SM. Basic psychopharmacology of antidepressants, part I: anti-depressants have seven distinct mechanisms of action. J Clin Psychiatry 1998;59:5–14.

[146] Yeon W, Yooseok K, Jun H. Antipsychotic induced sexual dysfunction and its management. World J Mens Health 2012;30:153–9.

[147] Mailman RB, Murthy V. Third generation antipsychotic drugs: partial agonism or receptor functional selectivity? Curr Pharm Des 2010;16:488–501.

[148] Smals AG, Weusten JJ, Benraad TJ, Kloppenborg PW. The HMG-CoA reductase inhibitor simvastatin suppresses human testicular testosterone synthesis *in vitro* by a selective inhibitory effect on 17-ketosteroid-oxidoreductase enzyme activity. J Steroid Biochem Mol Biol 1991;38:465–8.

[149] Trivedi D, Kirby M, Norman F, Przybytniak I, Ali S, Wellsted DM. Can simvastatin improve erectile function and health-related quality of life in men aged ≥ 40 years with erectile dysfunction? Results of the Erectile Dysfunction and Statins Trial [ISRCTN66772971]. BJU Int 2013;111:324–33.

[150] Schooling CM, Yeung SLA, Freeman G, Cowling BJ. The effect of statins on testosterone in men and women, a systematic review and meta-analysis of randomized controlled trials. BMC Med 2013;11:57. http://www.biomedcentral.com/1741-7015/11/57.

[151] Gupta S, Salimpour P, Saenzde-Tejada I, Daley J, Gholami S, Daller M, Krane RJ, Traish AM, Goldstein I. A possible mechanism for alteration of human erectile function by digoxin: inhibition of corpus cavernosum sodium/potassium adenosine triphosphatase activity. J Urol 1998;159:1529–36.

[152] Berterö C. Altered sexual patterns after treatment for prostate cancer. Cancer Pract 2001;9:245–51.

[153] Smith S. Drugs that cause sexual dysfunction. Psychiatry 2007;6:111–4.

Chapter 5.1

Herbal medicine used to treat andrological problems: Americas

Gustavo F. Gonzales[a,b], Manuel Gasco[a,b], Cinthya Vasquez-Velasquez[a,b], Diego Fano-Sizgorich[a], and Dulce Esperanza Alarcón-Yaquetto[a,b]

[a]*Endocrinology and Reproduction Unit, Research and Development Laboratories (LID), Department of Biological and Physiological Sciences, Faculty of Sciences and Philosophy, Universidad Peruana Cayetano Heredia, Lima, Peru*, [b]*High Altitude Research Institute, Universidad Peruana Cayetano Heredia, Lima, Peru*

1 Introduction

Diseases have plagued humans throughout history. Using trial and error, native cultures worldwide have used herbal remedies alone or in admixture to treat these maladies. During the last century, the modern pharmaceutical industry used individual active compounds obtained from plants to develop pharmaceutical products [1].

In different countries, many plants are used as part of traditional medicine, but only a small proportion of them have been scientifically investigated to demonstrate their efficacy. Science has contributed to demonstrate or deny the impact of plants on relieving or preventing diseases [2–4]. For example, a prospective association of total and subtypes of fruit and vegetable intake with the incidence of prostate cancer was studied in 142,239 European men from eight countries. The main finding of the study was that a higher fruit intake was associated with a small reduction in prostate cancer risk. However, whether or not there is a causal association between high fruit intake and reduced risk of prostate cancer remains unclear [5].

American traditional medicine was unknown to Europe, Asia, or Africa until the discovery of the New World. At the time of the European contact, in 1492 by Christopher Columbus, the splinting of broken bones and the cleaning and treatment of wounds were well advanced in the native population [6]. In the last decades, the use of herbal remedies in andrology has increased worldwide [7]. Although most of the remedies are used only locally, some of them have aroused worldwide interest. Examples are *Tribulus terrestris* for fertility [8], *Serenoa repens* [9] for prostate diseases; *Lepidium meyenii* (maca) for sexual desire, male infertility, and prostate diseases; or Korean red ginseng for erectile dysfunction [10].

After Europeans colonized the Americas, an opportunity for the development of new medicines based on numerous plants native to the New World was raised. These plants had been used by native cultures for centuries or millennia. The plants and, eventually, isolated drugs derived from them were incorporated into the *materia medica* of the Europeans both in Europe and in the new colonies. Many became official in the United States Pharmacopeia (USP) [11].

After the Spanish conquest of Peru, several medicinal plants from the Americas like ipecacuanha, guaiacum, sarsaparilla, jalap root, and cinchona moved with relative ease into Europe and Asia by the late 18th century. This explains the causes of the global 'spread' of American remedies [12]. Other plants such as *Smallanthus sonchifolius* (yacon*), Plukenetia volubilis* (sacha inchi), *Uncaria tomentosa* (uña de gato), *Myrciaria dubia* (camu camu), and *Lepidium meyenni* (maca), some considered as novel foods, have aroused interest in Europe [13].

Chroniclers of the Peruvian conquest have detailed many of the plants used for food and also as remedies to relieve several diseases. One of them was Bernabe Cobo who described several medicinal plants from Mexico and Peru used by natives at the time of the conquest [14]. In the 16th century, Cobo described one of the most important fertility-enhancing plants, named maca (*Lepidium meyenii*). This plant grows in hardish conditions at more than 4000 m above sea level in the Peruvian Central Andes. Currently, it is famous worldwide since scientific evidence have shown its effects in enhancing male sexual desire and improving male fertility [15].

Approximately 1400 plant species are thought to be used in Peruvian traditional medicine; however, only a few have undergone scientific investigation [16]. The plant that draws more attention worldwide and currently holds the record of being the most exported Peruvian medicinal plant is *L. meyenii* (maca). This is an example in which science has contributed to increase the interest for a plant described initially by the chroniclers of the conquest during the 16th century and that once was in danger of extinction in the 20th century [17].

Herbal Medicine in Andrology. https://doi.org/10.1016/B978-0-12-815565-3.00005-9

This chapter is devoted to gather scientific evidence of plants native to the Americas that have proven andrological properties.

2 Male infertility

Infertility is the failure to conceive a child after 1 year of regular, unprotected sexual intercourse [18]. Half of the cases seems to be due to male factor infertility [18]. Infertility largely affects society and has a negative impact on the social and emotional aspects of the patient.

Male factor infertility is a multifactorial disorder that affects a significant percentage of couples; however, it is not always treated. Despite considerable efforts to determine the pathophysiology of the male factor, the underlying etiology or the mechanisms of approximately half of the cases remain unknown. These cases are named *"idiopathic infertility"* [19].

In the event that couples fail to achieve a pregnancy despite a young female partner displaying a normal ovulation profile with patent tubes and a male partner with adequate semen parameters, the diagnosis of *"unexplained infertility"* is applied. This situation is observed in up to 30% of couples who are unable to reproduce [20, 21].

3 Herbal medicine for male infertility

The use of herbal medicine is still widespread despite the insurgence of mass produced chemically synthesized drugs [22]. A vast number of people from countries where ancient civilizations once thrived such as China, India, or Peru still rely on traditional medicine for their primary health care. The use of herbal medicine is so widespread in these countries that hospitals have units devoted to the use of traditional medicine (examples are China and Peru) [22].

Since conventional medicine is expensive and might be out of reach for a large proportion of the population, fertility is one of the areas where people recourse to herbal medicines the most [23]. In recent years, a considerable number of infertile men has sought 'herbal remedies' as an effective way of treatment [24].

Since oxidative stress (OS) is an important factor for male infertility as demonstrated by several studies [25, 26], it is possible that many cases regarded as "idiopathic male infertility" could actually be due to alterations in OS including methylation status [27]. Medicinal plants have been assessed in clinical trials for the treatment of idiopathic male infertility with good results and could be an important source for treating male infertility [28].

In several cases of OS, an abnormal seminal pattern is observed due to the decreased antioxidant status [27]. These observations led investigators to improve antioxidant levels in cases of male infertility associated with OS as a way to recover fertility [29]. Many plants have potent antioxidant activities and this could be one of the ways plants are used to treat male infertility. For such reason, epidemiological studies confirm that the incidence of OS-related conditions is lowered by the consumption of fruits and vegetables rich in compounds with high antioxidant activity [30, 31]. Thus, foods containing antioxidants and antioxidant nutrients may play an important role in preventing infertility.

Pomegranate, a plant with the highest antioxidant activity among the studied plants, has long been used to increase fertility [32]. In a placebo-controlled clinical trial, after 3 months of active treatment with pomegranate fruit extract and galangal rhizome, the average total number of motile sperm increased by 62% while for the placebo group, the number of motile sperm increased by 20%. Sperm morphology was not affected by the treatment [33].

Treatment with omega-3 polyunsaturated fatty acid in a placebo-controlled study may improve semen profile in infertile men with idiopathic oligoasthenoteratozoospermia [34]. A positive association between strong adherence to a healthy dietary pattern and semen parameters in men with good semen quality was observed. On the other hand, a Western dietary pattern may increase the risk of abnormal semen parameters [35]. Some plants have been found to correct the deficient intake of omega-3 essential fatty acids, which correlates with impaired sperm motility in infertile men [36], for example, linseed (flaxseed) oil that contains α-linolenic acid and lignans. Lignans are precursors of enterolacton, which inhibits aromatase and reduces the ratio of 16-OH over 2-OH estrogen metabolites. This may favorably influence Sertoli cell function [36].

Other causes of infertility are the exposure to some substances or pollutants. For example, bisphenol-A, an endocrine disruptor found in polycarbonate plastics and food packaging [37]. *Eruca sativa* aqueous extract protects toward in vitro bisphenol-A BPA-mediated toxicity and it is suggested as a complementary treatment for reproductive disorders in men [38].

There are some plants with a controversial role on male fertility, like *Tribulus terrestris*, a herbaceous plant from the Zygophyllaceae family. Flavonoids, alkaloids, saponins, lignin, amides, and glycosides are its main active phytoconstituents [8]. However, although many articles have been published, the exact role of this plant in male infertility is still controversial [8].

Many supplements have been proposed claiming to have fertility-enhancing effects. Favorable effects on male fertility as demonstrated in a small, randomized controlled trial (RCT) have been shown for aescin, coenzyme Q 10, glutathione,

Korean red ginseng, L-carnitine, *Nigella sativa*, omega-3 fatty acids, selenium, a combination of zinc and folate, and the Menevit antioxidant. However, there is no support for the use of vitamin C or vitamin E. In conclusion, the exact role of different plants in male infertility is still controversial and needs future double-blinded, placebo-controlled studies that deploy larger cohorts.

3.1 Overview of American herbs used to treat infertility

Due to a variety of microclimates, the Americas have a great biodiversity. The Amazon region is rich in plants used for traditional medicine [39–43]. It is generally agreed that the prospects of encountering enhanced small organic-molecule chemical diversity are better if tropical rather than temperate species are investigated in drug discovery efforts [44].

In the Americas, two big cultures were highly developed, the Mayas in Central America [45, 46] and the Incas in South America. They developed important traditional medicines in which plants were part of the remedies used against diseases. The Americas comprise North America, Central America, and South America. Central and South America are also named Latin America with a wealth of medicinal plants [47–49].

This in-depth review presents several studies that evaluate the role of American plants used to treat male infertility. The forthcoming sections are divided by geographical zones as used by the United Nations geoscheme for the Americas [50]. According to this classification, Mexico is considered as a part of Central America.

Both native plants and those introduced but widely used by locals are included. Table 1 provides an overview of plants used to treat male infertility. Despite infertility being a multifactorial problem, the majority of studies using plants focus on effects in sperm quality and sexual dysfunction. In some cases, where plants are used by local populations to treat male infertility but no evidence is found in the literature, a search for the main constituent was done, to assess the probable reasons behind these properties and to recommend more research.

3.2 Herbs with effects on sperm quality

The effects of fertility-enhancing herbs are mainly assessed based on the effects these plants exert on sperm quality variables such as motility and normal sperm morphology as well as seminal volume, which are considered the cornerstones of andrological tests.

3.2.1 North America

American ginseng (*Panax quinquefolius*) is a perennial herb of the Araliaceae family that grows in North America. It is one of the eight species of ginseng in the world and one of the three with known therapeutic applications. Although Asian ginseng (*P. ginseng*) is more widely known for its effects on male health, there is evidence which supports that *P. quinquefolius* might as well provide andrological benefits to its consumers.

Treating male rats with American ginseng diluted in saline for 6 weeks increased sperm count compared with the control group. Furthermore, the extract was able to revert the deleterious effects of cyclophosphamide on sperm cells [52]. The active compounds exerting these properties might be triterpenoid saponins exclusively found in the genus *Panax* and henceforth baptized as ginsenosides. There are two groups of ginsenosides, 20(S)-protopanaxatriol and 20(S)-protopanaxadiol [78]. Ginsenoside Re is the most abundant ginsenoside found in ginseng and belongs to the 20(S)-protopanaxatriol group alongside ginsenosides Rg1, Rg2, and Rb3, while Rb1, Rb2, Rc, and Rd. are ginsenosides that belong to the 20(S)-protopanaxadiol group [78]. Most American ginseng populations exhibit low Rg1 and high Re ginsenosides [79]. Re has been found to enhance fertile and infertile sperm motility by inducing nitric oxide synthase [51].

Amaranth (*Amaranthus hypochondriacus*) is a pseudocereal belonging to the Amaranthaceae family that grows mainly in North America although it is also seen in some parts of South America. Singhal and Kulkarni report that besides being a great source of vitamins and minerals, amaranth is also characterized by its high squalene concentration [80]. Squalene is a natural organic compound, which has shown effects on sperm quality such as improvement of semen volume and sperm motility in boars [81]. These effects may be attributed to the reported antioxidant activity [82] that should be studied further.

Goldenseal (*Hydrastis canadensis*) is also a widely used herb in North American traditional medicine. Although its traditional use is not related to andrological problems, one of its main constituents, the alkaloid berberine [83], is effective in increasing sperm motility rate and viability in vitro [84]. Further studies should focus on gathering more evidence on the effect of these American herbs on sperm motility.

TABLE 1 Herbs used to improve sperm quality and enhance sexual behavior in the Americas.

Scientific name	Common name	Zone	Properties	In-vitro studies	Animal studies	Uncontrolled human studies	RCT	Comment
Panax quinquefolius	American ginseng	North America	Increases sperm quality	Main component, ginsenoside Re increases sperm motility [51]	Increased sperm count and reverted toxicity effects on sperm cells [52]		RCTs were conducted to test other properties of the plant. Safety and tolerability have been established [53, 54]. No RCTs on male fertility properties	More evidence of fertility enhancing properties is found in Korean ginseng
			Increases sexual behavior		Decrease mount, intromission, and ejaculation latencies [55]			
Bertholletia excelsa	Castanha, Brazilian nuts, chestnut	South America	Constituents might protect sperm from oxidative damage	Selenium protects against ROS-mediated sperm damage [56]				Also contains squalene
Amaranthus hypochondriacus	Amaranth	North America	Main constituent increased sperm count		Enhanced sperm quality in boars			Main constituent squalene used in animal study
Hydrastis canadensis	Goldenseal	North America	Main constituent increased sperm quality and quantity	Increased sperm motility and viability				Main constituent berberine used on in vitro study
Carica papaya	Papaya	Central America	Sperm quality (divergent effects of rape fruit and seeds)			Fermented fruit increased sperm count in men with asthenozoospermia when given with other natural antioxidants [57]		Seeds and leafs contain papain, proteolytic enzyme with antispermatogenic effects
Mucuna pruriens	Cowitch	Introduced. Caribbean	Improves sperm parameters and recovers sperm function		Revert the effects of aging in sperm DNA [58], recovered sperm function in diabetic rats [59], and enhances sperm quality, motility and concentration in rabbits [60]	Infertile men had increased sperm motility and decreased psychological stress following treatment with plant extract [61]. Regulates steroidogenesis and improves sperm parameters in infertile men [62]	Two RCTs assessing its effect to treat Parkinson's disease showed safety and long-term tolerability of seed powder [63, 64]	

Scientific name	Common name	Region	Effect				Notes
Lepidium meyenii	Maca	South America	Improves sperm parameters	Increased sperm count, motility, viability [65, 66]	Increased sperm parameters in healthy men [67]	Both on infertile men: increased sperm volume and motility [68]. Only increased motility but no changes in morphology [69]	Confronting evidence regarding its effects on sexual hormones
			Long-term usage increased libido	Increased sexual behavior in rodents [70–72]		Libido enhancement effects only seen after at least 3-week consumption. Safety and tolerability warranted [73]	Maca is wrongly marketed as Viagra. No immediate effect seen on sexual behavior and libido
Achillea millefolium	Yarrow	North America	Antispermatogenic		Severely affects spermatogenesis [74]		Used for other therapeutic properties
Tropaeolum tuberosum	Mashua	South America	Antispermatogenic		Diminishes daily sperm production and increases abnormal sperm morphology [75]		Used since ancient times to reduce sexual behavior
Chrysactinia mexicana	Damianita	Central America	Libido enhancer		Increased capacity to restart copulation after ejaculation [76]		Damiana and Damianita are used interchangeably by native Central American populations to treat sexual dysfunction due to their morphological resemblance despite no botanical relation
Turnera diffusa	Damiana	Central America	Libido enhancer		Increased sexual performance and reduces intromission and ejaculation latencies [77]		

Geographical divisions correspond to the United Nations geoscheme for the Americans, Mexico is included as Central America. RCT, randomize controlled trial.

3.2.2 Mexico and Central America

Papaya (*Carica papaya*) is a tree belonging to the Caricaceae family. Originally coming from Central America, mainly Costa Rica and Mexico, nowadays it is also grown in North and South America and other parts of the world. The fresh, ripe fruit is part of the everyday diet of many people around the globe and has been proven to be a protector against oxidative damage [85]. Fermented papaya fruit increases sperm quality in asthenoteratozoospermic men when given alongside vitamin C and E, lactoferrin, and β-glucan [57]. The effect of the ripe fruit alone is not properly investigated.

Nevertheless, papaya seeds and leaves contain proteolytic enzymes, mainly papain and chemopapain [86], which have antispermatogenic effects in animal models and spermicidal activity in humans [87]. *C. papaya* seed extract markedly affects sperm motility parameters essential for reproduction [88]. Some authors argue that the ability of papain to reduce seminal viscosity is a remarkable feature of high economic importance for assisted reproduction technologies in animals. These authors have shown that using papain alongside its inhibitor E64 led to reduced viscosity without damaging sperm integrity in alpacas [89], while others have stated it might be a good candidate for male contraception [88].

3.2.3 The Caribbean

Mucuna pruriens is a tropical legume originally coming from India that has been introduced in Caribbean countries where it now has a widespread distribution. It is also called Bengal velvet bean or "Cowitch" by locals and is used in traditional medicine. In an animal study, the ethanolic extract of *M. pruriens* reduced the production of reactive oxygen species and lipid peroxidation in sperm cells. The plant extract also increased enzymatic antioxidants, which reduced loss of chromosomal integrity and decreased sperm DNA damage in aged rats [58]. The same research group used a diabetic rat model to assess the effects of *M. pruriens*. In streptozotocin-induced diabetic rats, sperm parameters were altered, but treatment with the plant extract recovered sperm function, preserved sperm DNA integrity, chromosomal integrity, and mitochondrial membrane potential [59]. A recent study has shown the beneficial properties of *M. pruriens* mixed with the standard chow in rabbits. The treatment resulted in an improvement in semen quality, sperm motility, and concentration [90].

The fertility-enhancing properties of *M. pruriens* not only have been assessed in animal experiments, but also in a study with infertile men where treatment with the plant led to diminished psychological stress and an improvement in seminal parameters [91]. According to the authors, the effects on psychological stress alongside an improvement of the antioxidant defense system makes this plant ideal to treat male infertility since there is enough evidence linking psychological stress with male infertility [92].

Several researchers have tried to identify the metabolite responsible for the biological properties of *M. pruriens* on the testicular function of an organism. In a study, treating rats with L-dopa, the major constituent of the plant, had the same effects as that of this leguminous plant [93], mainly a reduction in ROS levels, an increase in the number of germ cells, and regulation of apoptosis.

3.2.4 South America

Brazil nuts, *Bertholletia excelsa,* are marketed as a sexual performance enhancer. Despite there are no studies using extracts of the plant in in vitro or in vivo models, the nuts are famous for its high selenium concentration [94, 95], and this inorganic element is effective in protecting the sperm of asthenoteratozoospermic men from ROS damage in in vitro studies [56]. These nuts also contain high quantities of squalene [96], an organic compound with apparent sperm quality enhancement property [81, 82].

Lepidium meyenii is a prodigious crop that grows exclusively in the Central Andean Region, specifically in the Highlands of Junin, Peru. Ancient Peruvians used it widely for therapeutic reasons and were aware of its fertility-enhancing properties, so that when the Spanish started populating these areas and were unable to conceive, local Peruvians recommended this plant. Fortunately, this information is preserved until today in several chronicles from this epoch [17]. *L. meyenii* or "maca" as it is widely known is arguably the most studied Peruvian plant and its effects on male fertility were the first to be scientifically proven. The edible part of the plant are the hypocotyl (Fig. 1) that can be found in several phenotypes distinguishable by color.

The improvement in sperm quality seen after maca treatment has been observed in several animal models. An increase in length and frequency of stages IX–XIV of spermatogenesis was observed after treating male rats with aqueous extract of *L. meyenii* [97]. Maca is also able to reverse the detrimental effects of chemically and physically induced testicular dysfunction with the resultant subfertility and deteriorated seminal parameters as was evidenced by Valdivia Cuya et al. [98]. In the same way, when subfertility was induced in mice by cyclophosphamide, treatment with maca improved gonadal insufficiency and testicular morphology [99]. In a recent study, maca improved fertilization rates by increasing sperm motility and inducing acrosome reaction using oocytes of mouse and human sperm [100].

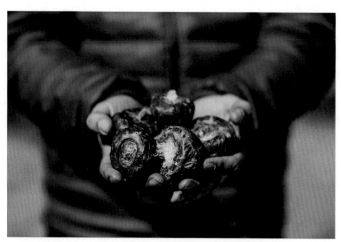

FIG. 1 Hypocotyls of *Lepidium meyenii* (maca), a Peruvian plant with fertility-enhancing effects.

Recently, studies have aimed to figure out which fraction of the hydroalcoholic extract contains the bioactive compounds with properties to enhance sperm quality. Inoue determined that the methanolic fraction of maca had higher biological activity than the butanolic fraction as determined by epididymal and vas deferens sperm count increase [101].

There are also several reports on the effects of maca on sperm quality in humans. In an uncontrolled observational study conducted in healthy participants, Gonzales et al. found increased seminal volume, motile sperm count, and sperm motility after a 4-month treatment with tablets of maca (1500 mg or 3000 mg /day). There was no difference between the doses [67]. In a randomized, placebo-controlled trial (RCT), where gelatinized maca in capsules were given for 12 weeks, the total sperm count and sperm concentration were not significantly different than the control group (milled apple fiber), but normal morphology, semen volume, and progressive sperm motility increased in the maca-treated group [68].

There is also one RCT conducted on 60 infertile men where a pill containing 1 g of maca extract was given twice a day for 90 days. Seminal analysis was conducted at the beginning of the study and after 30, 60, and 90 days. Maca increased sperm motility, but no changes were seen in sperm morphology [69].

3.2.5 Herbs with antispermatogenic effects

There are also plants that affect sperm parameters in a negative way and that are worth discussing further. *Achillea millefolium* subspecies *lanulosa* (Nutt.), commonly known as yarrow, is a native plant from North America widely used by populations that once resided in Boreal Canada for treating wounds and for other health issues including respiratory and digestive problems [102]. Nevertheless, Montanari et al. showed that both the ethanolic and hydroalcoholic extracts of yarrow flowers severely altered spermatogenesis in mice [74].

Tropaeolum tuberosum (mashua), an Andean edible crop, is known by locals to have fertility-reducing properties. According to ancient chronists, Father Bernabé Cobo and Inca Garcilaso de la Vega, mashua was used to make soldiers "forget" their women [103]. These anecdotal claims have been confirmed by research in rats. Mashua lowered daily sperm production values and increased the percentage of abnormal sperm morphology and delay in sperm transit. This effect was reversed 24 h after discontinuation of the treatment [75].

3.3 Sexual desire and behavior

Sexual dysfunction is defined by the International Classification of Diseases Volume 10 (ICD-10) as the inability to participate in a sexual relationship as one would wish. This condition can be caused by psychological or somatic processes [104]. Lack of desire, arousal, or orgasm are categories of male sexual dysfunction characterized by erectile dysfunction, premature or delayed ejaculation or anorgasmia [105].

Erectile dysfunction or the "inability to maintain an erection for satisfactory sexual performance" is a condition that has affected men throughout history with evidence of its occurrence even in Ancient Egypt [106]. This is why it is not surprising that many ancient civilizations tried to ameliorate the condition using herbal medicine.

3.3.1 North America

Over-the-counter products containing American ginseng are sold as sexual performance boosters. Yet, there is not much scientific evidence that support this fact, at least in comparison to Korean ginseng, for which placebo-controlled studies in infertile men have shown efficacy of its use as treatment for male sexual dysfunction [10, 107, 108]. On the other hand, it is well known that ginsenosides are the substances behind the aphrodisiac effect of *P. ginseng* by increasing the synthesis of NO [109]. Nevertheless, there are several ginsenosides present in both species of ginseng and the NO-increasing effect has not been individualized for a particular type of ginsenoside. Much more studies are needed to affirm that the libido-enhancing properties of American ginseng are comparable to those of Asian ginseng.

3.3.2 Mexico and Central America

Turnera diffusa is a plant of the Passifloraceae family with its origin in Central America and Mexico but can also be found in South America. It is locally called "damiana" and is used in traditional Mexican medicine as a sort of panacea. The Mayas used to call this plant *mis kok*, which means "creature that fights bad wind." Bad wind was thought to be the cause of respiratory problems, which are nowadays referred to as asthma, alongside depression and impotency [77]. There is evidence supporting these claims. In a model of sexually impotent rats, Arletti et al. found that fluid extracts of the plant were effective in increasing sexual performance of animals. Furthermore, the highest dose (1 mL/kg BW) reduced mount, intromission, and ejaculation latency [110]. Also, a single dose of aqueous *T. diffusa* extract was effective, recovering copulation in rats that were induced to exhaustion by repeated ejaculation [111].

False damiana or "damianita" (*Chrysactinia mexicana*) is also used in folk Mexican medicine as a sexual function enhancer. This Asteraceae strikes a morphological resemblance to *T. diffusa*, thus the vulgar name. The aqueous extract of the aerial parts of *C. mexicana* has been proven to enhance sexual function and thus recover from sexual exhaustion in an animal model. This effect is dose dependent since only the highest dose (320 mg/kg) showed an effect increasing the number of rats that restarted copulation after ejaculation [76]. This study compared the effects of *C. mexicana* with those exhibited by *T. diffusa* in an attempt to validate folk medicine knowledge that uses both plants to treat sexual dysfunction interchangeably. Results show that their biological properties are equivalent [76]. Randomized, controlled interventions are still missing to further corroborate what has already been proven by animal studies.

3.3.3 South America

Peruvian maca (*L. meyenii*) first gained widespread attention due to its alleged properties as a sexual enhancer. It was called "Andean Viagra" as a witty way to introduce the herb to international markets.

One of the first studies of maca back in 2000 was aimed at testing the effects of its lipidic extract on sexual behavior. It was found that maca extracts increased the number of complete intromissions and decreased the latent period of erection [112]. Pulverized maca extract improved performance during copulation in inexperienced male rats and these effects were not associated to its high nutritional value since the spontaneous locomotor activity remained unchanged [70]. Another study found only a very discrete effect on male sexual behavior following maca administration [71].

A double-blinded, placebo-controlled trial in healthy men showed that maca is able to enhance libido, but only after at least a 3-week treatment [113]. Therefore, the alleged "Viagra-like" properties attributed to maca are not supported by evidence.

The methanolic extract of leaves and stem of *Jatropha macrantha*, a Peruvian plant used in folk medicine as a libido enhancer, has shown properties to treat erectile dysfunction in a rat model, thereby the number of intromissions increased in a dose-dependent manner, being even similar to the treatment with sildenafil at a dose of 157.1 mg/kg. This was further confirmed when the plasma concentration of NO was evaluated [114]. Hence, a potent vasodilation effect on the corpora cavernosa of the penis is evident.

3.4 American plants affecting sexual hormones

3.4.1 Plants from North America

Dioscorea villosa, also called wild yam, is a North American plant of the family Dioscoreaceae. It is known for reducing serum concentrations of luteinizing hormone (LH). A systematic review of different plants with beneficial effects on menopause symptoms found that the effects of *D. villosa* were not conclusive. Nonetheless, the mixed treatment with *Hypericum perforatum* (St. John's wort) has a more significant effect in hormonal regulation. In addition, *D. villosa* extract decreases the estrogen catabolism into the genotoxic metabolite 16-αOH-estrone.

3.4.2 Plants from South America

One of the most popular plants in South America is *Mauritia flexuosa* L., an Arecaceae, also known as *buriti* in Brasil or *aguaje* in Peru or moriche palm in the United States. There is controversy surrounding the use of this plant, because it is believed that its use is linked to the development of feminine behavior in men. Traditionally, it is consumed as a beverage or the pulp of the fruit is directly eaten. There is not much research involving this plant's effects over sexual hormones or reproductive outcomes, and the few devoted to it have focused on its antioxidant potential. Campos Correa and Gutierrez Landa in 2013 [115] showed that the hydroalcoholic extract of *M. flexuosa* has estrogenic activity in ovariectomized rats, with significant increase in osteoblast count at a treatment dose of 100 mg/kg. Yet, no estrogenic activity was found in the uterus regardless of the doses.

There is mixed information regarding the effect of maca on sexual hormones. In a rat model, a long-term feeding with maca extract enhanced steroidogenesis in Leydig cells, a sort of antiaging effect, although it may cause only a transient increase in blood testosterone levels in sexually maturing male rats [116].

A cumulative effect over testosterone levels in male mice was also seen when *L. meyenii* was used in admixture with *Jatropha macrantha*, a Peruvian Euphorbiaceae, known as Huanarpo macho, in which the group treated with maca alone presented a serum testosterone concentration of 4.37 ng/mL, while in the mixed treatment levels marked 4.92 ng/mL [117].

On the other hand, in a double-blinded, clinical, placebo-controlled trial, in which maca was given for 12 weeks, no differences were detected for LH, FSH, prolactin, 17-α hydroxyprogesterone, testosterone, and 17-β estradiol. This means that the aphrodisiac effect of maca is sex-hormone independent, guaranteeing that maca does not produce hormonal disorders, thus no pathologies [118].

An experimental study with ovariectomized rats found that long-term consumption of maca modulates the endocrine hormone balance, especially decreasing enhanced FSH levels [119], suggesting maca as a novel therapeutic for women in the postmenopause period. This was previously seen in a study by Gonzales et al. in 2010, in which black and red maca regenerate bone structure in ovariectomized rats [120].

4 Male reproductive tract diseases

The male reproductive tract is composed of the testicles, genital ducts, the urethra, accessory glands as well as the prostate and seminal vesicles, and finally the penis. In order of appearance, they accomplish the following functions: steroids and spermatogenesis, fluid transport (urine or semen), production and release of seminal components, and copulation.

Each of the abovementioned structures have a specific function in order to assure reproductive success. The accessory glands must also produce and secrete seminal fluid containing fructose, citric acid, proteases, etc., while the ducts are needed for sperm transportation. All these structures are prone to develop different diseases, leading not only to infertility, but compromising patient's life and life quality.

The etiology of male infertility can be divided into three categories: pretesticular, testicular, and posttesticular causes [121]. The first one involves a dysfunction in the first two components of the hypothalamus-pituitary-testicular axis. For example, a decreased production of the gonadotropin-releasing hormone (GnRH) will cause diminished production of LH and FSH, thus leading to lower testosterone production and testicular development, resulting in hypogonadotropic hypogonadism, a condition that can also be seen with normal GnRH levels but lower levels of LH and FSH due to hypophysis malfunction [122]. This could be the result of an inadequate interplay of hormones like in the case of hyperprolactinemia in which the pulsatile release of GnRH is interrupted, causing infertility [122].

The testicular causes can be attributed to structural malformations; for instance, cryptorchidism is characterized by a failed descent of the testicles from the abdominal cavity during infancy. If not treated, this could lead to impaired spermatogenesis due to the high production of ROS and low expression of antioxidant enzymes such as superoxide dismutase (SOD) [123]. Nonetheless, this can be redressed with plant extract treatment as with *Moringa oleifera* that have proved to reduce germ cell apoptosis in an induced unilateral cryptorchidism rat model [124].

Testicular function can also be affected by the exposure to different toxins or components, with a higher relevance in occupational health, for example, workers in the plastic industries in the past century were exposed to high levels of bisphenol-A (BPA), a potent endocrine disruptor that alters testicular function [125, 126]. Another example is DuPont's Teflon plant where workers exposed to perfluorooctanoic acid (PFOA) during the 1950s developed different kinds of cancers including testicular cancer [127, 128].

Fortunately, perhaps due to the antioxidant properties of different plants, the effects of this exogenous components are attenuate, like in a recent experimental study that evaluated an *Aloe vera* extract, showing a higher diameter and thickness of the seminiferous tubules and higher spermatid, primary spermatocyte, and spermatogonia in the BPA-positive *Aloe vera* group compared with the BPA group [129]. Other causes that can damage the testes or epididymal function are bacterial and viral infections, which can further produce epididymitis and duct obstruction, in which a combined treatment of antibiotic with an extract of a given natural product like Korean ginseng, as shown in an experimental study of *E. coli*-induced epidydimo-orchitis [130].

Finally, other diseases of the male reproductive tract are posttesticular. These involves obstruction in the ejaculatory conducts, leading to ejaculatory abnormalities such as low semen volume or fructose negative; nonetheless, this does not necessarily imply abnormal hormone levels. One of the most common causes for obstruction in the ejaculatory ducts is benign prostatic hyperplasia (BPH), a nonmalignant growth of the prostate gland with an enormous impact, not only on public health, but also economically. In the United States alone, BPH-related urology visits amount to 23% and its treatment amounts to four billion dollars annually [131].

Although the etiology of BPH is not clear, it is evident that it is an age-related disease given the higher prevalence with age, ranging from 50% to 75% in 50–70-years olds [132], and that the hormonal component is the key to understand it. There is large evidence about the effectiveness of different plant extracts to treat BPH, that is, why we consider it necessary a special section on this topic.

Albeit the majority of studies are related to Asian plants, there are also species original from the Americas that are also effective. This brief description helps as an introduction to review the different documented plants used in traditional medicine in the Americas to treat the many diseases that compromise the male reproductive tract.

4.1 Overview of American herbs used to treat male reproductive tract diseases

Table 2 presents a summary of the information of the American herbs presented in this chapter. We have divided the table according to pathology.

4.2 Benign prostatic hyperplasia

Benign prostatic hyperplasia (BPH) is perhaps one of the most concerning male reproductive tract diseases due to its increasing prevalence with age. It has a reported prevalence of 50% in 50-year-old men [147], with an increasing prevalence of up to 80% in 90-year-olds [148], which is indistinguishable between races [148–150]. This means that, along with the increasing lifespan, almost every male is likely to suffer from it. Thus, BPH is a public health concern [151].

During the embryo stage, the prostate is divided and grows into five different clusters around the urethra [152]. Due to this arrangement, during the progression of BPH, characterized by the macroscopic enlargement of the transition zone of the prostate and a microscopic increase in the stromal area and epithelial cells, a narrowing of the urethral conduct is observed, leading to the development of lower urinary tract symptoms (LUTS). LUTS includes nocturia, increased urinary frequency, pain during urination, and low urine flow [153], thus severely affecting the patient's quality of life.

Conventionally, since 1990, BPH is treated with finasteride [154], a drug that inhibits the action of the enzyme 5-α-reductase. This enzyme catalyzes the conversion of testosterone to its most active form dihydrotestosterone (DHT), which activates the androgen receptor (AR) in the prostate, thus promoting prostatic growth [155]. Although finasteride is capable of reducing prostate size, thus treating LUTS, it has been linked to several side effects such as erectile dysfunction, sexual impotence, decreased libido, and ejaculatory disorders. Nonetheless, there is still no consensus about these side effects [156]. Other common treatments include α-blockers such as tamsulosin, which causes prostate smooth muscle cell relaxation, thus relieving LUTS. Nonetheless, this inability to control the muscular tone could provoke ejaculatory problems [157]. However, this is debatable [158].

Androgens and AR have a crucial role in normal prostate maintenance, but overstimulation could result in BPH. In addition, one needs to keep in mind that the prostate has a particular behavior in contrast to other androgen-dependent organs, because it maintains its sensitivity to androgens for life [159], thus promoting the expression of growth factors in the prostate, as the epidermal growth factor, keratinocyte growth factor, and insulin-like growth factor [153, 160]. Additionally, the AR has a critical role in immune and inflammatory pathways, involving macrophage recruitment and chemokine (C-C motif) ligand 3 (CCL3) cytokine expression, which promotes prostatic stroma growth [151, 160] and deregulation of the growth/apoptosis balance through the NF-κB, which induce the expression and release of proinflammatory cytokines [161].

Other hormonal factors, although less studied, involve the role play between estrogen receptors α and β (ER α/β) and an interplay of both with AR. Normal function of ERα is important for the normal development of the prostate. A halt in this synthesis results in the suppression of prostate growth in the early life [162]. It is noteworthy that ERα is differentially expressed in different stages of the disease, with higher levels during the medium growth (40–80 mL) and decreasing levels in an advanced stage (>80 mL) [163].

TABLE 2 Summary of American herbs used to treat male reproductive tract diseases.

Disease	Plant	In vitro studies	Animal studies	RCTs
Benign prostatic hyperplasia	*Serenoa repens*	Different extracts of the plant inhibit 5α reductase I and II on epithelial and fibroblast cells [133]. Pro-inflammatory phenotype in rat peritoneal macrophages diminished after treatment [134]		Several. Mild-to-moderate improvement in UFM [135]
	Lepidium meyenii		Reduced prostate size with ethanolic extracts of the red variety [136]	None
	Urtica dioica		Prostate/body weight ratio, histological analyses and urine flow were	Better IPSS scores and UFM than placebo [137] In admixture with Sabal palm, improvement of obstructive symptoms in those with severe and moderate symptomatology [138] In admixture with *P. africanum*, no effect compared to placebo [139]
	Cucurbita pepo		Seed oil reduces prostate size in rat model [140]	In admixture with *E. parviflorum*, lycopene, *P. africanum*, and *S. repens* shown to have good effects on BPH symptoms after 3 month treatment [141]
	Roystonea regia		Extract prevents the impairment of micturition and histological prostate changes induced by phenylephrine [142]	
Prostatic carcinoma	*Serenoa repens*	Extract in admixture with carotenoid axthathanthin inhibit 5α reductase in prostatic carcinoma cell line LNCap-FGC [143]. Extract decreased expression of anti-inflammatory related genes in 2 PC cell lines LNCaP and PC3 [144]		
	Tillandsia recurvata	Inhibit proliferation of cancer cell lines [145] Flavonone HLBT-100 showed broad effect against prostate cancer at doses as low as 0.003 μg/mL [146]		

RCT, randomized controlled trial.

ERβ exerts an antiproliferative and proapoptotic TNFα-mediated function [164]. In a rat BPH model, contrary to ERα a reduction in ERβ expression was shown. However, the treatment with 3-α-andriol, a potent ERβ agonist, resulted in a higher expression of ERβ and a further stabilization of the ERβ/ERα ratio similar to the control [165].

The search for new BPH treatments, along with the purpose to validate the ancient knowledge about herbal medicine, encouraged different research groups to establish how natural products exert their action against this disease; thus, leading to a better understanding of the etiology of BPH.

4.2.1 North America

One of the most studied plants is saw palmetto (*Serenoa repens*), a member of the Arecaceae family, and native of the United States and the Northern Mexico, with long known use by native Americans [166]. This plant is widely used to treat genitourinary problems, especially BPH, and also to treat prostate cancer [167].

The hexane extract of *Serenoa repens*, commercially known as Permixon, has a potent anti-inflammatory effect, decreasing the levels of cytokines CCR7, CXCL6, IL6, and IL17 in a mouse model [168]. A recent meta-analysis has evaluated the effect of Permixon in observational studies and randomized clinical trials, finding a better outcome of Permixon compared with other drugs as α-blockers and the placebo group with regard to the maximum urinary flow rate, the international prostate symptom score (IPSS), and prostate volume, with no sexual dysfunctions associated to it [169]. The effects of the hexanic extract has also been evaluated in prostate biopsies; in the second biopsy, 6 months after the first one, there was a significant decrease in the inflammation grading and aggressiveness score, and also significant lower levels of cytokines CD3, CD8, CD20, and CD163, tested by immunohistochemistry, compared with the control group [170].

For the ethanolic extract a dose-dependent effect, similar to the hexanic extract, to inhibit the action of 5-α-reductase in a coculture in vitro model of fibroblast and epithelial cells from a patient with BPH has been demonstrated [171]. The effects of the ethanolic extract were also evaluated in a clinical trial in patients aged between 40 and 79 years, resulting in lower prostate volume and a better urinary flow compared with the control group [172]. This indicates how different types of extracts of the same plant can have a similar effect.

4.2.2 Central America

Cucurbita pepo, commonly named as pumpkin, is a widely distributed plant that can be found in Central American territories. *C. pepo* contains different fatty compounds such as avenasterol, spinasterol, sitosterol, stigmasterol, linoleic and oleic acid, and vitamin E, among others. Although compounds such as tocopherols (vitamin E) show a potent antioxidant effect that help relieve BPH symptoms and reduce prostate growth, the first two sterols are the main active compound of the plant that decreases DHT levels [141]. Considering the effect of the fatty components, there are commercial products being distributed in the form of *C. pepo* seed oil, demonstrating a reduction in prostate size in a testosterone-induced-BPH model in rats in a dose-response manner [140].

Different studies have assessed the usefulness of different extracts and parts of *C. pepo*. The seeds have potent anti-inflammatory effects evidenced by the lower level of lipid peroxidation and inhibited inflammatory routes. Considering that the molecular pathways are linked to androgens promotes cell growth and inflammation. It has been shown that the seed extract inhibits the action of the enzyme 5-α-reductase-type II converting testosterone into dihydrotestosterone, a 10 times more potent androgen. Consequently, although it has been demonstrated that the action of *C. pepo* is not mediated through sex hormone receptors, as seen in prostate cell line experiments, this will halt prostate growth and reduce its size [173].

A recent review by Damiano et al. in 2016 [174] listed different clinical studies using *C. pepo* as a treatment showing an average 40% improvement in the quality of life score and a greater decrease in the international prostate symptom score, with almost no side effects, around 4% of participants in one study [175].

Unfortunately, phytotherapy is not suitable for all patients; some patients can be resistant to treatments with a particular plant extract. Nonetheless, a mixture of different plant extracts with demonstrated BPH relief effect, such as *S. repens*, *C. pepo* seed oil, and *P. africana*, among others, could be adequate, as shown in a phase-II clinical trial. In this trial, a mixture of the latter plants with *Epilobium parviflorum* and lycopene showed that both daytime and nighttime urinary frequencies had an outstanding decrease compared with the placebo group [141].

4.2.3 The Caribbean

Emblematic Cuban tree (*Roystonea regia*) extract has shown potential as a BPH treatment in animals with BPH induced by phenylephrine. The extract prevented the impairment of micturition and histological prostate changes [142].

Although a beneficial effect on BPH has not been shown yet, *Tillandsia recurvata*, commonly known as Jamaican Ball Moss, which belongs to the Bromeliaceae family, has demonstrated to inhibit human cancer cell-line proliferation (IC50) at low concentrations of 3.75 µg/mL [145]. The in vitro anticancer effects were also tested in a rat model, in which 75% of Kaposi sarcoma were inhibited at a dosage of 200 mg/kg with no toxic effect [176].

In a recent study, a flavonone named as HLBT-100 was extracted from *T. recurvata*, showing a broad effect against different kinds of cancers such as brain cancer, breast cancer, and leukemia, among others, including prostate cancer at doses as low as 0.003 µg/mL [146].. This compound should be also tested for BPH-cell lines and in in vivo models too.

4.2.4   South America

The following plants have been studied for more than 15 years, but they are not usually found in reviews about phytotherapy for BPH. Nonetheless, their use has been proven effective for several reproductive impairments, not only in animals but also in humans [15].

Lepidium meyenii (maca) has a huge impact on male fertility, especially the black phenotype [177] while the red phenotype has effects on female fertility [178]. Nonetheless, in 2007, the red maca phenotype showed beneficial effects against BPH in a rat model [179] in a dose-dependent manner [136].

It is still not clear how does red maca reduce prostate size, but a recent study has shown that the methanolic and ethanolic extracts of red maca were effective against BPH. When separating the extract into its aqueous and butanolic fractions, only the butanolic fraction showed effects. Both fractions modulate the expression of ERβ returning it to similar levels as those found on the control group. Nonetheless, the aqueous fraction had a potent androgenic effect increasing AR levels, which augmented the ERα levels [180], ultimately inhibiting the effect of red maca. AR overactivation not only promotes the expression of ERα, but inhibits the action of ERβ [181], hence promoting cell growth and inflammation.

The *Annona muricata* fruit called soursop in English and guanábana in Latin America is part of the Annonaceae family. The effects of *A. muricata* have recently been studied. In a BPH-1 cell line, an IC50 of 1.36 mg/mL of *A. muricata* extract was observed. Also, using immunohistochemistry methods, an upregulation of the proapoptotic Bax protein was observed with a downregulation of Bcl-2 protein along with a reduction of prostate size [182]. In addition, expression of the tumor suppressor protein p53 was restored [183].

Recently, in a rat model in which BPH was induced by testosterone propionate, treatment with the hexane fraction of *A. muricata* seeds resulted in a reduction of prostate weight by 22%. This was enhanced with a combination treatment with finasteride and the hexane fraction by 34%. This fraction had also an antioxidant effect seen as a higher activity of superoxide dismutase enzyme compared to the BPH group. Nonetheless, this activity was not higher compared to the treatment with finasteride only. Furthermore, it seems to reestablish the expression of androgen receptors [183], which is also observed in red maca [180]. Thus, the regulation of hormone activity is the key to control the progression of this disease.

5   Concluding remarks

The American continent is home to a wide diversity of plant species that Native American populations have been using to treat and cure diseases including infertility. This chapter aimed to gather the most representative American herbs used to treat andrological problems. In Section 3, we reviewed plants that exhibit sperm quality enhancing effects. The majority of studies assessing these effects are conducted with good results in animal models, but there is a concerning lack of human studies and even more of randomized, controlled trials (see Table 1).

Lepidium meyenii is largely the most studied plant with its effects on sperm quality improvement proven in animal models and in a couple of RCTs. Nevertheless, some other effects attributed to this plant such as libido enhancement are not backed up by evidence. The inherent difficulties and costs of performing high-quality RCTs is a hurdle that research on medicinal herbs must overcome. Taking as an example the case of red ginseng, its fame came after systematic reviews using results of at least six RCTs with a sample size of more than 300 men and even then, the authors did not draw definite conclusions. Not as many studies have been performed with maca. American ginseng is not as intensely studied as the Korean one and, apparently, its effects on male sexuality have not attracted much interest from the academic community, despite its relationship with *P. ginseng* and the presence of ginsenosides which might infer similar properties.

The other hurdle faced by herbal medicine is that the mechanisms of actions are not fully understood. The case of *Lepidium meyenii* stands out, mainly because of the wide array of properties attributed to its consumption. Several pathways have been proposed but have not reached conclusive results. The conflicting evidence regarding the effect of *L. meyenii* on sexual hormones needs to be clarified.

When it comes to herbs used to treat benign prostatic hyperplasia—reviewed in Section 4—the picture is quite clearer for some species such as saw palmetto. Two systematic reviews found effectiveness of the treatment based on several RCTs.

Unfortunately, for other species, the same problem is seen: an apparent stagnation on in vitro and in vivo studies, but few to no human trials to confirm their properties.

Some of the herbs reviewed in this chapter have other attributed therapeutic uses besides andrological ones, and have been assessed for tolerability and safety which is important to note when recommending them to patients. These herbs include *P. quinquefolius*, *L. meyenii*, *S. repens*.

This review highlights some herbs for which only a small number of studies (in vitro or in vivo) with promising results are available. Therefore, we urge researchers to start looking at these species as new opportunities for the development of complementary medicine. Among these species is Mexican *Turnera diffusa* for male infertility and Cuban Royal Tree for benign prostatic hyperplasia.

Plants have been used for millennia in the Americas to treat maladies affecting male sexual and reproductive health. Since in vitro and in vivo evidence is promising, this justifies further research. Existing studies ought to be the stepping stone for what should be a fully backed by evidence to complement conventional medicine with herbs. What has been done with Korean red ginseng and saw palmetto might serve as an example for other herbs.

References

[1] Li F-S, Weng J-K. Demystifying traditional herbal medicine with modern approach. Nat Plants 2017;3(8):17109. https://doi.org/10.1038/nplants.2017.109.

[2] Tandon N, Yadav SS. Contributions of Indian Council of Medical Research (ICMR) in the area of medicinal plants/traditional medicine. J Ethnopharmacol 2017;197:39–45. https://doi.org/10.1016/j.jep.2016.07.064.

[3] Thomford N, Senthebane D, Rowe A, et al. Natural products for drug discovery in the 21st century: innovations for novel drug discovery. Int J Mol Sci 2018;19(6):1578. https://doi.org/10.3390/ijms19061578.

[4] Schwabl H, Vennos C. From medical tradition to traditional medicine: a Tibetan formula in the European framework. J Ethnopharmacol 2015;167:108–14. https://doi.org/10.1016/j.jep.2014.10.033.

[5] Perez-Cornago A, Travis RC, Appleby PN, et al. Fruit and vegetable intake and prostate cancer risk in the European Prospective Investigation into Cancer and Nutrition (EPIC). Int J Cancer 2017;141(2):287–97. https://doi.org/10.1002/ijc.30741.

[6] Verano JW. Health and medical practices in the pre-Columbian Americas. Perspect Health 1999;4(1):9–12.

[7] Gonzales GF, Tambi MI. Foreword to complementary medicine in andrology—special issue Andrologia. Andrologia 2016;48(8):849. https://doi.org/10.1111/and.12704.

[8] GamalEl Din SF. Role of *Tribulus terrestris* in male infertility: is it real or fiction? J Diet Suppl 2018;15(6):1010–3. https://doi.org/10.1080/19390211.2017.1402843.

[9] Novara G, Giannarini G, Alcaraz A, et al. Efficacy and safety of hexanic lipidosterolic extract of *Serenoa repens* (Permixon) in the treatment of lower urinary tract symptoms due to benign prostatic hyperplasia: systematic review and meta-analysis of randomized controlled trials. Eur Urol Focus 2016;2(5):553–61. https://doi.org/10.1016/j.euf.2016.04.002.

[10] Choi HK, Seong DH, Rha KH. Clinical efficacy of Korean red ginseng for erectile dysfunction. Int J Impot Res 1995;7(3):181–6.

[11] Blumenthal M. New world plants; new world drugs. Allergy Proc 1992;13(6):345–52.

[12] Gänger S. World trade in medicinal plants from Spanish America, 1717–1815. Med Hist 2015;59(01):44–62. https://doi.org/10.1017/mdh.2014.70.

[13] Valerio LG, Gonzales GF. Toxicological aspects of the South American herbs cat's claw (*Uncaria tomentosa*) and Maca (*Lepidium meyenii*) : a critical synopsis. Toxicol Rev 2005;24(1):11–35.

[14] Cobo B. History of the New World. Biblioteca de autores españoles: Sevilla, ed. EHESS: España; 1956. https://doi.org/10.4000/nuevomundo.566.

[15] Gonzales GF. Ethnobiology and ethnopharmacology of *Lepidium meyenii* (Maca), a plant from the Peruvian highlands. Evid-Based Complem Altern Med 2012;2012:1–10. https://doi.org/10.1155/2012/193496.

[16] Lock O, Perez E, Villar M, Flores D, Rojas R. Bioactive compounds from plants used in Peruvian traditional medicine. Nat Prod Commun 2016;11(3):315–37. http://www.ncbi.nlm.nih.gov/pubmed/27169179. [Accessed 30 September 2018].

[17] Gonzales GF, Alarcón-Yaquetto DE. Maca, a nutraceutical from the Andean highlands. Therapeut Foods 2017;373–96.

[18] Vander Borght M, Wyns C. Fertility and infertility: definition and epidemiology. Clin Biochem 2018;62:2–10. https://doi.org/10.1016/j.clinbiochem.2018.03.012.

[19] Gunes S, Arslan MA, Hekim GNT, Asci R. The role of epigenetics in idiopathic male infertility. J Assist Reprod Genet 2016;33(5):553–69. https://doi.org/10.1007/s10815-016-0682-8.

[20] Gunn DD, Bates GW. Evidence-based approach to unexplained infertility: a systematic review. Fertil Steril 2016;105(6):1566–74. e1 https://doi.org/10.1016/j.fertnstert.2016.02.001.

[21] O'Neill CL, Parrella A, Keating D, Cheung S, Rosenwaks Z, Palermo GD. A treatment algorithm for couples with unexplained infertility based on sperm chromatin assessment. J Assist Reprod Genet 2018;35(10):1911–7. https://doi.org/10.1007/s10815-018-1270-x.

[22] Wachtel-Galor S, Benzie IFF. Herbal medicine: an introduction to its history, usage, regulation, current trends, and research needs. CRC Press/Taylor & Francis; 2011.

[23] Lans C, Taylor-Swanson L, Westfall R. Herbal fertility treatments used in North America from colonial times to 1900, and their potential for improving the success rate of assisted reproductive technology. Reprod Biomed Soc Online 2018;5:60–81. https://doi.org/10.1016/j.rbms.2018.03.001.

[24] Safarinejad MR, Shafiei N, Safarinejad S. A prospective double-blind randomized placebo-controlled study of the effect of saffron (*Crocus sativus* Linn.) on semen parameters and seminal plasma antioxidant capacity in infertile men with idiopathic oligoasthenoteratozoospermia. Phyther Res 2011;25(4):508–16. https://doi.org/10.1002/ptr.3294.

[25] Wright C, Milne S, Leeson H. Sperm DNA damage caused by oxidative stress: modifiable clinical, lifestyle and nutritional factors in male infertility. Reprod Biomed Online 2014;28(6):684–703. https://doi.org/10.1016/j.rbmo.2014.02.004.

[26] Darbandi M, Darbandi S, Agarwal A, et al. Oxidative stress-induced alterations in seminal plasma antioxidants: is there any association with *keap-1*gene methylation in human spermatozoa? Andrologia 2019;51(1). https://doi.org/10.1111/and.13159.

[27] Darbandi M, Darbandi S, Agarwal A, et al. Reactive oxygen species-induced alterations in H19-Igf2 methylation patterns, seminal plasma metabolites, and semen quality. J Assist Reprod Genet 2019;36(2):241–53. https://doi.org/10.1007/s10815-018-1350-y.

[28] Kolangi F, Shafi H, Memariani Z, et al. Effect of *Alpinia officinarum* Hance rhizome extract on spermatogram factors in men with idiopathic infertility: a prospective double-blinded randomised clinical trial. Andrologia 2019;51(1). https://doi.org/10.1111/and.13172.

[29] Busetto GM, Agarwal A, Virmani A, et al. Effect of metabolic and antioxidant supplementation on sperm parameters in oligo-astheno-teratozoospermia, with and without varicocele: a double-blind placebo-controlled study. Andrologia 2018;50(3). https://doi.org/10.1111/and.12927.

[30] Jansen E, Ruskovska T. Serum biomarkers of (anti)oxidant status for epidemiological studies. Int J Mol Sci 2015;16(11):27378–90. https://doi.org/10.3390/ijms161126032.

[31] Romieu I, Trenga C. Diet and obstructive lung diseases. Epidemiol Rev 2001;23(2):268–87.

[32] Leiva KP, Rubio J, Peralta F, Gonzales GF. Effect of *Punica granatum*(pomegranate) on sperm production in male rats treated with lead acetate. Toxicol Mech Methods 2011;21(6):495–502. https://doi.org/10.3109/15376516.2011.555789.

[33] Fedder MDK, Jakobsen HB, Giversen I, Christensen LP, Parner ET, Fedder J. An extract of pomegranate fruit and galangal rhizome increases the numbers of motile sperm: a prospective, randomised, controlled, double-blinded trial. Kim S, ed. PLoS ONE 2014;9(10):e108532. https://doi.org/10.1371/journal.pone.0108532.

[34] Safarinejad MR. Effect of omega-3 polyunsaturated fatty acid supplementation on semen profile and enzymatic anti-oxidant capacity of seminal plasma in infertile men with idiopathic oligoasthenoteratospermia: a double-blind, placebo-controlled, randomised study. Andrologia 2011;43(1):38–47. https://doi.org/10.1111/j.1439-0272.2009.01013.x.

[35] Danielewicz A, Przybyłowicz K, Przybyłowicz M. Dietary patterns and poor semen quality risk in men: a cross-sectional study. Nutrients 2018;10(9):1162. https://doi.org/10.3390/nu10091162.

[36] Comhaire F, Mahmoud A. The role of food supplements in the treatment of the infertile man—PubMed—NCBI. Reprod Biomed Online 2003;7(4):385–91.

[37] Cariati F, D'Uonno N, Borrillo F, Iervolino S, Galdiero G, Tomaiuolo R. Bisphenol a: an emerging threat to male fertility. Reprod Biol Endocrinol 2019;17(1):6. https://doi.org/10.1186/s12958-018-0447-6.

[38] Grami D, Rtibi K, Selmi S, et al. Aqueous extract of *Eruca sativa* protects human spermatozoa from mitochondrial failure due to bisphenol A exposure. Reprod Toxicol 2018;82:103–10. https://doi.org/10.1016/j.reprotox.2018.10.008.

[39] Breitbach UB, Niehues M, Lopes NP, Faria JEQ, Brandão MGL. Amazonian Brazilian medicinal plants described by C.F.P. von Martius in the 19th century. J Ethnopharmacol 2013;147(1):180–9. https://doi.org/10.1016/j.jep.2013.02.030.

[40] Ruiz L, Ruiz L, Maco M, Cobos M, Gutierrez-Choquevilca A-L, Roumy V. Plants used by native Amazonian groups from the Nanay River (Peru) for the treatment of malaria. J Ethnopharmacol 2011;133(2):917–21. https://doi.org/10.1016/j.jep.2010.10.039.

[41] Polesna L, Polesny Z, Clavo MZ, Hansson A, Kokoska L. Ethnopharmacological inventory of plants used in Coronel Portillo Province of Ucayali Department. Peru Pharm Biol 2011;49(2):125–36. https://doi.org/10.3109/13880209.2010.504927.

[42] Rodrigues E. Plants and animals utilized as medicines in the Jaú National Park (JNP), Brazilian Amazon. Phyther Res 2006;20(5):378–91. https://doi.org/10.1002/ptr.1866.

[43] Blanchard DS, Bean A. Healing practices of the people of Belize. Holist Nurs Pract 2001;15(2):70–8.

[44] Henkin JM, Ren Y, Soejarto DD, Kinghorn AD. The search for anticancer agents from tropical plants. In: Progress in the chemistry of organic natural products, vol. 107; 2018. p. 1–94. https://doi.org/10.1007/978-3-319-93506-5_1.

[45] Andrade-Cetto A, Heinrich M. Introduction to the special issue: the Centre of the Americas—an ethnopharmacology perspective. J Ethnopharmacol 2016;187:239–40. https://doi.org/10.1016/j.jep.2016.04.026.

[46] Kufer J, Heinrich M, Förther H, Pöll E. Historical and modern medicinal plant uses—the example of the Ch'orti' Maya and Ladinos in Eastern Guatemala. J Pharm Pharmacol 2005;57(9):1127–52. https://doi.org/10.1211/jpp.57.9.0008.

[47] Calixto JB. Twenty-five years of research on medicinal plants in Latin America: a personal view. J Ethnopharmacol 2005;100(1–2):131–4. https://doi.org/10.1016/j.jep.2005.06.004.

[48] Leonti M, Vibrans H, Sticher O, Heinrich M. Ethnopharmacology of the Popoluca, Mexico: an evaluation. J Pharm Pharmacol 2001;53(12):1653–69.

[49] Cruz EC, Andrade-Cetto A. Ethnopharmacological field study of the plants used to treat type 2 diabetes among the Cakchiquels in Guatemala. J Ethnopharmacol 2015;159:238–44. https://doi.org/10.1016/j.jep.2014.11.021.[50]United Nations. Standard country or area codes for statistical use.United Nations. Standard country or area codes for statistical use.

[51] Zhang H, Zhou Q-M, Li X-D, et al. Ginsenoside R(e) increases fertile and asthenozoospermic infertile human sperm motility by induction of nitric oxide synthase. Arch Pharm Res 2006;29(2):145–51.

[52] Akram H, Ghaderi Pakdel F, Ahmadi A, Zare S. Beneficial effects of american ginseng on epididymal sperm analyses in cyclophosphamide treated rats. Cell J 2012;14(2):116–21.

[53] Vohra S, Johnston BC, Laycock KL, et al. Safety and tolerability of North American ginseng extract in the treatment of pediatric upper respiratory tract infection: a phase II randomized, controlled trial of 2 dosing schedules. Pediatrics 2008;122(2):e402–10. https://doi.org/10.1542/peds.2007-2186.

[54] McElhaney JE, Gravenstein S, Cole SK, et al. A placebo-controlled trial of a proprietary extract of North American ginseng (CVT-E002) to prevent acute respiratory illness in institutionalized older adults. J Am Geriatr Soc 2004;52(1):13–9.

[55] Murphy LL, Cadena RS, Chávez D, Ferraro JS. Effect of American ginseng (*Panax quinquefolium*) on male copulatory behavior in the rat. Physiol Behav 1998;64(4):445–50.

[56] Ghafarizadeh AA, Vaezi G, Shariatzadeh MA, Malekirad AA. Effect of in vitro selenium supplementation on sperm quality in asthenoteratozoospermic men. Andrologia 2018;50(2). https://doi.org/10.1111/and.12869.

[57] Piomboni P, Gambera L, Serafini F, Campanella G, Morgante G, De Leo V. Sperm quality improvement after natural anti-oxidant treatment of asthenoteratospermic men with leukocytospermia. Asian J Androl 2008;10(2):201–6. https://doi.org/10.1111/j.1745-7262.2008.00356.x.

[58] Suresh S, Prithiviraj E, Prakash S. Effect of *Mucuna pruriens* on oxidative stress mediated damage in aged rat sperm. Int J Androl 2010;33(1):22–32. https://doi.org/10.1111/j.1365-2605.2008.00949.x.

[59] Suresh S, Prithiviraj E, Venkata Lakshmi N, Karthik Ganesh M, Ganesh L, Prakash S. Effect of *Mucuna pruriens* (Linn.) on mitochondrial dysfunction and DNA damage in epididymal sperm of streptozotocin induced diabetic rat. J Ethnopharmacol 2013;145(1):32–41. https://doi.org/10.1016/j.jep.2012.10.030.

[60] Mutwedu VB, Ayagirwe RBB, Bacigale SB, et al. Effect of dietary inclusion of small quantities of Mucuna pruriens seed meal on sexual behavior, semen characteristics, and biochemical parameters in rabbit bucks (*Oryctolagus cuniculus*). Tropl Anim Health Prod 2019. https://doi.org/10.1007/s11250-019-01808-2.

[61] Shukla KK, Mahdi AA, Ahmad MK, Jaiswar SP, Shankwar SN, Tiwari SC. Mucuna pruriens reduces stress and improves the quality of semen in infertile men. Evid Based Complement Alternat Med 2010;7(1):137–44. https://doi.org/10.1093/ecam/nem171.

[62] Shukla KK, Mahdi AA, Ahmad MK, Shankhwar SN, Rajender S, Jaiswar SP. *Mucuna pruriens* improves male fertility by its action on the hypothalamus–pituitary–gonadal axis. Fertil Steril 2009;92(6):1934–40. https://doi.org/10.1016/j.fertnstert.2008.09.045.

[63] Katzenschlager R. *Mucuna pruriens* in Parkinson's disease: a double blind clinical and pharmacological study. J Neurol Neurosurg Psychiatry 2004;75(12):1672–7. https://doi.org/10.1136/jnnp.2003.028761.

[64] Cilia R, Laguna J, Cassani E, et al. *Mucuna pruriens* in Parkinson disease. Neurology 2017;89(5):432–8. https://doi.org/10.1212/WNL.0000000000004175.

[65] Yucra S, Gasco M, Rubio J, Nieto J, Gonzales GF. Effect of different fractions from hydroalcoholic extract of Black Maca (*Lepidium meyenii*) on testicular function in adult male rats. Fertil Steril 2008;89(5):1461–7. https://doi.org/10.1016/j.fertnstert.2007.04.052.

[66] Gasco M, Aguilar J, Gonzales GF. Effect of chronic treatment with three varieties of *Lepidium meyenii* (Maca) on reproductive parameters and DNA quantification in adult male rats. Andrologia 2007;39(4):151–8. https://doi.org/10.1111/j.1439-0272.2007.00783.x.

[67] Gonzales GF, Cordova A, Gonzales C, Chung A, Vega K, Villena A. *Lepidium meyenii* (Maca) improved semen parameters in adult men. Asian J Androl 2001;3(4):301–3. http://www.ncbi.nlm.nih.gov/pubmed/11753476. [Accessed 30 September 2018].

[68] Melnikovova I, Fait T, Kolarova M, Fernandez EC, Milella L. Effect of *Lepidium meyenii* Walp. on semen parameters and serum hormone levels in healthy adult men: a double-blind, randomized, placebo-controlled pilot study. Evid Based Complem Altern Med 2015;2015:324369. https://doi.org/10.1155/2015/324369.

[69] Poveda C, Rodriguez R, Chu EE, Aparicio LE, Gonzales IG, Moreno CJ. A placebo-controlled double-blind randomized trial of the effect of oral supplementation with spermotrend, maca extract (*Lepidium meyenii*) or L-carnitine in semen parameters of infertile men. Fertil Steril 2013;100(3):S440. https://doi.org/10.1016/j.fertnstert.2013.07.560.

[70] Cicero AFG, Bandieri E, Arletti R. *Lepidium meyenii* Walp. improves sexual behaviour in male rats independently from its action on spontaneous locomotor activity. J Ethnopharmacol 2001;75(2–3):225–9.

[71] Lentz A, Gravitt K, Carson CC, Marson L. Acute and chronic dosing of *Lepidium meyenii* (Maca) on male rat sexual behavior. J Sex Med 2007;4(2):332–40. https://doi.org/10.1111/j.1743-6109.2007.00437.x.

[72] Zhang Y, Yu L, Jin W, Ao M. Effect of *Lepidium meyenii* (maca) extracts on sexual performance in mice, and the seminal vesicle weight and serum testosterone levels in castrated mice. Eur J Biomed Pharm Sci 2016;3(5):624–7.

[73] Gonzales-Arimborgo C, Yupanqui I, Montero E, et al. Acceptability, safety, and efficacy of oral administration of extracts of black or red maca (*Lepidium meyenii*) in adult human subjects: a randomized, double-blind, placebo-controlled study. Pharmaceuticals 2016;9(3):49. https://doi.org/10.3390/ph9030049.

[74] Montanari T, de Carvalho JE, Dolder H. Antispermatogenic effect of *Achillea millefolium* L. in mice. Contraception 1998;58(5):309–13. https://doi.org/10.1016/S0010-7824(98)00107-3.

[75] Leiva-Revilla J, Cárdenas-Valencia I, Rubio J, et al. Evaluation of different doses of mashua (*Tropaeolum tuberosum*) on the reduction of sperm production, motility and morphology in adult male rats. Andrologia 2012;44:205–12. https://doi.org/10.1111/j.1439-0272.2011.01165.x.

[76] Estrada-Reyes R, Ferreyra-Cruz OA, Jiménez-Rubio G, Hernández-Hernández OT, Martínez-Mota L. Prosexual effect of *Chrysactinia mexicana* A. gray (Asteraceae), false damiana, in a model of male sexual behavior. Biomed Res Int 2016;2016:2987917. https://doi.org/10.1155/2016/2987917.

[77] Szewczyk K, Zidorn C. Ethnobotany, phytochemistry, and bioactivity of the genus *Turnera* (Passifloraceae) with a focus on damiana—*Turnera diffusa*. J Ethnopharmacol 2014;152(3):424–43. https://doi.org/10.1016/j.jep.2014.01.019.

[78] Peng D, Wang H, Qu C, Xie L, Wicks SM, Xie J. Ginsenoside Re: its chemistry, metabolism and pharmacokinetics. Chin Med 2012;7:2. https://doi.org/10.1186/1749-8546-7-2.

[79] Qi L-W, Wang C-Z, Yuan C-S. Ginsenosides from American ginseng: chemical and pharmacological diversity. Phytochemistry 2011;72(8):689–99. https://doi.org/10.1016/j.phytochem.2011.02.012.

[80] Singhal RS, Kulkarni PR. Amaranths—an underutilized resource. Int J Food Sci Technol 2007;23(2):125–39. https://doi.org/10.1111/j.1365-2621.1988.tb00559.x.

[81] Zhang W, Zhang X, Bi D, et al. Feeding with supplemental squalene enhances the productive performance in boars. Anim Reprod Sci 2008;104(2–4):445–9. https://doi.org/10.1016/j.anireprosci.2007.08.003.

[82] Awolu OO, Osemeke RO, Ifesan BOT. Antioxidant, functional and rheological properties of optimized composite flour, consisting wheat and amaranth seed, brewers' spent grain and apple pomace. J Food Sci Technol 2016;53(2):1151–63. https://doi.org/10.1007/s13197-015-2121-8.

[83] Zeiger E, Tice R. Goldenseal (*Hydrastis canadensis* L.) and two of its constituent alkaloids berberine [2086-83-1] and hydrastine [118-08-1] review of toxicological literature; 1997.

[84] Chen L, Wang T, Liu J. AB229. Effect of berberine on human sperm parameters in vitro. Transl Androl Urol 2016;5(S1):AB229. https://doi.org/10.21037/tau.2016.s229.

[85] Aruoma OI, Colognato R, Fontana I, et al. Molecular effects of fermented papaya preparation on oxidative damage, MAP Kinase activation and modulation of the benzo[a]pyrene mediated genotoxicity. Biofactors 2006;26(2):147–59. https://doi.org/10.1002/biof.5520260205.

[86] Chávez-Quintal P, González-Flores T, Rodríguez-Buenfil I, Gallegos-Tintoré S. Antifungal activity in ethanolic extracts of *Carica papaya* L. cv. maradol leaves and seeds. Indian J Microbiol 2011;51(1):54–60. https://doi.org/10.1007/s12088-011-0086-5.

[87] Lohiya NK, Kothari LK, Manivannan B, Mishra PK, Pathak N. Human sperm immobilization effect of *Carica* papaya seed extracts: an in vitro study. Asian J Androl 2000;2(2):103–9.

[88] Ghaffarilaleh V, Fisher D, Henkel R. Carica papaya seed extract slows human sperm. J Ethnopharmacol 2019;241:111972. https://doi.org/10.1016/j.jep.2019.111972.

[89] Kershaw CM, Evans G, Rodney R, Maxwell WMC. Papain and its inhibitor E-64 reduce camelid semen viscosity without impairing sperm function and improve post-thaw motility rates. Reprod Fertil Dev 2017;29(6):1107. https://doi.org/10.1071/RD15261.

[90] Mutwedu VB, Ayagirwe RBB, Bacigale SB, et al. Effect of dietary inclusion of small quantities of *Mucuna pruriens* seed meal on sexual behavior, semen characteristics, and biochemical parameters in rabbit bucks (*Oryctolagus cuniculus*). Tropl Anim Health Prod January 2019. https://doi.org/10.1007/s11250-019-01808-2.

[91] Shukla KK, Mahdi AA, Ahmad MK, Jaiswar SP, Shankwar SN, Tiwari SC. *Mucuna pruriens* reduces stress and improves the quality of semen in infertile men. Evid-Based Complem Altern Med 2010;7(1):137–44. https://doi.org/10.1093/ecam/nem171.

[92] Nargund VH. Effects of psychological stress on male fertility. Nat Rev Urol 2015;12(7):373–82. https://doi.org/10.1038/nrurol.2015.112.

[93] Singh AP, Sarkar S, Tripathi M, Rajender S. *Mucuna pruriens* and its major constituent L-DOPA recover spermatogenic loss by combating ROS, loss of mitochondrial membrane potential and apoptosis. Vavvas D, ed. PLoS ONE 2013;8(1):e54655. https://doi.org/10.1371/journal.pone.0054655.

[94] Chunhieng T, Pétritis K, Elfakir C, Brochier J, Goli T, Montet D. Study of selenium distribution in the protein fractions of the Brazil nut, *Bertholletia excelsa*. J Agric Food Chem 2004;52(13):4318–22. https://doi.org/10.1021/jf049643e.

[95] Strunz CC, Oliveira TV, Vinagre JCM, Lima A, Cozzolino S, Maranhão RC. Brazil nut ingestion increased plasma selenium but had minimal effects on lipids, apolipoproteins, and high-density lipoprotein function in human subjects. Nutr Res 2008;28(3):151–5. https://doi.org/10.1016/j.nutres.2008.01.004.

[96] Ryan E, Galvin K, O'Connor TP, Maguire AR, O'Brien NM. Fatty acid profile, tocopherol, squalene and phytosterol content of brazil, pecan, pine, pistachio and cashew nuts. Int J Food Sci Nutr 2006;57(3–4):219–28. https://doi.org/10.1080/09637480600768077.

[97] Gonzales GF, Ruiz A, Gonzales C, Villegas L, Cordova A. Effect of *Lepidium meyenii* (maca) roots on spermatogenesis of male rats. Asian J Androl 2001;3(3):231–3. http://www.ncbi.nlm.nih.gov/pubmed/11561196. [Accessed 30 September 2018].

[98] Valdivia Cuya M, Yarasca De La Vega K, Lévano Sánchez G, et al. Effect of *Lepidium meyenii* (maca) on testicular function of mice with chemically and physically induced subfertility. Andrologia 2016;48(8):927–34. https://doi.org/10.1111/and.12682.

[99] Onaolapo AY, Oladipo BP, Onaolapo OJ. Cyclophosphamide-induced male subfertility in mice: an assessment of the potential benefits of Maca supplement. Andrologia 2018;50(3). https://doi.org/10.1111/and.12911.

[100] Aoki Y, Tsujimura A, Nagashima Y, et al. Effect of *Lepidium meyenii* on in vitro fertilization via improvement in acrosome reaction and motility of mouse and human sperm. Reprod Med Biol 2019;18(1):57–64. https://doi.org/10.1002/rmb2.12251.

[101] Inoue N, Farfan C, Gonzales GF. Effect of butanolic fraction of yellow and black maca (*Lepidium meyenii*) on the sperm count of adult mice. Andrologia 2016;48(8):915–21. https://doi.org/10.1111/and.12679.

[102] Applequist WL, Moerman DE. Yarrow (*Achillea millefolium* L.): a neglected Panacea? A review of ethnobotany, bioactivity, and biomedical research. Econ Bot 2011;65(2):209–25.

[103] Johns T, Kitts WD, Newsome F, Towers GH. Anti-reproductive and other medicinal effects of *Tropaeolum tuberosum*. J Ethnopharmacol 1982;5(2):149–61.[104]World Health Organization. International Statistical Classification of Diseases and Related Health Problems 10th Revision (ICD-10). International Statistical Classification of Diseases and Related Health Problems 10th Revision (ICD-10).World Health Organization. International Statistical Classification of Diseases and Related Health Problems 10th Revision (ICD-10). International Statistical Classification of Diseases and Related Health Problems 10th Revision (ICD-10).

[105] Rösing D, Klebingat K-J, Berberich HJ, Bosinski HAG, Loewit K, Beier KM. Male sexual dysfunction: diagnosis and treatment from a sexological and interdisciplinary perspective. Dtsch Arztebl Int 2009;106(50):821–8. https://doi.org/10.3238/arztebl.2009.0821.

[106] Gurtner K, Saltzman A, Hebert K, Laborde E. Erectile dysfunction: a review of historical treatments with a focus on the development of the inflatable penile prosthesis. Am J Mens Health 2017;11(3):479–86. https://doi.org/10.1177/1557988315596566.

[107] Hong B, Ji YH, Hong JH, Nam KY, Ahn TY. A double-blind crossover study evaluating the efficacy of korean red ginseng in patients with erectile dysfunction: a preliminary report. J Urol 2002;168(5):2070–3. https://doi.org/10.1097/01.ju.0000034387.21441.87.

[108] de Andrade E, de Mesquita AA, de Almeida CJ, et al. Study of the efficacy of Korean Red Ginseng in the treatment of erectile dysfunction. Asian J Androl 2007;9(2):241–4. https://doi.org/10.1111/j.1745-7262.2007.00210.x.

[109] Kotta S, Ansari SH, Ali J. Exploring scientifically proven herbal aphrodisiacs. Pharmacogn Rev 2013;7(13):1–10. https://doi.org/10.4103/0973-7847.112832.

[110] Arletti R, Benelli A, Cavazzuti E, Scarpetta G, Bertolini A. Stimulating property of *Turnera diffusa* and *Pfaffia paniculata* extracts on the sexual-behavior of male rats. Psychopharmacology (Berl) 1999;143(1):15–9.

[111] Estrada-Reyes R, Ortiz-López P, Gutiérrez-Ortíz J, Martínez-Mota L. Turnera diffusa Wild (Turneraceae) recovers sexual behavior in sexually exhausted males. J Ethnopharmacol 2009;123(3):423–9. https://doi.org/10.1016/j.jep.2009.03.032.

[112] Zheng BL, He K, Kim CH, et al. Effect of a lipidic extract from *Lepidium meyenii* on sexual behavior in mice and rats. Urology 2000;55(4):598–602. http://www.ncbi.nlm.nih.gov/pubmed/10736519. [Accessed 30 September 2018].

[113] Gonzales-Arimborgo C, Yupanqui I, Montero E, et al. Acceptability, safety, and efficacy of oral administration of extracts of black or red maca (*Lepidium meyenii*) in adult human subjects: a randomized, double-blind, placebo-controlled study. Pharmaceuticals 2016;9(3). https://doi.org/10.3390/ph9030049.

[114] Tinco A, Arroyo J, Bonilla P. Anales de La Facultad de Medicina. vol. 72. Facultad de Medicina San Fernando de la Universidad Nacional Mayor de San Marcos; 2011.

[115] Campos Correa K, Gutiérrez C. Actividad estrogénica del extracto hidroalcohólico del fruto de aguaje *Mauritia flexuosa* L en ratas ovariectomizadas. Rev Peru Investig Matern Perinat 2013;2(1):14–8.

[116] Yoshida K, Ohta Y, Kawate N, et al. Long-term feeding of hydroalcoholic extract powder of *Lepidium meyenii* (maca) enhances the steroidogenic ability of Leydig cells to alleviate its decline with ageing in male rats. Andrologia 2018;50(1). https://doi.org/10.1111/and.12803.

[117] Oshima M, Gu Y, Tsukada S. Effects of *Lepidium meyenii* Walp and *Jatropha macrantha* on blood levels of estradiol-17 beta, progesterone, testosterone and the rate of embryo implantation in mice. J Vet Med Sci 2003;65(10):1145–6. http://www.ncbi.nlm.nih.gov/pubmed/14600359. [Accessed 30 September 2018].

[118] Gonzales GF, Córdova A, Vega K, Chung A, Villena A, Góñez C. Effect of *Lepidium meyenii* (Maca), a root with aphrodisiac and fertility enhancing properties, on serum reproductive hormone levels in adult healthy men. J Endocrinol 2003;176(1):163–8. http://www.ncbi.nlm.nih.gov/pubmed/12525260. [Accessed 30 September 2018].

[119] Zhang Y, Yu L, Jin W, Ao M. Effect of ethanolic extract of *Lepidium meyenii* Walp on serum hormone levels in ovariectomized rats. Indian J Pharmacol 2014;46(4):416. https://doi.org/10.4103/0253-7613.135955.

[120] Gonzales C, Cárdenas-Valencia I, Leiva-Revilla J, Anza-Ramirez C, Rubio J, Gonzales GF. Effects of different varieties of Maca (*Lepidium meyenii*) on bone structure in ovariectomized rats. Forschende Komplementärmedizin/Res Complement Med 2010;17(3):4. https://doi.org/10.1159/000315214.

[121] Fode M, Sonksen J, Ohl D. Disorders of the male reproductive tract. In: Fielding A, Lebowitz H, editors. Pathophysiology of disease: an introduction to clinical medicine. 8th ed. New York: McGraw-Hill Education; 2019. p. 656–63.

[122] Donato Jr J, Frazão R. Interactions between prolactin and kisspeptin to control reproduction. Arch Endocrinol Metab 2016;60(6):587–95. https://doi.org/10.1590/2359-3997000000230.

[123] Vigueras-Villaseñor RM, Ojeda I, Gutierrez-Pérez O, et al. Protective effect of α-tocopherol on damage to rat testes by experimental cryptorchidism. Int J Exp Pathol 2011;92(2):131–9. https://doi.org/10.1111/j.1365-2613.2010.00757.x.

[124] Tekayev M, Bostancieri N, Saadat KASM, et al. Effects of *Moringa oleifera* Lam extract (MOLE) in the heat shock protein 70 expression and germ cell apoptosis on experimentally induced cryptorchid testes of rats. Gene 2019;688:140–50. https://doi.org/10.1016/j.gene.2018.11.091.

[125] Desdoits-Lethimonier C, Lesné L, Gaudriault P, et al. Parallel assessment of the effects of bisphenol A and several of its analogs on the adult human testis. Hum Reprod 2017;32(7):1465–73. https://doi.org/10.1093/humrep/dex093.

[126] Chianese R, Troisi J, Richards S, et al. Bisphenol A in reproduction: epigenetic effects. Curr Med Chem 2017;24(6):748–70. https://doi.org/10.2174/0929867324666171009121001.

[127] Steenland K, Fletcher T, Savitz DA. Epidemiologic evidence on the health effects of perfluorooctanoic acid (PFOA). Environ Health Perspect 2010;118(8):1100–8. https://doi.org/10.1289/ehp.0901827.

[128] Barry V, Winquist A, Steenland K. Perfluorooctanoic acid (PFOA) exposures and incident cancers among adults living near a chemical plant. Environ Health Perspect 2013;121(11–12):1313–8. https://doi.org/10.1289/ehp.1306615.

[129] Behmanesh MA, Najafzadehvarzi H, Poormoosavi SM. Protective effect of *Aloe vera* extract against bisphenol A induced testicular toxicity in wistar rats. Cell J 2018;20(2):278–83. https://doi.org/10.22074/cellj.2018.5256.

[130] Eskandari M, Ghalyanchi Langeroudi A, Zeighami H, et al. Co-administration of ginseng and ciprofloxacin ameliorates epididymo-orchitis induced alterations in sperm quality and spermatogenic cells apoptosis following infection in rats. Andrologia 2017;49(3). https://doi.org/10.1111/and.12621.

[131] Vuichoud C, Loughlin KR. Benign prostatic hyperplasia: epidemiology, economics and evaluation. Can J Urol 2015;22(Suppl 1):1–6.

[132] Egan KB. The epidemiology of benign prostatic hyperplasia associated with lower urinary tract symptoms. Urol Clin North Am 2016;43(3):289–97. https://doi.org/10.1016/j.ucl.2016.04.001.

[133] Scaglione F, Lucini V, Pannacci M, Caronno A, Leone C. Comparison of the potency of different brands of *Serenoa repens* extract on 5α-reductase types I and II in prostatic co-cultured epithelial and fibroblast cells. Pharmacology 2008;82(4):270–5. https://doi.org/10.1159/000161128.

[134] Bonvissuto G, Minutoli L, Morgia G, et al. Effect of *Serenoa repens*, *Lycopene*, and *Selenium* on proinflammatory phenotype activation: an in vitro and in vivo comparison study. Urology 2011;77(1):248.e9–248.e16. https://doi.org/10.1016/j.urology.2010.07.514.

[135] Wilt T, Ishani A, MacDonald R. *Serenoa repens* for benign prostatic hyperplasia. In: Tacklind J, editor. Cochrane database of systematic reviews. Chichester, UK: John Wiley & Sons, Ltd.; 2002. p. CD001423. https://doi.org/10.1002/14651858.CD001423.

[136] Gasco M, Villegas L, Yucra S, Rubio J, Gonzales GF. Dose–response effect of Red Maca (*Lepidium meyenii*) on benign prostatic hyperplasia induced by testosterone enanthate. Phytomedicine 2007;14(7–8):460–4. https://doi.org/10.1016/j.phymed.2006.12.003.

[137] Safarinejad MR. *Urtica dioica* for treatment of benign prostatic hyperplasia: a prospective, randomized, double-blind, placebo-controlled, crossover study. J Herb Pharmacother 2005;5(4):1–11.

[138] Lopatkin NA, Sivkov AV, Medvedev AA, et al. Combined extract of Sabal palm and nettle in the treatment of patients with lower urinary tract symptoms in double blind, placebo-controlled trial. Urologiia 2006;2(12):14–9.

[139] Melo EA, Bertero EB, Rios LAS, Mattos D. Evaluating the efficiency of a combination of *Pygeum africanum* and stinging nettle (*Urtica dioica*) extracts in treating benign prostatic hyperplasia (BPH): double-blind, randomized, placebo controlled trial. Int Braz J Urol. 2002 28(5):418–425.

[140] Gossell-Williams M, Davis A, O'Connor N. Inhibition of testosterone-induced hyperplasia of the prostate of Sprague-Dawley rats by pumpkin seed oil. J Med Food 2006;9(2):284–6. https://doi.org/10.1089/jmf.2006.9.284.

[141] Coulson S, Rao A, Beck SL, Steels E, Gramotnev H, Vitetta L. A phase II randomised double-blind placebo-controlled clinical trial investigating the efficacy and safety of ProstateEZE Max: a herbal medicine preparation for the management of symptoms of benign prostatic hypertrophy. Complement Ther Med 2013;21(3):172–9. https://doi.org/10.1016/j.ctim.2013.01.007.

[142] Arruzazabala ML, Más R, Molina V, Noa M, Carbajal D, Mendoza N. Effect of D-004, a lipid extract from the cuban royal palm fruit, on atypical prostate hyperplasia induced by phenylephrine in rats. Drugs R D 2006;7(4):233–41. https://doi.org/10.2165/00126839-200607040-00003.

[143] Anderson ML. A preliminary investigation of the enzymatic inhibition of 5alpha-reduction and growth of prostatic carcinoma cell line LNCap-FGC by natural astaxanthin and Saw Palmetto lipid extract in vitro. J Herb Pharmacother 2005;5(1):17–26.

[144] Silvestri I, Cattarino S, Aglianò A, et al. Effect of *Serenoa repens* (Permixon®) on the expression of inflammation-related genes: analysis in primary cell cultures of human prostate carcinoma. J Inflamm 2013;10(1):11. https://doi.org/10.1186/1476-9255-10-11.

[145] Lowe HIC, Toyang NJ, Bryant J. In vitro and in vivo anti-cancer effects of *Tillandsia recurvata* (ball moss) from Jamaica. West Indian Med J 2013;62(3):177–80.

[146] Lowe H, Toyang N, Watson C, Ayeah K, Bryant J. HLBT-100: a highly potent anti-cancer flavanone from *Tillandsia recurvata* (L.) L. Cancer Cell Int 2017;17:38. https://doi.org/10.1186/s12935-017-0404-z.

[147] Isaacs JT, Coffey DS. Etiology and disease process of benign prostatic hyperplasia. Prostate Suppl 1989;2:33–50.

[148] Bin LK. Epidemiology of clinical benign prostatic hyperplasia. Asian J Urol 2017;4(3):148–51. https://doi.org/10.1016/j.ajur.2017.06.004.

[149] Hoke GP, McWilliams GW. Epidemiology of benign prostatic hyperplasia and comorbidities in racial and ethnic minority populations. Am J Med 2008;121(8):S3–S10. https://doi.org/10.1016/j.amjmed.2008.05.021.

[150] Martinez M, Maislos S, Rayford W. How to engage the Latino or African American patient with benign prostatic hyperplasia: crossing socioeconomic and cultural barriers. Am J Med 2008;121(8):S11–7. https://doi.org/10.1016/j.amjmed.2008.05.022.

[151] Izumi K, Li L, Chang C. Androgen receptor and immune inflammation in benign prostatic hyperplasia and prostate cancer. Clin Investig (Lond) 2014;4(10):935–50. https://doi.org/10.4155/cli.14.77.

[152] McNeal JE. Anatomy of the prostate: an historical survey of divergent views. Prostate 1980;1(1):3–13.

[153] Nicholson TM, Ricke WA. Androgens and estrogens in benign prostatic hyperplasia: past, present and future. Differentiation 2011;82(4–5):184–99. https://doi.org/10.1016/j.diff.2011.04.006.

[154] Ho CKM, Habib FK. Estrogen and androgen signaling in the pathogenesis of BPH. Nat Rev Urol 2011;8(1):29–41. https://doi.org/10.1038/nrurol.2010.207.

[155] Grino PB, Griffin JE, Wilson JD. Testosterone at high concentrations interacts with the human androgen receptor similarly to dihydrotestosterone. Endocrinology 1990;126(2):1165–72. https://doi.org/10.1210/endo-126-2-1165.

[156] Shin YS, Karna KK, Choi BR, Park JK. Finasteride and erectile dysfunction in patients with benign prostatic hyperplasia or male androgenetic alopecia. World J Mens Health 2018;36. https://doi.org/10.5534/wjmh.180029.

[157] Kaplan SA. Side effects of alpha-blocker use: retrograde ejaculation. Rev Urol 2009;11(Suppl 1):S14–8.

[158] Kim SW, Lee WC, Kim MT, et al. Effects of low-dose Tamsulosin on sexual function in patients with lower urinary tract symptoms suggestive of benign prostatic hyperplasia. Korean J Urol 2013;54(10):697. https://doi.org/10.4111/kju.2013.54.10.697.

[159] Roehrborn CG. Pathology of benign prostatic hyperplasia. Int J Impot Res 2008;20(S3):S11–8. https://doi.org/10.1038/ijir.2008.55.

[160] Izumi K, Mizokami A, Lin W-J, Lai K-P, Chang C. Androgen receptor roles in the development of benign prostate hyperplasia. Am J Pathol 2013;182(6):1942–9. https://doi.org/10.1016/j.ajpath.2013.02.028.

[161] Khurana N, Sikka S. Targeting crosstalk between Nrf-2, NF-κB and androgen receptor signaling in prostate cancer. Cancers (Basel) 2018;10(10):352. https://doi.org/10.3390/cancers10100352.

[162] Zhang Y, Zhang J, Lin Y, et al. Role of epithelial cell fibroblast growth factor receptor substrate 2 in prostate development, regeneration and tumorigenesis. Development 2008;135(4):775–84. https://doi.org/10.1242/dev.009910.

[163] Zhang P, Hu W-L, Cheng B, et al. Which play a more important role in the development of large-sized prostates (≥80 ml), androgen receptors or oestrogen receptors? A comparative study. Int Urol Nephrol 2016;48(3):325–33. https://doi.org/10.1007/s11255-015-1181-z.

[164] McPherson SJ, Hussain S, Balanathan P, et al. Estrogen receptor-beta activated apoptosis in benign hyperplasia and cancer of the prostate is androgen independent and TNFalpha mediated. Proc Natl Acad Sci U S A 2010;107(7):3123–8. https://doi.org/10.1073/pnas.0905524107.

[165] Mizoguchi S, Mori K, Wang Z, et al. Effects of estrogen receptor β stimulation in a rat model of non-bacterial prostatic inflammation. Prostate 2017;77(7):803–11. https://doi.org/10.1002/pros.23320.

[166] Geavlete P, Multescu R, Geavlete B. Serenoa repens extract in the treatment of benign prostatic hyperplasia. Ther Adv Urol 2011;3(4):193–8. https://doi.org/10.1177/1756287211418725.

[167] Suzuki M, Ito Y, Fujino T, et al. Pharmacological effects of saw palmetto extract in the lower urinary tract. Acta Pharmacol Sin 2009;30(3):227–81. https://doi.org/10.1038/aps.2009.1.

[168] Bernichtein S, Pigat N, Camparo P, et al. Anti-inflammatory properties of lipidosterolic extract of *Serenoa repens* (Permixon®) in a mouse model of prostate hyperplasia. Prostate 2015;75(7):706–22. https://doi.org/10.1002/pros.22953.

[169] Vela-Navarrete R, Alcaraz A, Rodríguez-Antolín A, et al. Efficacy and safety of a hexanic extract of *Serenoa repens* (Permixon®) for the treatment of lower urinary tract symptoms associated with benign prostatic hyperplasia (LUTS/BPH): systematic review and meta-analysis of randomised controlled trials and obser. BJU Int 2018;122(6):1049–65. https://doi.org/10.1111/bju.14362.

[170] Gravas S, Samarinas M, Zacharouli K, et al. The effect of hexanic extract of *Serenoa repens* on prostatic inflammation: results from a randomized biopsy study. World J Urol July 2018. https://doi.org/10.1007/s00345-018-2409-1.

[171] Buonocore D, Verri M, Cattaneo L, Arnica S, Ghitti M, Dossena M. *Serenoa repens* extracts: in vitro study of the 5α-reductase activity in a co-culture model for Benign Prostatic Hyperplasia. Arch Ital di Urol e Androl 2018;90(3):199. https://doi.org/10.4081/aiua.2018.3.199.

[172] Saidi S, Stavridis S, Stankov O, Dohcev S, Panov S. Effects of *Serenoa repens* alcohol extract on benign prostate hyperplasia. Prilozi 2017;38(2):123–9. https://doi.org/10.1515/prilozi-2017-0030.

[173] Medjakovic S, Hobiger S, Ardjomand-Woelkart K, Bucar F, Jungbauer A. Pumpkin seed extract: cell growth inhibition of hyperplastic and cancer cells, independent of steroid hormone receptors. Fitoterapia 2016;110:150–6. https://doi.org/10.1016/j.fitote.2016.03.010.

[174] Damiano R, Cai T, Fornara P, Franzese CA, Leonardi R, Mirone V. The role of *Cucurbita pepo* in the management of patients affected by lower urinary tract symptoms due to benign prostatic hyperplasia: a narrative review. Arch Ital di Urol e Androl 2016;88(2):136. https://doi.org/10.4081/aiua.2016.2.136.

[175] Friederich M, Theurer C, Schiebel-Schlosser G. Prosta Fink Forte-Kapseln in der Behandlung der benignen Prostatahyperplasie. Eine multizentrische Anwendungsbeobachtung an 2245 Patienten. Complement Med Res 2000;7(4):200–4. https://doi.org/10.1159/000021344.

[176] Lowe HI, Toyang NJ, Watson C, Badal S, Bahado-Singh P, Bryant J. In vitro anticancer activity of the crude extract and two dicinnamate isolates from the Jamaican Ball Moss (*Tillandsia recurvata* L.). Am Int J Contemp Res 2013;3(1):93–6.

[177] Gonzales GF, Gonzales-Castañeda C, Gasco M. A mixture of extracts from Peruvian plants (black maca and yacon) improves sperm count and reduced glycemia in mice with streptozotocin-induced diabetes. Toxicol Mech Methods 2013;23(7):509–18. https://doi.org/10.3109/15376516.2013.785656.

[178] Gonzales GF, Villaorduña L, Gasco M, Rubio J, Gonzales C. Maca (*Lepidium meyenii* Walp), a review of its biological properties. Rev Peru Med Exp Salud Publica 2014;31(1):100–10.

[179] Gonzales GF, Miranda S, Nieto J, et al. Red maca (*Lepidium meyenii*) reduced prostate size in rats. Reprod Biol Endocrinol 2005;3:5. https://doi.org/10.1186/1477-7827-3-5.

[180] Fano D, Vásquez-Velásquez C, Gonzales-Castañeda C, Guajardo-Correa E, Orihuela PA, Gonzales GF. N-butanol and aqueous fractions of red maca methanolic extract exerts opposite effects on androgen and oestrogens receptors (alpha and beta) in rats with testosterone-induced benign prostatic hyperplasia. Evid-Based Complement Altern Med 2017;2017. https://doi.org/10.1155/2017/9124240.

[181] Wu X, Gu Y, Li L. The anti-hyperplasia, anti-oxidative and anti-inflammatory properties of Qing Ye Dan and swertiamarin in testosterone-induced benign prostatic hyperplasia in rats. Toxicol Lett 2017;265:9–16. https://doi.org/10.1016/j.toxlet.2016.11.011.

[182] Asare GA, Afriyie D, Ngala RA, et al. Antiproliferative activity of aqueous leaf extract of *Annona muricata* L. on the prostate, BPH-1 cells, and some target genes. Integr Cancer Ther 2015;14(1):65–74. https://doi.org/10.1177/1534735414550198.

[183] Adaramoye OA, Oladipo TD, Akanni OO, Abiola OJ. Hexane fraction of *Annona muricata* (Sour sop) seed ameliorates testosterone-induced benign prostatic hyperplasia in rats. Biomed Pharmacother 2019;111:403–13. https://doi.org/10.1016/j.biopha.2018.12.038.

Chapter 5.2

Herbal medicine used to treat andrological problems: Middle East

Roodabeh Bahramsoltani[a,b] and Roja Rahimi[a,b]

[a]Department of Traditional Pharmacy, School of Persian Medicine, Tehran University of Medical Sciences, Tehran, Iran, [b]PhytoPharmacology Interest Group (PPIG), Universal Scientific Education and Research Network (USERN), Tehran, Iran

1 Middle East and medicinal plants: The history

The Middle East is a transcontinental area comprising countries surrounding the southern and eastern parts of the Mediterranean Sea including Egypt in Africa, Iran, Turkey, Lebanon, Iraq, Cyprus, Syria, Jordan, and Saudi Arabia in Asia; however, some definitions consider a longer list of countries in the Middle East [1].

The history of the use of medicinal plants in the Middle East for health benefits dates back thousands of years. Ancient Egypt made a great contribution to the development of different fields in medicine, including the knowledge on the use of medicinal plants. The Ebers Papyrus, an ancient text of Egyptian medicine and pharmacy, which dates back to the 17th and 16th century BC, introduces several medicinal plants such as opium, cannabis, fennel, frankincense, senna, and castor oil, as well as multicomponent medicinal prescriptions. Also, explorations in the tombs of pharaohs such as Tutankhamen revealed that ancient Egyptians used to put some medicinal plants like garlic in the burial sites. It should be mentioned that popularity of mummification procedure in ancient Egypt made Egyptians the pioneers in anatomy [2].

The use of medicinal plants in Iraq dates back to the Sumerian civilization from 3000 to 1970 BC followed by the Babylonian and Assyrians (1970–580 BC) and is still used by local people in different parts of Iraq [3, 4]. Nowadays, the tradition of using ancient medicinal plants in Iraq is overshadowed by the teachings of the Prophet Muhammad (PBUH), so many spices mentioned in the Holy Quran are widely used by people due to their belief in the benefits of these plants for the indications mentioned in religious texts [3].

The geographical features of Pakistan provide a great botanical biodiversity in which numerous plants with medicinal properties grow. As a result, Pakistan is among the major exporters of medicinal plants [5]. Ethnobotanical studies revealed the use of 600–1000 plant species with medicinal properties by local people, of which 350–400 plants are commercially available in herbal drugs [6].

Persian medicine as one of the most important medical doctrines in the Middle East has an ancient history, which dates back about 10,000 years. Medieval Persian physicians such as Rhazes and Avicenna had great contributions to the development of medicine and pharmacy, evident from their books "*Al-Havi*" or *Liber Continens*(AD 10th century) and "*Al-Qanoon-Fil-Tib*" or *The Canon of Medicine* (AD 11th century), respectively. These two books were the main text books of medicine until 17th century [7]. Both books, as well as several other ancient text books of Persian medicine, devoted some parts of their main chapters to the principles and practice of the use of individual medicinal plants and multicomponent herbal preparations. In the Sassanid era, there were physicians called *urvarō baēšaza*, meaning a physician who works with medicinal herbs or the so-called pharmacist [8]. Although Persian physicians used animal and minerals along with herbs, medicinal plants were the most popular category of natural compounds used in Persian medicine. Different forms of plant materials including herbal exudates [9], herbal oils [10], different extracts obtained by the maceration of plant material in liquids like vinegar or wine, powdered plants, and aromatic waters were used in a wide variety of dosages for internal and external applications [11].

Persian physicians have also paid specific attention to libido and sexual problems. Rhazes has discussed sexual dysfunctions and related topics in two chapters of *Liber* and a specific manuscript, "*Fil-Bah*," which is about aphrodisia. Additionally, Avicenna devoted one chapter of *The Canon of Medicine* to male urogenital disorders. There are also discussions about premature ejaculation, as well as other types of sexual problems in the manuscripts of other ancient Persian physicians such as "*Zakhireh Khwarazmshahi*" (Treasures of the Khwarazm Shah) by Hakim Ismaeil Jorjani (CE 1042–1137)

Herbal Medicine in Andrology. https://doi.org/10.1016/B978-0-12-815565-3.00013-8

and "*Kamil al-sinaa al-tibbiya*" (The Perfect Book of the Art of Medicine) by Haly Abbas (CE 949–982) highlighting the role of Persian physicians in the development of treatment approaches for this category of disorders [12].

In Persian medicine, the type of remedy administered for the treatment of andrological problems depend on the cause of the disease. Aphrodisiac plants, which were known as *Adviah-al-Bahia*, were mostly aromatic and spicy plants of hot and dry nature, whereas the treatment of infertility or other sexual problems consisted of medicinal plants with both hot and cold nature. *Nigella sativa* seeds, date (*Phoenix dactylifera*) pollen, cinnamon bark, *Withania somnifera*, and ginger rhizome (*Zingiber officinale*) are some examples of medicinal plants administered as sex tonic in Persian medicine [13], some of which are also reported in folk medicine of other countries of the Middle East (Table 1). In fact, Persian medicine introduces a long list of medicinal plants to manage impotence and ejaculation dysfunction, which were reviewed in a previous publication [38]. It is interesting to know that some of the folk recipes for sexual problems suggest the addition of milk and honey to boost the effect of the medicinal plants (Table 1). This is also recommended in several prescriptions of Persian medicine.

TABLE 1 Ethnopharmacological reports on the use of medicinal plants for andrological problems in Middle East.

Plant	Part used	Preparation	Location	Use	Reference
Acacia modesta Wall.	Leaves or gum	Powdered, orally with milk	Northwest Pakistan	Sex tonic	[14]
Acacia modesta Wall.	Fruits, bark	ND	Karak, Pakistan	Sex tonic (in animals)	[15]
Acacia nilotica (L.) Delile	Young shoots	ND	Northwest Pakistan	Increase in sperm flow	[14]
Acacia nilotica (L.) Delile	Unripe fruits	Powder	Lakki Marwat District of Pakistan	Aphrodisiac	[16]
Acacia nilotica (L.) Delile	Fruits, flowers	Powder with cow milk	District Bhimber, Azad Jammu and Kashmir, Pakistan	Premature ejaculation and spermatoria	[17]
Albizia lebbeck Benth	Seeds	ND	District Bhimber, Azad Jammu and Kashmir, Pakistan	Sexual problems	[17]
Allium cepa L.	Fresh fruit	Orally	Darab, South of Iran	Aphrodisiac	[18]
Avicenna marina (Forssk.) Vierh.	Fruit, root, resin	Orally	Hormozgan province, Iran	Sex tonic	[19]
Biebersteinia multifida DC.	Root, tuber	Decoction	South East of Iran	Sex tonic	[20]
Capparis decidua (Forssk.)	Flowers, stems, roots, fruits	Decoction or powder	Hafizabad district, Punjab, Pakistan	Sexual dysfunction	[21]
Capparis decidua (Forssk.) Edgew	Flowers, young stems	Powder, with water before breakfast	District Bhimber, Azad Jammu and Kashmir, Pakistan	Sexual problems	[17]
Cerasus mahaleb (L.) Miller	Seeds	Infusion	East Anatolia, Turkey	Aphrodisiac	[22]
Chenopodium murale L.	Whole plant, leaves	Decoction or powder	Hafizabad district, Punjab, Pakistan	Infertility	[21]
Cichorium intybus L.	Roots, leaves	Decoction	Sulaymaniyah Province, Kurdistan, Iraq	Prostate problems	[3]
Coriandrum sativum L.	Aerial parts	ND	Lakki Marwat District of Pakistan	Premature ejaculation	[16]

Continued

TABLE 1 Ethnopharmacological reports on the use of medicinal plants for andrological problems in Middle East—cont'd

Plant	Part used	Preparation	Location	Use	Reference
Crocus sativus L.	Stigmas	Spice	Sulaymaniyah Province, Kurdistan, Iraq	Sex tonic	[3]
Cuscuta reflexa Roxb.	Whole plant	ND	District Bhimber, Azad Jammu and Kashmir, Pakistan	Sexual disorders especially premature ejaculation	[17]
Datura innoxia Mill.	Seeds	Two seeds, wrapped in silver cover is daily used for 1 month	District Bhimber, Azad Jammu and Kashmir, Pakistan	Sexual disorders especially premature ejaculation	[17]
Euphorbia hirta L.	Milk (exudate)	Fresh plant is washed with water and is placed in freshwater overnight. Next day early morning the plant is removed and water is taken	District Bhimber, Azad Jammu and Kashmir, Pakistan	Sexual problems	[17]
Ficus benghalensis L.	Latex	ND	Lakki Marwat District of Pakistan	Increase in sperm count, aphrodisiac	[16]
Ficus palmata Forssk.	Fruit	With milk	District Sargodha, Punjab, Pakistan	Sexual tonic	[23]
Gundelia tournefortii L var. *tournefortii* L.	Roots	Decoction, orally and externally	Antakya, Hatay, Turkey	Aphrodisiac, impotence	[24]
Hibiscus rosa-sinensis L.	Flowers, leaves	Juice or powder	Hafizabad district, Punjab, Pakistan	Sexual dysfunction	[21]
Kigelia africana (Lam.) Benth.	Bark, fruit	Decoction	District Sargodha, Punjab, Pakistan	Impotency, Aphrodisiac, syphilis	[23]
Lallemantia royleana Benth.	Seeds	Orally	Northwest Pakistan	Increase in sperm capability	[14]
Lawsonia alba Lam.	Flower	Cooking the flowers with meat	Northwest Pakistan	Increase in sexual power	[14]
Lepidium sativum L.	Seeds	Decoction	Tafila region, Jordan	Sexual tonic	[25]
Medicago monantha (C. A. Mey.) Trautv.	Whole plant	ND	Lakki Marwat District of Pakistan	Aphrodisiac	[16]
Mirabilis jalapa L.	Roots	Cooking the roots with meat	Northwest Pakistan	Increase in sperm production	[14]
Mirabilis jalapa L.	Leaves	ND	Karamar valley Swabi, Pakistan	Aphrodisiac	[26]
Nerium oleander L.	Roots	Boiled in milk for oral use	Northwest Pakistan	Strengthening the penis	[14]
Onobrychis altissima Grossh.	Aerial parts	Topical liniment	South of Kerman, Iran	Prostate problems	[27]
Petroselinum crispum (Mill.) Fuss	Leaves	Decoction, vegetables	Sulaymaniyah Province, Kurdistan, Iraq	Sexual problems	[3]

Continued

TABLE 1 Ethnopharmacological reports on the use of medicinal plants for andrological problems in Middle East—cont'd

Plant	Part used	Preparation	Location	Use	Reference
Petroselinum crispum (Mill.) Fuss	Aerial parts	Orally	Darab, South of Iran	Aphrodisiac	[18]
Phoenix dactylifera L.	Fruits, leaves, seeds	ND	Northern and Southern provinces of Oman	Aphrodisiac	[28]
Phoenix dactylifera L.	Unripe fruit	Boiled in water and milk	Lakki Marwat District of Pakistan	Aphrodisiac	[16]
Raphanus sativus L.	Seeds and leaves	Decoction	Northern Badia, Jordan	Female and male infertility and aphrodisiac	[29]
Rosa canina L.	Fruit	Boiled in water and mixed with honey	Central Anatolia of Turkey	Aphrodisiac	[30]
Rosa canina L.	Fruit	Decoction, one tea glass two times a day	Çatak, Van, Turkey	Aphrodisiac	[31]
Salvia aegyptiaca L.	Small grains	Orally	Northwest Pakistan	Male infertility, increase in sperm count, thickening the sexual fluid	[14]
Salvia officinalis L.	Leaves, flowers	Decoction	Sulaymaniyah Province, Kurdistan, Iraq	Infertility	[3]
Silybum marianum (L.) Gaertn	Seed	Powder, orally	Peshawar valley, Pakistan	Sexual problems	[32]
Smilax aspera L.	Fruits, leaves	Pads form	Shobak, Jordan	Aphrodisiac	[33]
Tamarix aphylla (L.) H. Karst.	Bark, gals	ND	Traditional medicine of Pakistan	Aphrodisiac, treatment of syphilis	[34]
Trigonella foenum-graecum L.	Seeds	Orally	Urmia, West Azerbaijan, Iran	Aphrodisiac	[35]
Valeriana jatamansi Jones	Root	Powder	Koh-e-Safaid Range, northern Pakistani-Afghan borders	Aphrodisiac	[36]
Withania somnifera (L.) Dunal	Whole plant	ND	District Rajanpur, Punjab, Pakistan	Aphrodisiac	[37]
Withania somnifera (L.) Dunal	Roots	Decoction, powder mixed with honey every night for 2–3 weeks	District Bhimber, Azad Jammu and Kashmir, Pakistan	Sex organ weakness, premature ejaculation, sexual debility, syphilis	[17]
Ziziphus jujuba Mill.	Fruits	ND	Lakki Marwat District of Pakistan	Aphrodisiac	[16]

Abbreviations: *ND*, not determined.

2 Medicinal plants used for andrological problems in the Middle East: Traditional and folk medicines

Aside from traditional medicines, which were handed down from the ancient physicians to new generations, people of different areas may discover some health benefits of medicinal plants by trial and error, and thus obtain some new herbal remedies for different health problems. This is the main reason for designing ethnopharmacological studies, in which the folk knowledge of local people regarding medicinal plants is collected.

Several medicinal plants have been reported to be used for andrological problems in different countries of the Middle East (Table 1). In East and Central Anatolia in Turkey, seeds of *Cerasus mahaleb* and fruits of *Rosa canina* are used as aphrodisiacs [22, 30]. In Jordan, *Raphanus sativus* seeds and leaves are used to treat infertility [29]. Species of genus *Acacia*, a plant from the Fabaceae family, seems to be among the most popular plants used as sex tonic in Pakistan. Nearly all aerial parts of the plant, especially the fruits (pods or legumes), are orally taken as a sex tonic and to increase sperm flow [14]. *Acacia modesta* is also used as a sex tonic in animals [15]. Fruits and young shoots of *Capparis decidua* from the Capparaceae family is another herbal medicine used for sexual problems in both Punjab and Azad Jammu and Kashmir regions of Pakistan [17, 21]. *Mirabilis jalapa* mostly known as an ornamental plant is also used as an aphrodisiac. Both roots and leaves of the plant are taken to increase sperm production [14, 26]. *W. somnifera* is also used for sexual debility and premature ejaculation [17, 37]. *Salvia aegyptiaca* is used to increase sperm count and to treat infertility in Northwest Pakistan [14]. In Sulaymaniyah province of Iraq, another species of the genus *Salvia*, *S. officinalis* is used to treat male infertility [3]. Parsley (*Petroselinum crispum*), which is a member of Apiaceae family, is reported to be used for sexual problems in both Iraq and Iran [3, 18]. *Crocus sativus* or saffron is another sex tonic used as a spice by people in Iraq. Since saffron is a plant native to Iran and this country is the number one producer of saffron, the plant was well recognized by ancient Persian physicians, and thus was used as a potent ingredient in several medicinal products, including those with aphrodisiac effects [39]. In the Hormozgan province of Iran, the fruits, roots, and resin from *Avicenna marina*, one of the species of mangroves, are used as sex tonic. Fresh onion fruit (*Allium cepa*) is also used by people of Darab as aphrodisiac [18]. *Trigonella foenum-graecum* and *Biebersteinia multifida* are other medicinal plants with aphrodisiac activity used by people in Iran.

All parts of the Middle East are rich in a wide variety of medicinal plants; however, only a limited number of ethnopharmacological studies have been performed, possibly due to the economic limitations and war in several countries of this region or because of national/international political problems, which have put these countries in a critical situation. Therefore, there are still several undiscovered folk remedies used by local people in Middle East countries, which can open new avenues to the complementary and alternative treatments for andrological problems.

3 Current evidence on the beneficial effect of traditionally used medicinal plants to treat andrological problems

There are several investigations that investigated the effect of medicinal plants introduced by traditional and folk medicines in animal models of andrological problems, as well as some clinical studies on the safety and efficacy of these plants, as summarized in Table 2.

A. cepa L. (onion) as one of the traditional aphrodisiac plants has been assessed in several animal studies. The onion bulb is the most consumed medicinal part of the plant; however, other parts such as the seeds are also used. In rats infected with *Toxoplasma gondii*, a parasitic protozoon that infects both male and female reproductive system, the administration of the bulb juice for 1 month significantly improved the negative effects of this parasite on the testis weight, sperm quality, and testosterone level [46]. Onion juice could also reverse aluminum-induced and cadmium-induced toxicity in reproductive system of rats [47, 48]. The antioxidant activity of onion is mostly attributed to its flavonoids such as quercetin [46]; however, it is also rich in sulfur compounds and seleno-compounds, which are responsible for its pharmacological activities [89].

P. dactylifera (date) pollen is another traditionally used medicinal plant for andrological problems. The pollens are rich in several minerals such as zinc, selenium, manganese, and iron, vitamins C, E, and A, and amino acids including lysine and leucine and thus can act as a general tonic [90]. Powdered pollen of date palm increased sperm count and motility, as well as serum level of testosterone, luteinizing hormone (LH), and estradiol after 5 weeks of administration in rats [63]. Date palm pollen showed a significant beneficial effect on the testicular toxicity of cadmium, a heavy metal with toxic effects on endocrine system mainly due to the induction of oxidative stress [62]. The ethanolic extract of the pollen reversed cadmium-induced impairments in spermatogenesis, histology of sex glands, and hormonal changes. Additionally, it reduced glutathione and lipid peroxidation, which indicates that oxidative damage reached normal level in date pollen-treated animals [62]. Hamed et al. performed a fingerprinting of male flowers of the date palm, which showed the presence of several saponins with steroidal structure [64]. Administration of these saponins, extracted from the methanolic extract, resulted in a remarkable increase in sperm count and quality, as well as increased testosterone levels in rats [64] demonstrating the important role of these compounds of date pollen in the biological activities of the reproductive system.

C. sativus (saffron) is the most expensive spice in the world and is also known as "red gold" [91]. In male rats, aqueous saffron extract demonstrated aphrodisiac activity evidenced by increased mounting and erection frequency [55]. The extract also reduced the negative impact of sodium valproate and cadmium on the reproductive system of rats (Table 2). Crocin, a

TABLE 2 Pharmacological and clinical evidences regarding the effect of traditionally-used medicinal plants in Middle East for andrological problems.

Plant	Parts used/ extract or active component	Model	Results	Reference
Albizia lebbeck	Pod/triterpenes	Antifertility activity in rats with the dose of 50 mg/rat/day	↓Weight of testis, epididymides, seminal vesicle, and ventral prostate, ↓sperm count and motility, ↓testosterone ↓primary and secondary spermatocytes, ↓Sertoli, and Leydig cells	[40]
Albizia lebbeck	Bark/saponins	Antifertility activity in rats with the dose of 50 mg/kg/day	↓Weight of testis, epididymides, seminal vesicle and ventral prostate, ↓sperm count, and motility, ↓preleptotene spermatocytes, secondary spermatocytes, and spermatogonia, ↓Sertoli and Leydig cells	[41]
Albizia lebbeck	Bark/MeOH ext	Antifertility activity in rats with the dose of 100 mg/rat/day	↓Weight of testis, epididymides, seminal vesicle, and ventral prostate, ↓sperm count and motility, ↓preleptotene, pachytene, secondary spermatocytes, and step-19 spermatid, ↓Sertoli and Leydig cells	[42]
Biebersteinia multifida	Root/MeOH ext	Protective effect on testicular torsion-induced reperfusion injury in rats with the dose of 75 and 150 mg/kg	Improvement in histological changes of testis	[43]
Allium cepa	Bulb/fresh juice	Protective effect on *Toxoplasma gondii* infected rats with the dose of 1 mL/rat/day	↑Testis weight, ↑sperm viability and motility, ↑testosterone	[44]
Allium cepa	Seed/50% EtOH ext	Antifertility activity in rats with the dose of 50 mg/rat/day	↓Weight of testis, epididymides, seminal vesicle, and ventral prostate, ↓fertility, ↓fructose concentration of seminal vesicle, and glycogen concentration of testis	[45]
Allium cepa	Bulb/fresh juice	Protective effect on reproductive system of rats with the dose of 0.5 and 1 g/rat/day	↑Sperm concentration, viability, and motility, ↑Testosterone and LH, No difference in sexual organ weight, sperm morphology, and FSH	[46]
Allium cepa	Bulb/fresh juice	Protective effect on cadmium-induced testicular toxicity in rat with the dose of 1 mL/100 g/day	↑Testis weight, ↑sperm count and motility, ↑CAT and SOD activity, Improvement of sperm morphology, ↓LPO	[47]

Plant	Part/extract	Study	Effects	Ref.
Allium cepa	Bulb/fresh juice	Protective effect on aluminum-induced testicular toxicity in rat with the dose of 1 mL/100 g/day	↑Sperm count, viability, and motility, ↑testosterone and LH, FSH, ↓LPO	[48]
Cichorium intybus	Aerial parts/EtOH ext	Antifertility activity in rats with the dose of 125–500 mg/kg/day	↓Weight of testis, epididymides, seminal vesicle and ventral prostate, ↓sperm count, motility and viability, ↓FSH and LH, ↑prolactin	[49]
Coriandrum sativum	Seed/aqueous and EtOH ext	Protective effect on lead-induced testicular toxicity in mice with the dose of 250–600 mg/kg/day	↑Sperm density, ↑CAT activity only with the high dose, ↑SOD and GSH nonsignificantly, Improvement in histological changes of testis	[50]
Coriandrum sativum	Seed/powder	Antifertility activity in rats with the dose of 0.05 g/100 g/day	↑Testicular weight and diameter of seminiferous tubules (nonsignificant), ↓diameter of Leydig cells (nonsignificant), ↓LH	[51]
Coriandrum sativum	Leaf/aqueous ext	Antifertility activity in mice with the dose of 125 and 250 mg/kg/day	↓Testis weight, ↓sperm count, motility, and viability, ↓testosterone, ↑abnormal sperms, Degeneration in histological view	[52]
Crocus sativus	Crocin	Protective effect on cyclophosphamide-induced testicular toxicity in rat with the dose of 10 and 20 mg/kg/day	↑Testis weight, ↑sperm count and motility, ↓abnormal sperms, ↑testosterone and LH, ↑activity of sorbitol dehydrogenase, LDH-X, γ glutamyl transpeptidase and ß glucoronidase in the testis and epididymis, ↓Casp-3 activity	[53]
Crocus sativus	Crocin	Protective effect on nicotine-induced reproductive toxicity in mice with the dose of 12.5–50 mg/kg/day	↑Testis weight and diameter of seminiferous tubules, ↑sperm viability, and motility, ↑testosterone	[54]
Crocus sativus	Stigma/aqueous ext, safranal and crocin	Protective effect on reproductive system of rat with the dose of: Ext: 80–320 mg/kg/day Crocin: 100–400 mg/kg/day Safranal: 0.1–0.4 mL/kg/day	↑Mounting frequency, intromission frequency, erection frequency, ↓mount latency, intromission latency, and ejaculation latency by crocin and ext, No aphrodisiac effect by safranal	[55]
Crocus sativus	Stigma/powder	Open, pilot clinical study in 20 male patients with erectile dysfunction, treated with 200 mg/day of saffron	Improvement in tip rigidity, tip tumescence, base rigidity, and base tumescence, ↑IIEF-15 total scores	[56]
Crocus sativus	Stigma	Randomized, double-blinded clinical trial in 50 diabetic patients with erectile dysfunction treated with the topical saffron gel	↑IIEF-15 total scores	[57]

Continued

TABLE 2 Pharmacological and clinical evidences regarding the effect of traditionally-used medicinal plants in Middle East for andrological problems—cont'd

Plant	Parts used/ extract or active component	Model	Results	Reference
Crocus sativus	Stigma/aqueous ext	Protective effect on sodium valproate-induced testicular toxicity in rat with the dose of 20mg/kg/day	↓Abnormal sperms, ↓LPO, ↑CAT and RAP, Improvement in histological changes	[58]
Crocus sativus	Stigma	Randomized, double-blinded clinical trial in 260 infertile patients with idiopathic Oligoasthenoteratozoospermia treated with 60mg/day of saffron	No significant change in semen quality and sperm parameters	[59]
Crocus sativus	Stigma/aqueous ext	Protective effect on cadmium-induced testicular toxicity in rat with the dose of 100mg/kg/day	↑Sperm count, viability, and Johnsen Scores, ↑testosterone, ↓LPO	[60]
Cuscuta reflexa	Stem/MeOH ext	Antifertility activity in mice with the dose of 25–75mg/kg/day	↓Weight of testis and epididymides, ↓fertility, ↑adrenal gland weight, ↓sperm count, and motility, ↓testosterone, ↓activity of LDH, MDH, and ascorbic acid oxidase, ↑carbonic anhydrase activity	[61]
Phoenix dactylifera	Pollen/EtOH ext	Protective effect on cadmium-induced testicular toxicity in rat with the dose of 40mg/kg/day	↓Weight of testis, epididymides, and accessory sex glands, ↑spermatogenesis, sperm count and motility, ↓abnormal sperms, ↑testosterone and GSH, ↓LPO, Improvement in histological changes of testis	[62]
Phoenix dactylifera	Pollen/powder	Protective effect on reproductive system of rat with the dose of 120–360mg/kg/day	↑Weight of testis, epididymides, and seminiferous tubules diameter, ↑sperm count and motility, ↑testosterone, LH, and estradiol, No difference in FSH	[63]
Phoenix dactylifera	Male flower/ steroidal saponins of MeOH ext	Protective effect on reproductive system of rat with the dose of 50–200mg/kg/day	↑Sperm count, viability, and motility, ↑testosterone	[64]
Euphorbia hirta	Leaf/aqueous ext	Antifertility effect on reproductive system of West African Dwarf Rams with the dose of 400mg/kg/day	↓Sperm count, viability, and motility	[65]
Euphorbia hirta	Leaf/aqueous ext	Antifertility effect on reproductive system of rat with the dose of 400mg/kg/day	Induction of testicular damage	[66]

Species	Part/extract	Effect description	Results	Reference
Hibiscus rosa-sinensis	Flower/aqueous ext	Antifertility effect on reproductive system of rat with the dose of 150 and 300 mg/kg/day	↓Testis weight, Induction of testicular damage	[67]
Hibiscus rosa-sinensis	Flower/benzene ext	Antifertility effect on reproductive system of rat with the dose of 200 mg/kg/day	↓Weight of testis and epididymides, ↓sperm count and motility	[68]
Hibiscus rosa-sinensis	Flower/aquesous ext	Antifertility effect on reproductive system of mice with the dose of 500 mg/kg/day	↓Weight of testis and epididymides, ↓sperm count, ↓testosterone, Induction of testicular damage	[69]
Kigelia africana	Fruit/powder	Protective effect on reproductive system of African Catfish with the dose of 50–200 g/kg of diet	↑Sperm count, motility, and fertilization ability, ↑milt volume	[70]
Kigelia africana	Fruit/EtOH	Protective effect on reproductive system of immature rat with the dose of 200–800 mg/kg/day	↓Onset of puberty, ↑weight of testis, epididymides, seminal vesicle, prostate, and vas deferens, ↑body growth and sexual organ development	[71]
Lepidium sativum	Seed/MeOH ext	Protective effect on reproductive system of rabbit with the dose of 32–96 mg/kg/day	↑Sperm count and motility	[72]
Lepidium sativum	Seed/EtOH	Protective effect on reproductive system of diabetic rat with the dose of 200 and 400 mg/kg/day	Improvement in epithelium height, interstitial volume density and fibro muscular thickness	[73]
Ziziphus jujuba	Fruit/aqueous ext	Protective effect on ethanol-induced testicular toxicity in rat with the dose of 200 mg/kg/day	↑Sperm count, motility, and plasma membrane integrity, ↑Gpx and SOD activity, ↓LPO	[74]
Petroselinum crispum	Aerial parts/EtOH ext	Protective effect on dioxin-induced testicular toxicity in rat with the dose of	↓Testis LPO, Pc, NO, TGF-β1, and CD95 cells, ↑SOD, CAT, GSH	[75]
Petroselinum crispum	Aerial parts/ hydroethanolic ext	Protective effect on reproductive system of mice with the dose of 100–200 mg/kg/day	↑Weight of testis and prostate, ↑sperm motility, ↑NO, No difference in sperm count, morphology, and seminiferous tubules	[76]
Raphanus sativus	Whole plant/ aqueous ext	Protective effect on zearalenone-induced reproductive toxicity of mice with the dose of 15 mg/kg/day	↑Sperm count and motility, ↑CAT, SOD, and Gpx activity, ↓LPO, ↑testosterone	[77]
Salvia officinalis	ND	Protective effect on reproductive system of breeder rooster 110–420 mg/kg/day	↑Sperm viability and plasma membrane integrity, ↑testosterone, ↓serum copper	[78]

Continued

TABLE 2 Pharmacological and clinical evidences regarding the effect of traditionally-used medicinal plants in Middle East for andrological problems—cont'd

Plant	Parts used/extract or active component	Model	Results	Reference
Silybum marianum	Seed/silymarin	Protective effect on Nickel chloride-induced reproductive toxicity of rabbit with the dose of 0.1 mg/100 g/day	↑Sperm count, viability, and motility, ↓abnormal sperms, ↑fertility	[79]
Silybum marianum	Seed/silymarin	Protective effect on cadmium-induced testicular toxicity in mice with the dose of 100 mg/kg/day	↑Testis diameter, wall thickness of the seminiferous tubules, and nucleus diameter of spermatogonia. Improvement in testis histological damage, ↑FRAP, CAT, SOD, and Gpx activity, ↑testosterone, ↓LPO	[80]
Trigonella foenum-graecum	Seed/furostanol glycosides	Protective effect on reproductive system of immature castrated and noncastrated rats with the dose of 10 and 35 mg/kg/day	No significant androgenic activity	[81]
Trigonella foenum-graecum	Seed	One-arm, open-labeled, multicenter clinical study in 50 male subjects treated with the dose of 500 mg/day	↑Sperm count, ↑testosterone, Improvement in sperm morphology and libido	[82]
Withania somnifera	Root	Pilot clinical study in 46 patients with oligospermia treated with the dose of 675 mg/day	↑Semen volume, sperm count and motility, ↑testosterone and LH	[83]
Withania somnifera	Root	Protective effect on reproductive system of diabetic prepubertal rat with the dose of 500 mg/kg/day	↑Testis weight, ↑thiol, GSH, SOD, CAT, Gpx, 3β-HSD activity, ↓ROS, LPO, LDH, G6PDH	[84]
Withania somnifera	Root	Clinical study in 180 male infertile patients treated with the dose of 5 g/day of the root powder taken with milk	↑Testosterone and LH, ↓FSH and prolactin, Improvement in the amino acid content of the seminal plasma	[85]
Withania somnifera	Root	Randomized, triple-blind, controlled clinical trial in 100 patients treated with 5 g/day of the root powder or pentoxifylline	↑Sperm count and motility, Improvement in sperm morphology	[86]
Withania somnifera	Root	Clinical study in 60 normozoospermic but infertile subjects treated with 5 g/day of the root powder	↑Sperm count and motility, ↑testosterone and LH, ↑SOD activity, GSH, and ascorbic acid, ↓LPO, ↓FSH and prolactin	[87]
Withania somnifera	Root	Clinical study in 75 infertile subjects treated with 5 g/day of the root powder	↑Sperm count and motility, ↑testosterone and LH, ↑SOD, CAT, and GSH, ↓LPO and Pc, ↓FSH and prolactin	[88]

acarotenoid pigment of saffron, and safranal, a volatile terpene responsible for the aroma of this spice, were also individually administered to rats in purified form. While crocin significantly increased mounting and erection, no such effect was observed with safranal [55]. Further, crocin exhibits protective effects on nicotine-induced and cyclophosphamide-induced testicular toxicity in animals (Table 2). Thus, the aphrodisiac activity of saffron, at least in part, is attributed to crocin. Therefore, this compound can be considered as an active compound for standardization of saffron commercial aphrodisiac products.

There are also some human studies on saffron. In a pilot study in male volunteers with erectile dysfunction, saffron was administered in the form of 200 mg tablets for 10 days. Based on the nocturnal penile tumescence (NPT) test and the international index of erectile function questionnaire (IIEF-15), results demonstrated significant improvement in the symptoms compared with the baseline scores [56]. Erectile dysfunction is one of the complications of diabetes, as well. In a clinical study in diabetic patients, saffron extract was administered as a topical starch-based gel for 1 month, which showed significant improvement in IIEF-15 scores compared with the placebo group [57]. Another clinical study assessed the effect of saffron in infertile subjects with idiopathic oligoasthenoteratozoospermia, a condition in which sperm count, morphology, and motility are impaired. Saffron at a dose of 60 mg/day was administered for a period of 26 weeks. There were no statistically significant improvements in the semen parameters of the treatment group in comparison to the placebo group [59]. A recent metaanalysis of six clinical studies regarding the andrological effects of saffron concluded that the effect of this spice on erectile dysfunction is successfully supported by the clinical studies, whereas current evidence regarding its impact on sperm parameters and male infertility is not yet conclusive [92]. Therefore, future studies are needed to clarify the effect of saffron on fertility.

W. somnifera (ashwagandha or Indian ginseng) is perhaps one of the most clinically studied medicinal plants regarding its effects on male reproductive system and infertility [93]. The plant belongs to the Solanaceae family, and due to its medicinal properties, the roots are the main used part [86]. Withanolides, the steroidal lactones of ashwagandha, are considered the major active ingredients responsible for the beneficial effects of this plant on male fertility [94]. In diabetic prepubertal rats, treatment with ashwagandha could improve the testis weight, as well as several biomarkers of oxidative damage [84]. There are several clinical studies that assessed the effect of ashwagandha on male fertility considering various mechanisms (Table 2). Improvement in biomarkers of oxidative stress such as superoxide dismutase (SOD), catalase (CAT), and GSH, reversal of hormonal imbalance, and improvement in sperm parameters are the main mechanisms by which ashwagandha improves male fertility (Table 2). A recent systematic review revealed that most studies demonstrated a positive role for ashwagandha in improving male fertility; though, there are some preclinical reports on the spermicidal activity of this plant [95]. A metaanalysis of clinical studies regarding the effect of ashwagandha on male infertility expressed that all included studies support the beneficial effects of this plant; however, due to the few number of eligible studies and small sample sizes, future clinical studies are still necessary to confirm the safety and efficacy of this plant in male infertility [95].

On the other hand, there is a series of pharmacological investigations on some medicinal plants, which do not confirm the traditional claims of the health benefits in andrological problems. For instance, *Albizia lebbeck* is used for some sexual problems in Pakistan. However, three animal studies on pods and bark of the plant demonstrated antifertility effects of this plant, evident from the decrease in the weight of sexual glands and semen parameters (Table 2). The same data is available for the flowers of *Hibiscus rosa-sinensis*, which also induced testicular damage in both mice and rats [63, 67]. Some other plants such as *Coriandrum sativum* (coriander) reportedly have controversial effects regarding their impact on the male reproductive system. The seeds showed protective effects against lead-induced testicular damage [50], whereas in healthy rats it demonstrated antifertility properties by decreasing the gonadal weight and sperm parameters [51, 52]. One of the possible explanations for these conflicting results is that in ethnopharmacological studies, the medicinal use of the plants is expressed with a general term such as "sexual dysfunction" or "sexual problems." In other words, the real andrological condition is not clearly defined as to what "sexual problem" exactly means. Another reason may be different diagnostic criteria by herbalists or traditional healers compared with those used in modern medicine, e.g., the same andrological problem in modern medicine may be defined as several different malfunctions and each of the traditionally used plants is only used for a limited specific forms of diseases. Thus, clinical trials in which the diagnostic criteria from both modern and traditional healers are considered and clearly described and defined can be helpful for further clarification of the effects of medicinal plants on the reproductive system.

4 Future developments in the use of Middle East herbs in andrology

There is only a limited number of ethnopharmacological studies from the Middle East available, which is possibly due to the complicated political and economic conditions of countries in this area. A number of indigenous communities are not yet investigated regarding their folk and ethnic use of medicinal plants for andrological problems and should be the subject of future studies. Ethnopharmacological studies are important not only because of their value as a historical and cultural record of local communities, but also because of the important information they provide about the medicinal properties of different natural agents including herbal materials, which can be a starting point for the discovery and development of new drugs based on the natural backbones. An example of such process can be seen in *Artemisia annua*, a medicinal plant that was traditionally used to treat fever [96]. Investigations on this plant finally lead to the isolation of artemisinin, an important agent for the treatment of chloroquine-resistant malarias, and the researcher who discovered this molecule was awarded Nobel Prize [96]. As evident from Table 1, there are several medicinal plants locally used for the treatment of different andrological problems that are not yet scientifically evaluated. Thus, researchers have a long list of potentially effective medicinal plants that can be investigated in animal models as well as in clinical studies. Additionally, as previously discussed, there are some controversies in the traditional uses and the results of pharmacological evaluations regarding the effects of some medicinal plants on male fertility. This shows the necessity for accurate investigations on each traditional medical doctrine, especially regarding the diagnostic criteria, in order to understand the exact conditions under which these plants are administered.

5 Conclusions

The Middle East includes a wide variety of climates, which is the reason why there is a high biodiversity with a high number of medicinal plants. There are several records regarding the ancient use of these plants by physicians, which were handed down to the current era via their valuable manuscripts. Based on their geographical location and their accessibility to medicinal plants, people of each country use a specific list of herbal remedies for medicinal purposes. There are animal studies and clinical trials supporting the traditionally reported beneficial effects of some of the medicinal plants used for andrological problems. On the other hand, for some plants conflicting data regarding their effects in this category of diseases have been reported. Future mechanistic pharmacological investigations and well-designed clinical studies with a suitable sample size and proper follow-up period are required to confirm the safety and efficacy of medicinal plants as complementary and alternative therapies for andrological problems.

References

[1] Britannica TEoE. Middle East. [cited 2019 April 15]; Available from: https://www.britannica.com/place/Middle-East; 2019.
[2] Aboelsoud NH. Herbal medicine in ancient Egypt. J Med Plants Res 2010;4(2):082–6.
[3] Ahmed HM. Ethnopharmacobotanical study on the medicinal plants used by herbalists in Sulaymaniyah Province, Kurdistan, Iraq. J Ethnobiol Ethnomed 2016;12(1):8.
[4] Naqishbandi A. Plants used in Iraqi traditional medicine in Erbil-Kurdistan region. Zanco J Med Sci 2014;18(3):811–5.
[5] Shaikh BT, Hatcher J. Complementary and alternative medicine in Pakistan: prospects and limitations. Evid Based Complement Alternat Med 2005;2(2):139–42.
[6] Khan H. Medicinal plants in light of history: recognized therapeutic modality. J Evid Based Complement Alternat Med 2014;19(3):216–9.
[7] Zargaran A. The Iranian National Collaboration for the History and Philosophy of Medicine. J Res Hist Med 2016;5(4):181–2.
[8] Zargaran A. Ancient Persian medical views on the heart and blood in the Sassanid era (224–637 AD). Int J Cardiol 2014;172(2):307–12.
[9] Zarshenas MM, Arabzadeh A, Tafti MA, Kordafshari G, Zargaran A, Mohagheghzadeh A. Application of herbal exudates in traditional Persian medicine. Galen Med J 2013;1(2):78–83.
[10] Hamedi A, Zarshenas MM, Sohrabpour M, Zargaran A. Herbal medicinal oils in traditional Persian medicine. Pharm Biol 2013;51(9):1208–18.
[11] Baranifard M, Khazaei M, Jamshidi S, Zarshenas M, Zargaran A. A critical comparison between dosage forms in traditional Persian pharmacy and those reported in current pharmaceutical sciences. Res J Pharmacogn 2017;4(3):67–74.
[12] Sharifi AR, Homayounfar A, Mosavat SH, Heydari M, Naseri M. Premature ejaculation and its remedies in medieval Persia. Urology 2016;90:225–8.
[13] Tahvilzadeh M, Hajimahmoodi M, Toliyat T, Karimi M, Rahimi R. An evidence-based approach to medicinal plants for the treatment of sperm abnormalities in traditional Persian medicine. Andrologia 2016;48(8):860–79.
[14] Adnan M, Ullah I, Tariq A, Murad W, Azizullah A, Khan AL, et al. Ethnomedicine use in the war affected region of northwest Pakistan. J Ethnobiol Ethnomed 2014;10:16.
[15] Khattak NS, Nouroz F, Inayat Ur R, Noreen S. Ethno veterinary uses of medicinal plants of district Karak, Pakistan. J Ethnopharmacol 2015;171:273–9.
[16] Ullah S, Khan MR, Shah NA, Shah SA, Majid M, Farooq MA. Ethnomedicinal plant use value in the Lakki Marwat District of Pakistan. J Ethnopharmacol 2014;158:412–22.
[17] Mahmood A, Mahmood A, Shaheen H, Qureshi RA, Sangi Y, Gilani SA. Ethno medicinal survey of plants from district Bhimber Azad Jammu and Kashmir, Pakistan. J Med Plants Res 2011;5(11):2348–60.
[18] Moein M, Zarshenas MM, Khademian S, Razavi AD. Ethnopharmacological review of plants traditionally used in Darab (south of Iran). Trends Pharm Sci 2015;1(1):39–43.

[19] Safa O, Soltanipoor MA, Rastegar S, Kazemi M, Dehkordi KN, Ghannadi A. An ethnobotanical survey on Hormozgan province, Iran. Avicenna J Phytomedicine 2013;3(1):64–81.

[20] Rajaei P, Mohamadi N. Ethnobotanical study of medicinal plants of Hezar mountain allocated in south east of Iran. Iran J Pharm Res 2012;11(4):1153–67.

[21] Umair M, Altaf M, Abbasi AM. An ethnobotanical survey of indigenous medicinal plants in Hafizabad district, Punjab-Pakistan. PloS One 2017;12(6):e0177912.

[22] Altundag E, Ozturk M. Ethnomedicinal studies on the plant resources of east Anatolia, Turkey. Procedia Soc Behav Sci 2011;19:756–77.

[23] Shah A, Rahim S, Bhatti K, Khan A, Din N, Imran M, et al. Ethnobotanical study and conservation status of trees in the district Sargodha, Punjab, Pakistan. Phyton Int J Exp Bot 2016;84(1):34–44.

[24] Güzel Y, Güzelşemme M, Miski M. Ethnobotany of medicinal plants used in Antakya: a multicultural district in Hatay Province of Turkey. J Ethnopharmacol 2015;174:118–52.

[25] Abdelhalim A, Aburjai T, Hanrahan J, Abdel-Halim H. Medicinal plants used by traditional healers in Jordan, the Tafila region. Pharmacogn Mag 2017;13(Suppl. 1):S95.

[26] Khalid M, Bilal M, Hassani D, Zaman S, Huang D. Characterization of ethno-medicinal plant resources of karamar valley Swabi, Pakistan. J Radiat Res Appl Sci 2017;10(2):152–63.

[27] Sadat-Hosseini M, Farajpour M, Boroomand N, Solaimani-Sardou F. Ethnopharmacological studies of indigenous medicinal plants in the south of Kerman, Iran. J Ethnopharmacol 2017;199:194–204.

[28] Divakar MC, Al-Siyabi A, Varghese SS, Al Rubaie M. The practice of ethnomedicine in the Northern and Southern provinces of Oman. Oman Med J 2016;31(4):245–52.

[29] Alzweiri M, Sarhan AA, Mansi K, Hudaib M, Aburjai T. Ethnopharmacological survey of medicinal herbs in Jordan, the Northern Badia region. J Ethnopharmacol 2011;137(1):27–35.

[30] Sezik E, Yesilada E, Honda G, Takaishi Y, Takeda Y, Tanaka T. Traditional medicine in Turkey X. Folk medicine in Central Anatolia. J Ethnopharmacol 2001;75(2–3):95–115.

[31] Mükemre M, Behçet L, Çakılcıoğlu U. Ethnobotanical study on medicinal plants in villages of Çatak (Van-Turkey). J Ethnopharmacol 2015;166:361–74.

[32] Bahadur S, Khan MS, Shah M, Shuaib M, Ahmad M, Zafar M, et al. Traditional usage of medicinal plants among the local communities of Peshawar valley, Pakistan. Acta Ecol Sin 2020;40(1):1–29.

[33] Al-Qura'n S. Ethnopharmacological survey of wild medicinal plants in Showbak, Jordan. J Ethnopharmacol 2009;123(1):45–50.

[34] Ahmad M, Zafar M, Sultana S. *Salvadora persica*, *Tamarix aphylla* and *Zizyphus mauritiana*—three woody plant species mentioned in Holy Quran and Ahadith and their ethnobotanical uses in north western part (DI Khan) of Pakistan. Pak J Nutr 2009;8:542–7.

[35] Miraldi E, Ferri S, Mostaghimi V. Botanical drugs and preparations in the traditional medicine of West Azerbaijan (Iran). J Ethnopharmacol 2001;75(2–3):77–87.

[36] Hussain W, Badshah L, Ullah M, Ali M, Ali A, Hussain F. Quantitative study of medicinal plants used by the communities residing in Koh-e-Safaid Range, northern Pakistani-Afghan borders. J Ethnobiol Ethnomed 2018;14(1):30.

[37] Aslam MS, Roy SD, Ghaffari MA, Choudhary BA, Uzair M, Ijaz AS, et al. Survey of ethno-medicinal weeds of district Rajhan Pur, Punjab, Pakistan. Indian Res J Pharm Sci 2014;1(2):38–45.

[38] Nimrouzi M, Jaladat AM, Zarshenas MM. A panoramic view of medicinal plants traditionally applied for impotence and erectile dysfunction in Persian medicine. J Tradit Complement Med 2020;10(1):7–12.

[39] Aghili M. In: Rahimi R, Shams Ardekani MR, Farjadmand F, editors. Makhzan-al-Adviah. Tehran: University of Medical Sciences Tehran; 1771. 2009.

[40] Chaudhary R, Gupta R, Kachhaw J, Singh D, Verma S. Inhibition of spermatogenesis by Triterpenes of *Albizia lebbeck* (L.) Benth pods in male albino rats. J Nat Rem 2007;7(1):86–93.

[41] Gupta R, Chaudhary R, Yadav RK, Verma SK, Dobhal M. Effect of saponins of *Albizia lebbeck* (L.) Benth bark on the reproductive system of male albino rats. J Ethnopharmacol 2005;96(1–2):31–6.

[42] Gupta R, Kachhawa J, Chaudhary R. Antispermatogenic, antiandrogenic activities of *Albizia lebbeck* (L.) Benth bark extract in male albino rats. Phytomedicine 2006;13(4):277–83.

[43] Kamali Y, Gholami S, Jahromi AR, Namazi F, Khorsand A. *Biebersteinia multifida* DC a potential savior against testicular torsion-induced reperfusion injury. Comp Clin Pathol 2016;25(5):1001–5.

[44] Khaki A, Farzadi L, Ahmadi S, Ghadamkheir E, Afshin Khaki A, Sahizadeh R. Recovery of spermatogenesis by *Allium cepa* in *Toxoplasma gondii* infected rats. Afr J Pharm Pharmacol 2011;5(7):903–7.

[45] Venkatesh V, Sharma J, Kamal R. A comparative study of effect of alcoholic extracts of *Sapindus emarginatus*, *Terminalia belerica*, *Cuminum cyminum* and *Allium cepa* on reproductive organs of male albino rats. Asian J Exp Sci 2002;16(1–2):51–63.

[46] Khaki A, Fathiazad F, Nouri M, Khaki A, Khamenehi H, Hamadeh M. Evaluation of androgenic activity of *Allium cepa* on spermatogenesis in the rat. Folia Morphol 2009;68(1):45–51.

[47] Ige SF, Olaleye SB, Akhigbe RE, Akanbi TA, Oyekunle OA, Udoh U-AS. Testicular toxicity and sperm quality following cadmium exposure in rats: ameliorative potentials of *Allium cepa*. J Hum Reprod Sci 2012;5(1):37–42.

[48] Ige SF, Akhigbe RE. The role of *Allium cepa* on aluminum-induced reproductive dysfunction in experimental male rat models. J Hum Reprod Sci 2012;5(2):200–5.

[49] Tatli-Çankaya I, Alqasoumi SA, Abdel-Rahman RF, Yusufoglu H, Anul SA, Akaydin G, Soliman GA. Evaluating the antifertility potential of the ethanolic extracts of *Bupleurum sulphureum* and *Cichorium intybus* in male rats. Asian J Pharm Clin Res 2014;7(1):211–8.

[50] Sharma V, Kansal L, Sharma A. Prophylactic efficacy of *Coriandrum sativum* (coriander) on testis of lead-exposed mice. Biol Trace Elem Res 2010;136(3):337 54.

[51] Firdous M, Nu'man A. A comparative study on the effect of *Coriandrum sativum*, *Nigella sativa*, and *Calendula officinalis* on the testis of rat. J Fac Med Baghdad Univ 2008;50(1):99–104.

[52] Al-Rubaye RHK. The inhibitory effect of aqueous extract of coriander (*Coriandrum sativum* L.) leaves on the activity of male reproductive system of albino mice. Iraqi J Sci 2016;57(1B):344–51.

[53] Potnuri AG, Allakonda L, Lahkar M. Crocin attenuates cyclophosphamide induced testicular toxicity by preserving glutathione redox system. Biomed Pharmacother 2018;101:174–80.

[54] Salahshoor MR, Khazaei M, Jalili C, Keivan M. Crocin improves damage induced by nicotine on a number of reproductive parameters in male mice. Int J Fertil Steril 2016;10(1):71–8.

[55] Hosseinzadeh H, Ziaee T, Sadeghi A. The effect of saffron, *Crocus sativus* stigma, extract and its constituents, safranal and crocin on sexual behaviors in normal male rats. Phytomedicine 2008;15(6–7):491–5.

[56] Shamsa A, Hosseinzadeh H, Molaei M, Shakeri MT, Rajabi O. Evaluation of *Crocus sativus* L. (saffron) on male erectile dysfunction: a pilot study. Phytomedicine 2009;16(8):690–3.

[57] Mohammadzadeh-Moghadam H, Nazari SM, Shamsa A, Kamalinejad M, Esmaeeli H, Asadpour AA, et al. Effects of a topical saffron (*Crocus sativus* L) gel on erectile dysfunction in diabetics: a randomized, parallel-group, double-blind, placebo-controlled trial. J Evid Based Complement Alternat Med 2015;20(4):283–6.

[58] Sakr SA, Zowail ME, Marzouk AM. Effect of saffron (*Crocus sativus* L.) on sodium valporate induced cytogenetic and testicular alterations in albino rats. Anat Cell Biol 2014;47(3):171–9.

[59] Safarinejad MR, Shafiei N, Safarinejad S. A prospective double-blind randomized placebo-controlled study of the effect of saffron (*Crocus sativus* Linn.) on semen parameters and seminal plasma antioxidant capacity in infertile men with idiopathic oligoasthenoteratozoospermia. Phytother Res 2011;25(4):508–16.

[60] Yari A, Sarveazad A, Asadi E, Raouf Sarshoori J, Babahajian A, Amini N, et al. Efficacy of *Crocus sativus* L. on reduction of cadmium-induced toxicity on spermatogenesis in adult rats. Andrologia 2016;48(10):1244–52.

[61] Pal D, Gupta M, Mazumder U. Effects of methanol extracts of *Cuscuta reflexa* Roxb. stem and *Corchorus olitorius* Linn. seed on male reproductive system of mice. Orient Pharm Exp Med 2009;9(1):49–57.

[62] El-Neweshy M, El-Maddawy Z, El-Sayed Y. Therapeutic effects of date palm (*Phoenix dactylifera* L.) pollen extract on cadmium-induced testicular toxicity. Andrologia 2013;45(6):369–78.

[63] Mehraban F, Jafari M, Toori MA, Sadeghi H, Joodi B, Mostafazade M, et al. Effects of date palm pollen (*Phoenix dactylifera* L.) and *Astragalus ovinus* on sperm parameters and sex hormones in adult male rats. Iran J Reprod Med 2014;12(10):705–12.

[64] Hamed AI, Ben Said R, Al-Ayed AS, Moldoch J, Mahalel UA, Mahmoud AM, et al. Fingerprinting of strong spermatogenesis steroidal saponins in male flowers of *Phoenix dactylifera* (date palm) by LC-ESI-MS. Nat Prod Res 2017;31(17):2024–31.

[65] Oyeyemi M, Olukole S, Taiwo B, Adeniji DA. Sperm motility and viability in west African dwarf rams treated with *Euphorbia hirta*. Int J Morphol 2009;27(2):459–62.

[66] Adedapo A, Abatan M, Akinloye A, Idowu S, Olorunsogo O. Morphometric and histopathological studies on the effects of some chromatographic fractions of *Phyllanthus amarus* and *Euphorbia hirta* on the male reproductive organs of rats. J Vet Sci 2003;4(2):181–5.

[67] Jana T, Das S, Ray A, Mandal D, Giri Jana S, Bhattacharya J. Study of the effects of *Hibiscus-rosa-sinensis* flower extract on the spermatogenesis of male albino rats. J Physiol Pharmacol Adv 2013;3(6):167–71.

[68] Kumar D, Agrawal P, Mishra DD, Singh V. Antifertility effect of benzene extract of flowers of *Hibiscus rosa sinensis* L. on reproductive system in male albino rats. Indian J Appl Pure Biol 2014;29:215–7.

[69] Mishra N, Tandon VL, Munjal A. Evaluation of medicinal properties of *Hibiscus rosa sinensis* in male swiss albino mice. Int J Pharm Clin Res 2009;1(3):106–11.

[70] Adeparusi EO, Dada AA, Alale OV. Effects of medicinal plant (*Kigelia africana*) on sperm quality of African catfish *Clarias gariepinus* (Burchell, 1822) broodstock. J Agric Sci 2010;2(1):193–9.

[71] Micheli V, Sanogo R, Mobilia MA, Occhiuto F. Effects of *Kigelia africana* (Lam.) Benth. fruits extract on the development and maturation of the reproductive system in immature male rats. Nat Prod Res 2020;34(1):162–6.

[72] Naji NS, Abood FN. Changes in sperm parameters of adult male rabbits by phenol extract of *Lepidium sativum* seeds. J Nat Sci Res 2013;3(8):17–22.

[73] Kamani M, Hosseini ES, Kashani HH, Atlasi MA, Nikzad H. Protective effect of *Lepidium sativum* seed extract on histopathology and morphology of epididymis in diabetic rat model. Int J Morphol 2017;35(2):603–10.

[74] Taati M, Alirezaei M, Meshkatalsadat M, Rasoulian B, Kheradmand A, Neamati S. Antioxidant effects of aqueous fruit extract of *Ziziphus jujuba* on ethanol-induced oxidative stress in the rat testes. Iran J Vet Res 2011;12(1):39–45.

[75] El-Gayar HA, El-Habibi E, Edrees G, Salem E, Gouida M. Role of alcoholic extracts of *Eruca sativa* or *Petroselinum crispum* on dioxin-induced testicular oxidative stress and apoptosis. Int J Sci Res 2016;5(1):1415–21.

[76] Jalili C, Salahshoor MR, Naderi T. The effect of hydroalcoholic extract of *P. crispum* on sperm parameters, testis tissue and serum nitric oxide levels in mice. Adv Biomed Res 2015;4:40.

[77] Salah-Abbès JB, Abbès S, Abdel-Wahhab MA, Oueslati R. *Raphanus sativus* extract protects against zearalenone induced reproductive toxicity, oxidative stress and mutagenic alterations in male Balb/c mice. Toxicon 2009;53(5):525–33.

[78] Ommati M, Zamiri M, Akhlaghi A, Atashi H, Jafarzadeh M, Rezvani M, et al. Seminal characteristics, sperm fatty acids, and blood biochemical attributes in breeder roosters orally administered with sage (*Salvia officinalis*) extract. Anim Prod Sci 2013;53(6):548–54.

[79] Ali WDA, Khudair ARN, AL-Masoudi EA. Ameliorative role of silymarin extracted from *Silybum marianum* seeds on nickel chloride induce changes in testicular functions in adult male rabbits. Basrah J Vet Res 2015;14(1):135–44.

[80] Faraji T, Momeni HR, Malmir M. Protective effects of silymarin on testis histopathology, oxidative stress indicators, antioxidant defence enzymes and serum testosterone in cadmium-treated mice. Andrologia 2019;51(5):e13242.

[81] Aswar U, Bodhankar SL, Mohan V, Thakurdesai PA. Effect of furostanol glycosides from *Trigonella foenum-graecum* on the reproductive system of male albino rats. Phytother Res 2010;24(10):1482–8.

[82] Maheshwari A, Verma N, Swaroop A, Bagchi M, Preuss HG, Tiwari K, et al. Efficacy of FurosapTM, a novel *Trigonella foenum-graecum* seed extract, in enhancing testosterone level and improving sperm profile in male volunteers. Int J Med Sci 2017;14(1):58–66.

[83] Ambiye VR, Langade D, Dongre S, Aptikar P, Kulkarni M, Dongre A. Clinical evaluation of the spermatogenic activity of the root extract of Ashwagandha (*Withania somnifera*) in oligospermic males: a pilot study. Evid Based Complement Alternat Med 2013;2013, 571420.

[84] Kyathanahalli CN, Manjunath MJ, Muralidhara. Oral supplementation of standardized extract of *Withania somnifera* protects against diabetes-induced testicular oxidative impairments in prepubertal rats. Protoplasma 2014;251(5):1021–9.

[85] Gupta A, Mahdi AA, Shukla KK, Ahmad MK, Bansal N, Sankhwar P, et al. Efficacy of *Withania somnifera* on seminal plasma metabolites of infertile males: a proton NMR study at 800 MHz. J Ethnopharmacol 2013;149(1):208–14.

[86] Nasimi Doost Azgomi R, Nazemiyeh H, Sadeghi Bazargani H, Fazljou SMB, Nejatbakhsh F, Moini Jazani A, et al. Comparative evaluation of the effects of *Withania somnifera* with pentoxifylline on the sperm parameters in idiopathic male infertility: a triple-blind randomised clinical trial. Andrologia 2018;50(7):e13041.

[87] Mahdi AA, Shukla KK, Ahmad MK, Rajender S, Shankhwar SN, Singh V, et al. *Withania somnifera* improves semen quality in stress-related male fertility. Evid Based Complement Alternat Med 2011;2011:576962.

[88] Ahmad MK, Mahdi AA, Shukla KK, Islam N, Rajender S, Madhukar D, et al. *Withania somnifera* improves semen quality by regulating reproductive hormone levels and oxidative stress in seminal plasma of infertile males. Fertil Steril 2010;94(3):989–96.

[89] Arnault I, Auger J. Seleno-compounds in garlic and onion. J Chromatogr A 2006;1112(1–2):23–30.

[90] Hassan HM. Chemical composition and nutritional value of palm pollen grains. Glob J Biotechnol Biochem 2011;6(1):1–7.

[91] Shahi T, Assadpour E, Jafari SM. Main chemical compounds and pharmacological activities of stigmas and tepals of 'red gold'; saffron. Trends Food Sci Technol 2016;58:69–78.

[92] Maleki-saghooni N, Mirzaeii K, Hosseinzadeh H, Sadeghi R, Irani M. A systematic review and meta-analysis of clinical trials on saffron (*Crocus sativus*) effectiveness and safety on erectile dysfunction and semen parameters. Avicenna J Phytomedicine 2018;8(3):198–209.

[93] Sengupta P, Agarwal A, Pogrebetskaya M, Roychoudhury S, Durairajanayagam D, Henkel R. Role of *Withania somnifera* (Ashwagandha) in the management of male infertility. Reprod Biomed Online 2018;36(3):311–26.

[94] Dar NJ, Hamid A, Ahmad M. Pharmacologic overview of *Withania somnifera*, the Indian Ginseng. Cell Mol Life Sci 2015;72(23):4445–60.

[95] Nasimi Doost Azgomi R, Zomorrodi A, Nazemyieh H, Fazljou SMB, Sadeghi Bazargani H, Nejatbakhsh F, et al. Effects of *Withania somnifera* on reproductive system: a systematic review of the available evidence. Biomed Res Int 2018;2018:4076430.

[96] Su X-Z, Miller LH. The discovery of artemisinin and the Nobel Prize in Physiology or Medicine. Sci China Life Sci 2015;58(11):1175–9.

Chapter 5.3

Herbal medicine used to treat andrological problems: Africa

Chinyerum S. Opuwari[a] and Paul F. Moundipa[b]

[a]Department of Pre-Clinical Sciences, University of Limpopo, Polokwane, South Africa, [b]Laboratory of Pharmacology and Toxicology, Department of Biochemistry, University of Yaounde I, Yaounde, Cameroon

1 Introduction

According to recent studies, the percentage of infertile men ranges from 2.5% to 12% with highest rates in Africa [1]. Environmental factors, lifestyle, and free radicals are correlated to male infertility [2]. Varicocele, azoospermia, oligozoospermia, asthenozoospermia and/or teratozoospermia, and sexual and ejaculatory dysfunctions are some factors responsible for infertility in several cases [3]. Although many synthetic drugs are available to treat some of these cases, numerous and severe side effects as well as high cost make treatment with natural remedies including plants an option for millions of people. Many plants are acclaimed for their effectiveness without scientific evidence. However, some of them have biological activity proven by scientific data. The present review is an attempt to gather the available scientific information on various herbal plants used in Africa, which have been assessed for their effect on male sexual performance and functionality. Studies on these plants focused on hormonal level, quantity and quality of semen, sexual performance, and/or erection. Medicinal plants used in male contraception are not discussed in this review. Table 1 presents a summary of the medicinal plants focused in this review [4–18].

1.1 *Aspalathus linearis*

Aspalathus linearis (rooibos) is indigenous to the Cederberg area in the Western Cape Province of South Africa (Fig. 1A) [19] and is produced as fermented and unfermented rooibos. Flavonoids such as aspalathin, quercetin, isoorientin, and nothofagin are major compounds present in rooibos [4, 5]. Both fermented and unfermented aqueous rooibos extract were shown to provide protection against induced oxidative damage in male rats by increasing the testicular SOD and GSH levels and reducing ROS and lipid peroxidation, thereby increasing sperm count and motility following a 60-day treatment [20, 21]. Rooibos tea extract (2%) was also shown to increase sperm motility in induced diabetic rats after a 7-week treatment [22]. Unfermented rooibos increased sperm motility, concentration, and viability, while fermented rooibos only increased sperm viability in male rats following a 52-day treatment [23]. However, another in vitro study showed antiandrogenic properties of rooibos by the reduced production of testosterone in TM3 Leydig cell [24].

1.2 *Basella alba*

Basella alba (Malabar spinach, Indian spinach, Ceylon spinach) is a popular tropical leafy-green vegetable found in tropical regions (Fig. 1B). It is an edible perennial vine [8, 25, 26]. Herbs such as *B. alba* and *Hibiscus macranthus* are traditionally used during the initiation ceremony for the new king in Cameroon. *B. alba* not only is a good source of calcium, iron, thiamine, riboflavin, niacin, and betacyanin, but also contains oxalic acid, phenolic acids, and vitamins A and C [7, 8]. Various compounds were isolated from the leaves including Basella saponins A, B, C, and D, ferulic acid, rutin, and amino acids (arginine, isoleucine, threonine tryptophan) [27].

Extracts from *B. alba* have been assessed in animal and cellular models for the assessment of their androgenic effect. Aqueous and methanol extracts of *B. alba* stimulated in vivo and in vitro testosterone production in rat and Leydig cells [28–30]. When treated with the methanol extract of *B. alba* leaves, 70-day-old Sprague-Dawley rats showed increased serum testosterone concentrations, testicular production of steroid, and aromatase mRNA [31]. These studies have validated the use of *B. alba* by traditional healers in the treatment of male infertility and sexual asthenia. Another study also

TABLE 1 List of medicinal plants studied with available scientific information.

Medicinal plants	Family	Distribution	Common names	Part used	Studied aspect	References
Aspalathus linearis	Fabaceae	South Africa	Rooibos	Tea	Preclinical	[4, 5]
Basella alba	Basellaceae	Cameroon	Vine spinach	Leaves	Preclinical	[6–8]
Fadogia agrestis	Rubiacaea	Western Africa	Baking again, Black aphrodisiac	Stem	Preclinical	[9]
Garcinia kola	Clusiacaea	Western and Central Africa	Bitter kola	Nuts	Preclinical	[10]
Mondia whitei	Apocynacaea	East, central west, south Africa	Nkang bongo (CMR) mbombongazi (Swahili)	Roots	Preclinical	[11, 12]
Moringa oleifera	Moringacaea	Africa		Leaves, seeds	Preclinical	[13, 14]
Typha capensis	Typhacaea	South Africa	Bulrush (Engl), papkuil (Afrikaans.), Ibhuma (Zulu, Swazi),	Rhizomes	Preclinical	[15, 16]
Pausinystalia johimbe	Rubiacaea	West, Central Africa	Yohimbe	Bark	Preclinical and clinical	[17, 18]

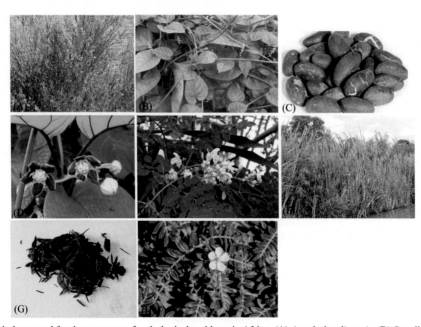

FIG. 1   Some medicinal plants used for the treatment of andrological problems in Africa. (A) *Aspalathus linearis*, (B) *Basella alba*, (C) *Garcinia kola*, (D) *Mondia whitei*, (E) *Moringa oleifera*, (F) *Typha capensis*, (G) *Yohimbe*, and (H) *Tribulus terrestris*.

demonstrated the androgenic effect of *B. alba* by increased level of testosterone production and enhancement of fecundity/fertility in rats exposed to flutamide (an androgen receptor antagonist) in utero as well as in normal rats [32]. *B. alba* is often found in testosterone booster products, and are used by bodybuilders to stimulate the development of their skeletal muscles [6]. In addition, studies conducted by Manfo et al. [33] illustrated the protective effect of the methanol extract of *B. alba* against an agropesticide (manganese ethylenebis)-induced adverse effects on fertility and testosterone levels in adult male rats. Manganese ethylenebis is one of the most commonly used fungicides in Cameroon [33].

1.3 *Fadogia agrestis*

Fadogia agrestis Schweinf. Ex Hiern (Black aphrodisiac) stem is commonly used in Nigeria in the treatment of erectile dysfunction [9]. The aqueous extract of *F. agrestis* stems contains alkaloids, saponins, flavonoids, and anthraquinones [34]. Administration of aqueous extract of *F. agrestis* stems (18, 50, and 100 mg/kg) to male rats for 7 days enhanced sexual activity by increasing mount frequency, intromission frequency with prolonged ejaculatory latency, followed by a decreased mount and intromission latency as well as increased serum testosterone [34]. The circulating increased testosterone level is thought to be the mechanism of action for the aphrodisiac activity of the plant [34]. Furthermore, following a 28-day treatment of male rats with aqueous extract of *F. agrestis* stems (18, 50, and 100 mg/kg), an increased testicular weights with increased testicular cholesterol, sialic acid, and glycogen concentrations was observed. On the other hand, testicular protein content, alkaline phosphatase, glutamate dehydrogenase, and acid phosphatase concentrations were reduced suggesting an adverse effect of *F. agrestis* stem on the functional capacity of the testes [35].

1.4 *Garcinia kola*

Garcinia kola (bitter kola) of the family Guttiferae is a plant found in the rain forests of Central and West Africa [10, 36]. *G. kola* (Fig. 1C) is commonly referred to as "bitter kola" due to its bitter taste and "male kola" for its traditional use as an aphrodisiac [10, 37, 38]. It is traditionally used for the treatment of erectile dysfunction [37, 38].

Akpantah et al. [39] demonstrated that the seeds of *G. kola* was found to have duration-dependent antispermatogenic properties in rats despite its acclaimed aphrodisiac activity [10, 38, 39]. The seed was shown to increase sexual behavior parameters such as mount frequency, number of ejaculations, and intromission frequency, with the low dose (200 mg/kg) being more effective compared to the high dose (400 mg/kg) [38]. However, some other studies showed increased libido, erection, ejaculation, testicular weight, sperm count, and testosterone levels after the administration of the seed extract (see summary in Table 2) [36, 38–45]. The discrepancies may be due to the quality of the nuts or seeds, the extraction solvents, the dosage used, and the experimental design, which should be normalized before any final conclusion can be taken.

Biflavonoids are the active compounds in *G. kola* [41]. Biflavonoid complex extracted from *G. kola* seeds are referred to as kolaviron [46]. Coadministration of kolaviron (200 mg) with nevirapine (18 and 36 mg/kg) showed an ameliorative effect of the isolated compound (kolaviron) toward the testicular toxicity effect induced by the drug such as decreased sperm motility, increased sperm with abnormality, and decreased testicular antioxidant activities [46]. Nevirapine is used in the treatment of HIV infections and has been demonstrated to be deleterious to the male reproductive system [46, 47]. Treatment of alloxan-diabetic animals with kolaviron (200 mg/kg) also showed the ameliorative effects of kolaviron by the restoration of the relative weights of testes, activities of antioxidant enzymes, and sperm and hormonal indices of the diabetic animals [47]. Following the testicular damage induced by lead II oxide (5 mg/kg), ethanolic extract of *G. kola* (100 mg/kg) also had a restorative effect after a 2-week coadministration [48].

1.5 *Mondia whitei*

Mondia whitei L. (White's ginger, tonic root) is a woody climber with a large tuberous root stock (Fig. 1D) and is widely distributed in tropical Africa [11, 12]. It is referred to as "ogombo" or "mukombelo" in the western part of Kenya, "mulondo" in Uganda, "mbombongazi" (Swahili) in Tanzania and "limte," "nkang bongo," "yang," or "la racine" in Cameroon [49, 50]. Its roots are used by traditional medical practitioners in Ghana and Cameroon in the management of erectile dysfunction and infertility, or for aphrodisiac purposes [11, 51].

According to scientific reports, the effect of aqueous extracts of the root bark of *M. whitei* on male reproductive function vary with the duration of treatment. For instance, chronic oral intake of aqueous extract of *M. whitei* (400 mg/kg/day) for 55 days resulted in testicular lesion (which included cessation of spermatogenesis, degenerative changes in the seminiferous tubules and epididymides), increased seminal weight, and no change in serum testosterone, even though the observed effects were reversible following a 55-day recovery period [52]. On the other hand, oral administration of the same extract (400 mg/kg/day) for 8 days caused a significant increase in the weight of testis, testosterone, testicular protein content, and sperm density (suggesting an androgenic effect of the plant), while the other parameters such as accessory gland weights, serum protein contents, testicular concentration of 17β-estradiol, and the fertility remained unchanged [53]. Aqueous extract of *M. whitei* (5, 10, 20, and 50 μL/mL) also greatly improved total and progressive motility in a time-dependent manner in human sperm in vitro after 2-h incubation, suggesting its benefit in the treatment of men affected by asthenozoospermia [54]. Furthermore, Tendwa et al. revealed that exposure of aqueous extract of *M. whitei* root (0.0185, 0.185, 1.85, 18.5, and 185 μg/mL) for 1 h to human sperm from either fertile or infertile men significantly increased total motility and

TABLE 2 Summary of studies on *Garcinia kola* nut extract on male reproduction in rats.

No	Extract	Dosage in mg/kg	Length of study	Reproductive organ	Sperm	Biochemical activities	References
1	Aqueous	200, 400	30 days	Decrease weight	Reduce	Decrease T	[38]
2	Ethanol	200, 400	28 days	No change in organ but increase sexual behavior	No change	Increase T	[40]
3	Aqueous	100	6 days/weeks, 2–8 weeks		Reduced	Increase T	[41]
4	Ethanol	100, 200	6 weeks	Testis degenerative changes	Increase		[42]
5	Kolaviron	100–800	8 weeks	Depletion and desquamation		Reduced cell in H & P	[43]
6	Ethanol	400	28 days		Reduction motility		[44]
7	Ethanol	100, 200, 400	56 days	Increase weight	Sperm count	Increase T	[45]
8	Corn oil	0, 250, 500, 1000	6 weeks			Increase T and antioxidant	[46]
9	Aqueous	25, 50, 100	3 hours	No change	No change	No change	[47]

H & P, hypothalamus and pituitary; *T*, testosterone.

mitochondrial membrane potential. It further increased progressive motility significantly in sperm from the infertile group [55]. This further suggests the beneficial effect of the plant in the treatment of men affected by asthenozoospermia.

Hexane extract of *M. whitei* (500 and 1000 mg/kg) increased relative weight of caput epididymides, ventral prostate, and seminal vesicle following a 30-day treatment [11]. It also enhanced sexual activity by considerably reducing mount latency in sexually inexperienced male rats following a 14-day treatment [50]. Aqueous, hexane and methylene chloride extracts of *M. whitei* also reduced α-adrenergically stimulated contraction in corpus cavernosum tissue in guinea pig and relaxes cavernous smooth muscles by inducing and maintaining penile erection [56].

1.6 *Moringa oleifera*

Moringa oleifera (Moringa, drum stick tree, horseradish tree, or ben oil tree), a member of the family of Moringaceae (Fig. 1E) grows in the tropical and subtropical regions [13, 14]. It is natural to sub-Himalayan region of Northwest India, Pakistan, Bangladesh, and Afghanistan and also cultivated in Africa, Arabia, Southeast Asia, South America, Pacific Islands, and Caribbean Islands [13, 14]. All parts of the plants are edible and possess nutritional and medicinal values. *M. oleifera* contains vitamins (A, B, C, E), calcium, protein, potassium, micronutrients (selenium and zinc), and phytochemicals (kaempferol, quercetin, rutin, caffeoylquinic acids) with potent antioxidant activities [57].

Dietary supplementation of *M. oleifera* leaves (120 and 140 g/day/h for 5 months) increased sperm parameters (sperm motility and viability) and testosterone level with a decrease in sperm abnormality and damaged acrosome in bulls [58], while 500 mg/kg body weight of the leaf extract significantly improved sperm count and levels of LH, FSH, and testosterone in rats [59, 60]. Administration of 200 or 400 mg/kg of aqueous or ethanolic leaf extract of *M. oleifera* to male rats for 8 weeks caused no substantial effect on reproductive parameters while the dose of 400 mg/kg hydroalcoholic extract greatly reduced sperm concentration, motility, and morphology while levels of testosterone and LH remained unchanged [61, 62]. Treatment of mice with hexane extract of *M. oleifera* leaves (0.5, 5, and 50 mg/30 g BW) for 21 days increased weight of testes, epididymis, seminal vesicles, diameter of seminiferous tubule, and thickness of epididymal wall, with no change in the level of LH and FSH [57].

With respect to seeds, the aqueous extract of *M. oleifera* at doses of 100, 200, and 500 mg/kg administered to male rats for 21 days augmented mounting frequency, intromission frequency, and ejaculation latency with decreased mounting latency, intromission latency, and postejaculatory interval, indicating an enhanced sexual behavior. It also greatly improved the libido, sperm count and viability, testosterone, FSH and LH levels, as well as reproductive organ weights [63–65]. Administration of 200 mg/kg methanolic extract of *M. oleifera* to cryptorchid male rats for 28 days significantly increased sperm count and germinal cell count [66]. A continuous intake of Moringa seeds was shown to improve sperm count in men [67].

A significant decrease in sperm parameters was observed in rats treated with 900 MHz mobile phone electromagnetic radiation (EMR) for 8 weeks; however, concurrent exposure to EMR and treatment with 200 mg/kg *M. oleifera* for 8 weeks demonstrated an ameliorative effect of the plant extract by significantly improving the sperm parameters (sperm count, motility, morphology) as well as in the restoration of the normal arrangement of the seminiferous tubules with Sertoli cells, Leydig cells, and different stages of spermatocytes [61]. Similarly, coadministration of paroxetine (10 mg/kg BW) and 400 mg/kg BW of *M. oleifera* ameliorated the reproductive toxicant effect induced by paroxetine [62]. Furthermore, concurrent administration of *M. oleifera* (50 mg/kg) with chromium (150 ppm) averted the induced reproductive toxicity induced by chromium by the enhancement of testicular morphology, improved sperm concentration, motility, and plasma testosterone with a decrease in the activity of GPx and testicular MDA [65].

1.7 *Typha capensis*

Typha capensis (Rohrb.) N.E.Br (commonly referred to as bulrush in English; Lesehu in Sepedi/North-Sotho, papkuil, matjiesriet or palmiet in Afrikaans; Ibhuma in Zulu/Swazi; Ingcongolo in Xhosa; Motsitla in Sesotho) is usually found in wet places of South Africa (Fig. 1F) [15, 16]. The Typha genus is shown to contain several flavones and other phenolic compounds [68]. *T. capensis* is used by traditional healers in South Africa to treat male fertility problems [69]. Medicinal uses of the rhizomes of *T. capensis* include prescription for easy child birth, dysmenorrhoea, venerea diseases, dysentery, diarrhea, and genital problems, and is also used to boost male potency and libido [70, 71]. Aqueous extract of Typha rhizome (1 μg/mL) considerably reduced human sperm motility, vitality, mitochondrial membrane potential, and ROS production following a 1-h incubation in vitro [69, 72]. In another study, Typha rhizome was shown to greatly enhance testosterone production in TM3 cells in a dose-dependent manner without causing change in cell viability or apoptosis [73].

1.8 *Pausinystalia yohimbe*

Pausinystalia yohimbe (commonly referred to as Yohimbe) is an evergreen tree that belongs to the family Rubiaceae [74]. It grows naturally in South, West, and Central Africa, and Asia [74]. Yohimbe was the first plant-derived drug accepted for the treatment of impotency by the US FDA and was referred to as the "herbal viagra." [18] The bark (Fig. 1G) is used as general tonic, performance enhancer for athletes, and as an aphrodisiac in West Africa [75]. The active compound in the yohimbe bark, yohimbine (a tryptamine alkaloid), is used to treat erectile dysfunction [76, 77]. The alkaloids present in yohimbe, which include isoyohimbine, allo-yohimbine, yohimbinine, yohimbane, yohimbenine, and corynanthein, cause vasodilation and penile erection by blocking α-2 adrenergic activity [18].

Yohimbine is orally administered in doses of 5–10 mg, two to three times daily, for about 8 weeks in the treatment of erectile dysfunction [75] or 5–15 mg daily [78] and 0.4 mg/kg (30 mg for the average man) for ejaculatory dysfunction, with an initial dose of 20 mg [79]. Treatment of male rats with *P. yohimbe* bark powder (2%, 4%, 6%, 8%, and 10%) for 30 days brought about a dose-dependent rise in testicular weights, semen volume, sperm counts, and motility, as well as a dose-dependent increase in primary, secondary, and total sperm abnormalities [74]. After the completion of treatment with 20 mg yohimbine, 16 men out of the 29 patients previously diagnosed with orgasmic dysfunction with different etiology could reach orgasm and ejaculate either during masturbation or sexual intercourse [79].

The mechanism of action for the aphrodisiac function of yohimbine is thought to be brought about by the improvement in sexual function through the displacement of epinephrine from alpha-2-adrenergic receptors in the pelvic area as well as increased tendency to arousal by the availability of epinephrine from the alpha-2-adrenergic receptors to the central nervous [18]. However, side effects such as nervousness, anxiety, insomnia, and mild hypertension have been described to be associated with the use of *P. yohimbe* [18]. Caution needs to be taken as the consumption of *P. yohimbe* (or its active compound yohimbine) in high dose is toxic and could lead to death as a result of its ability to excessively increase the mean arterial blood pressure [80].

1.9 *Miscellaneous plants*

Tribulus terrestris (goat's head, bullhead, bindii, burra gokharu, bhakhdi, caltrop, puncture vine, tackweed, devil's eyelashes) is a member of the Zygophyllaceae family (Fig. 1H) and is distributed in Africa and Asia [81]. *T. terrestris* is claimed to be an aphrodisiac and traditionally used for the treatment of sexual and erectile dysfunctions [82]. Oral administration of *T. terrestris* extract (2.5, 5, and 10 mg/kg) to rats and rabbits for 8 weeks increased testosterone, dihydrotestosterone, mount frequency, and intromission frequency with a decrease in mount latency and postejaculatory interval [83, 84]. The fruits' ethanolic extract insignificantly increased testosterone concentration in the treated rats as well as sperm motility in the treated cocks. However, sperm concentration significantly increased in the cocks [85].

Fagara tessmannii (Ewoungea; Bongo): It is a medicinal plant that is used in South Cameroon to improve reproductive function. Oral administration of the ethanolic extract of *F. tessmannii* (0.01, 0.1, and 1 g/kg BW/day) to sexually experienced male rats for 14 days resulted in a significant decrease in the weight of epididymis and seminal vesicle at low dose (0.01 g/kg) as well as decrease in the weight of prostate gland at all doses. The upper limit dose without any clinical sign of toxicity was 2 g/kg. However, a significant increase in the passage of spermatozoa in cauda epididymis was observed at the same lower dose. The length of stages IX–XI of the seminiferous tubule and serum testosterone level increased in a dose-dependent manner [86].

Zanthoxylum macrophylla (rue): The plant belongs to the family of Rutacaea, and is found in tropical region of Africa. The aqueous extract of leaves given to male rats for 14 days increased the daily sperm production, while the weight of seminal vesicle and prostate also increased, respectively, at dose of 200 and 400 mg/kg [87]. The serum testosterone level significantly increased at the same doses.

2 Conclusion

Although limited to animal models or in vitro studies, there have been good scientific evidence to validate the acclaimed reproductive properties of various traditional medicinal plants by traditional healers in the regions of Africa. However, other plants such as *Curtisia dentata* that is traditionally used as an aphrodisiac has not been scientifically proven. Despite the scientific findings, the mechanism of actions of most of the plants is poorly understood as there is a lack of human studies. Hence, more studies are needed to investigate the effects of these plants on humans as well as well as to understand the mechanism of actions.

References

[1] Agarwal A, Mulgund A, Hamada A, Chyatte MR. A unique view on male infertility around the globe. Reprod Biol Endocrinol 2015;13. [cited 2019 Sep 27]; Available from: https://www.ncbi.nlm.nih.gov/pmc/articles/PMC4424520/.

[2] Sharma A. Male infertility; evidences, risk factors, causes, diagnosis and management in human. Ann Clin Lab Res 2017;5(3). [cited 2019 Oct 21]; Available from: http://www.aclr.com.es/abstract/male-infertility-evidences-risk-factors-causes-diagnosis-and-management-inrnhuman-20252.html.

[3] Anon. WHO manual for the standardized investigation, diagnosis and management of the infertile male. WHO; 2000. [cited 2019 Oct 21]. Available from: https://www.who.int/reproductivehealth/publications/infertility/0521774748/en/.

[4] Kazuno S, Yanagida M, Shindo N, Murayama K. Mass spectrometric identification and quantification of glycosyl flavonoids, including dihydrochalcones with neutral loss scan mode. Anal Biochem 2005;347(2):182–92.

[5] Joubert E, Gelderblom WCA, Louw A, de Beer D. South African herbal teas: *Aspalathus linearis*, *Cyclopia spp.* and *Athrixia phylicoides*—a review. J Ethnopharmacol 2008;119(3):376–412.

[6] Adhikari R, Kumar H, Shruthi SD. A review on medicinal importance of *Basella alba* L. Int J Pharm Sci Drug Res 2012;4:110–4.

[7] Saroj V, Rao PS, Rao SK, Krunal S, Shah CU. Pharmacognostical study of *Basella alba* stem. Int J Res Pharmaceut Biomed Sci 2012;3(3):1093–4.

[8] Kumar S, Prasad AK, Iyer SV, Vaidya SK. Systematic pharmacognostical, phytochemical and pharmacological review on an ethno medicinal plant, *Basella alba* L. J Pharmacogn Phytother 2013;5(4):53–8.

[9] Irvine FR. Woody plants of Ghana—With special reference to their uses. Société Française d'Ethnopharmacologie; 1961. [cited 2019 Oct 21]. Available from: http://www.ethnopharmacologia.org/bibliotheque-ethnopharmacologie/woody-plants-of-ghana-with-special-reference-to-their-uses/.

[10] Uko OJ, Usman A, Ataja AM. Some biological activities of *Garcinia kola* in growing rats. Vet arhiv 2001;71(5):287–97.

[11] Watcho P, Donfack MM, Zelefack F, Nguelefack TB, Wansi S, Nguola F, et al. Effects of the hexane extract of *Mondia whitei* on the reproductive organs of male rat. Afr J Tradit Complement Altern Med 2005;2(3):302–11.

[12] Pratap SA, Rajender S. Potent natural aphrodisiacs for the management of erectile dysfunction and male sexual debilities. Front Biosci Sch Ed 2012;4:167–80.

[13] Iqbal S, Bhanger MI. Effect of season and production location on antioxidant activity of *Moringa oleifera* leaves grown in Pakistan. J Food Compos Anal 2006;19(6):544–51.

[14] Melo V, Vargas N, Quirino T, Calvo CM. *Moringa oleifera* L.—an underutilized tree with macronutrients for human health. Emir J Food Agric 2013;25(10):785–9.

[15] Masoko P, Mokgotho MP, Mbazima VG, Mampuru LJ. Biological activities of *Typha capensis* (Typhaceae) from Limpopo Province (South Africa). Afr J Biotechnol 2008;7(20). [cited 2019 Oct 21]; Available from: https://www.ajol.info/index.php/ajb/article/view/59423.

[16] van Wyk B-E, van Oudshoorn B, Gericke N. Medicinal plants of South Africa, 2nd edition. J S Afr Vet Assoc 2010;81(3):188.

[17] Duke J. Handbook of medicinal herbs. Boca Raton, FL; [cited 2019 Oct 22]. Available from: https://www.crcpress.com/Handbook-of-Medicinal-Herbs/Duke/p/book/9780849312847; 1985.

[18] Carey MP, Johnson BT. Effectiveness of yohimbine in the treatment of erectile disorder: four meta-analytic integrations. Arch Sex Behav 1996;25(4):341–60.

[19] Dahlgren R. Revision of the genus Aspalathus: Part II. The species with ericoid and pinoid leaflets: 7. Subgenus Nortieria. With remarks on rooibos tea cultivation; 1968. 44 pp.

[20] Awoniyi DO, Aboua YG, Marnewick JL, du Plesis S, Brooks NL. Protective effects of rooibos (*Aspalathus linearis*), green tea (*Camellia sinensis*) and commercial supplements on testicular tissue of oxidative stress-induced rats. Afr J Biotechnol 2011;10(75):17317–22.

[21] Awoniyi DO, Aboua YG, Marnewick J, Brooks N. The effects of rooibos (*Aspalathus linearis*), green tea (*Camellia sinensis*) and commercial rooibos and green tea supplements on epididymal sperm in oxidative stress-induced rats. Phytother Res 2012;26(8):1231–9.

[22] Ayeleso AO, Oguntibeju OO, Aboua YG, Brooks NL. Effects of red palm oil and rooibos on sperm motility parameters in streptozotocin-induced diabetic rats. Afr J Tradit Complement Altern Med 2014;11(5):8–15.

[23] Opuwari CS, Monsees TK. In vivo effects of *Aspalathus linearis* (rooibos) on male rat reproductive functions. Andrologia 2014;46(8):867–77.

[24] Opuwari C, Monsees T. Reduced testosterone production in TM3 Leydig cells treated with *Aspalathus linearis* (rooibos) or *Camellia sinensis* (tea). Andrologia 2015;47(1):52–8.

[25] Oboh G. Effect of blanching on the antioxidant properties of some tropical green leafy vegetables. LWT Food Sci Technol 2005;38(5):513–7.

[26] Ndangalasi HJ, Bitariho R, Dovie DBK. Harvesting of non-timber forest products and implications for conservation in two montane forests of East Africa. Biol Conserv 2007;134(2):242–50.

[27] Deshmukh SA, Gaikwad DK. A review of the taxonomy, ethnobotany, phytochemistry and pharmacology of *Basella alba* (Basellaceae). J Appl Pharm Sci 2014;4(01):153–65.

[28] Moundipa FP, Kamtchouing P, Koueta N, Tantchou J, Foyang NP, Mbiapo FT. Effects of aqueous extracts of *Hibiscus macranthus* and *Basella alba* in mature rat testis function. J Ethnopharmacol 1999;65(2):133–9.

[29] Moundipa PF, Beboy NSE, Zelefack F, Ngouela S, Tsamo E, Schill W-B, et al. Effects of *Basella alba* and *Hibiscus macranthus* extracts on testosterone production of adult rat and bull Leydig cells. Asian J Androl 2005;7(4):411–7.

[30] Nantia EA, Moundipa PF, Beboy NSE, Monsees TK, Carreau S. Etude de l'effet androgénique de l'extrait au méthanol de *Basella alba* L. (Basellaceae) sur la fonction de reproduction du rat mâle. Andrologie 2007;17(2):129.

[31] Nantia EA, Travert C, Manfo F-PT, Carreau S, Monsees TK, Moundipa PF. Effects of the methanol extract of *Basella alba* L (Basellaceae) on steroid production in Leydig cells. Int J Mol Sci 2011;12(1):376–84.

[32] Nantia EA, Manfo PFT, Beboy NE, Travert C, Carreau S, Monsees TK, et al. Effect of methanol extract of *Basella alba* L. (Basellaceae) on the fecundity and testosterone level in male rats exposed to flutamide in utero. Andrologia 2012;44(1):38–45.

[33] Manfo FPT, Nantia EA, Dechaud H, Tchana AN, Zabot M-T, Pugeat M, et al. Protective effect of *Basella alba* and *Carpolobia alba* extracts against mancb-induced male infertility. Pharm Biol 2014;52(1):97–104.

[34] Yakubu MT, Akanji MA, Oladiji AT. Aphrodisiac potentials of the aqueous extract of *Fadogia agrestis* (Schweinf. Ex Hiern) stem in male albino rats. Asian J Androl 2005;7(4):399–404.

[35] Yakubu MT, Akanji MA, Oladiji AT. Effects of oral administration of aqueous extract of *Fadogia agrestis* (Schweinf. Ex Hiern) stem on some testicular function indices of male rats. J Ethnopharmacol 2008;115(2):288–92.

[36] Abu A, Amuta P, Buba E, Inusa T. Evaluation of antispermatogenic effect of *Garcinia kola* seed extract in albino rats. Asian Pac J Reprod 2013;2(1):15–8.

[37] Malviya N, Malviya S, Jain S, Vyas S. A review of the potential of medicinal plants in the management and treatment of male sexual dysfunction. Andrologia 2016;48(8):880–93.

[38] Ralebona N, Sewani-Rusike C, Nkeh-Chungag B. Effects of ethanolic extract of *Garcinia kola* on sexual behaviour and sperm parameters in male Wistar rats. Afr J Pharm Pharmacol 2012;15:6.

[39] Akpantah AO, Oremosu AA, Ajala MO, Noronha CC, Okanlawon AO. The effect of crude extract of *Garcinia kola* seed on the histology and hormonal milieu of male Sprague-Dawley rats' reproductive organs. Niger J Health Biomed Sci 2003;2(1):40–6.

[40] Oluyemi K, Jimoh R, Adesanya O, Omotuyi O, Josiah S, Oyesola T. Effects of crude ethanolic extract of *Garcinia cambogia* on the reproductive system of male wistar rats (*Rattus novergicus*). Afr J Biotechnol 2007;1684-5315. 6(10).

[41] Augustine O, Nwoha P. Effects of kolaviron, the major constituent of *Garcinia kola*, on the histology of the hypothalamus, pituitary, and testes using adult male Wistar rats as a model organism. Forensic Med Anat Res 2014;02:80–7.

[42] Chikere OU, Gloria OC, Nnabuihe ED, Uchechi EE, Jesse AC. The effect of ethanolic extract of *Garcinia kola* on the sperm parameters and histology of the testis of male Wistar rats. Adv Life Sci Technol 2015;33:18–25.

[43] Sewani-Rusike CR, Ralebona N, Nkeh-Chungag BN. Dose- and time-dependent effects of *Garcinia kola* seed extract on sexual behaviour and reproductive parameters in male Wistar rats. Andrologia 2016;48(3):300–7.

[44] Farombi EO, Adedara IA, Oyenihi AB, Ekakitie E, Kehinde S. Hepatic, testicular and spermatozoa antioxidant status in rats chronically treated with *Garcinia kola* seed. J Ethnopharmacol 2013;146(2):536–42.

[45] Yakubu MT, Quadri AL. *Garcinia kola* seeds: is the aqueous extract a true aphrodisiac in male Wistar rats? Afr J Tradit Complement Altern Med 2012;9(4):530–5.

[46] Adaramoye OA, Akanni OO, Farombi EO. Nevirapine induces testicular toxicity in Wistar rats: reversal effect of kolaviron (biflavonoid from *Garcinia kola* seeds). J Basic Clin Physiol Pharmacol 2013;24(4):313–20.

[47] Adaramoye OA, Lawal SO. Effect of kolaviron, a biflavonoid complex from *Garcinia kola* seeds, on the antioxidant, hormonal and spermatogenic indices of diabetic male rats. Andrologia 2014;46(8):878–86.

[48] Dare B, Chukwu R, Oyewopo AO, Makanjuola V, Olayinka P, Akinrinade I, et al. Histological integrity of the testis of adult Wistar rats (*Rattus novergicus*) treated with *Garcinia kola*. Reprod Syst Sex Disord 2012;01. https://doi.org/10.4172/2161-038X.1000113.

[49] Oketch-Rabah HA. *Mondia whitei*, a medicinal plant from Africa with aphrodisiac and antidepressant properties: a review. J Diet Suppl 2012;9(4):272–84.

[50] Watcho P, Zelefack F, Nguelefack TB, Ngouela S, Telefo PB, Kamtchouing P, et al. Effects of the aqueous and hexane extracts of *Mondia whitei* on the sexual behaviour and some fertility parameters of sexually inexperienced male rats. Afr J Tradit Complement Altern Med 2006;4(1):37–46.

[51] Martey O, He X. Possible mode of action of *Mondia whitei*: an aphrodisiac used in the management of erectile dysfunction. J Pharmacol Toxicol 2010;5:460–8.

[52] Watcho P, Kamtchouing P, Sokeng S, Moundipa PF, Tantchou J, Essame JL, et al. Reversible antispermatogenic and antifertility activities of *Mondia whitei* L. in male albino rat. Phytother Res 2001;15(1):26–9.

[53] Watcho P, Kamtchouing P, Sokeng SD, Moundipa PF, Tantchou J, Essame JL, et al. Androgenic effect of *Mondia whitei* roots in male rats. Asian J Androl 2004;6(3):269–72.

[54] Lampiao F, Krom D, du Plessis SS. The in vitro effects of *Mondia whitei* on human sperm motility parameters. Phytother Res 2008;22(9):1272–3.

[55] Tendwa B, Morris A, Opuwari C, Henkel R. Effects of aqueous root extract of *Mondia whitei* on human sperm functions; 2017.

[56] Watcho P, Djoukeng CN, Zelefack F, Nguelefack TB, Ngouela S, Kamtchouing P, Tsamo E, Kamanyi A. Relaxant effect of Mondia whitei extracts on isolated guinea pig corpus cavernosum. Pharmacologyonline 2007;2:44–52.

[57] Cajuday L, Pocsidio G. Effects of *Moringa oleifera* Lam. (Moringaceae) on the reproduction of male mice (*Mus musculus*). J Med Plants Res 2010;4:1115–21.

[58] Wafa W, El-Nagar H, Gabr AA, Rezk M. Impact of dietary *Moringa oleifera* leaves supplementation on semen characteristics, oxidation stress, physiological response and blood parameters of heat stressed buffalo bulls. J Anim Poult Prod Mansoura Univ 2017;8:367–79.

[59] Priyadarshani N, Varma MC. Effect of *Moringa oleifera* leaf powder on sperm count, histology of testis and epididymis of hyperglycaemic mice *Mus musculus*. Am Int J Res Form Appl Nat Sci 2014;7(1):7–13.

[60] Ogunsola A, Joshua O, Sunday F, Nl N, As A. Moringa plant parts consumption had effects on reproductive functions in male and female rat models. IOSR J Dent Med Sci 2017;16:82–6.

[61] Bin-Meferij MM, El-Kott AF. The radioprotective effects of *Moringa oleifera* against mobile phone electromagnetic radiation-induced infertility in rats. Int J Clin Exp Med 2015;8(8):12487–97.

[62] El-Sheikh SMA, Khairy M, Fadil HA, Abo-Elmaaty AMA. Ameliorative effect of *Moringa oleifera* extract on male fertility in paroxetine treated rats. Zagazig Vet J 2016;44(3):244–50.

[63] Zade VS, Dabhadkar DK, Thakare VG, Pare SR. Effect of aqueous extract of *Moringa oleifera* seed on sexual activity of male albino rats. Int J Bio Forum 2013;5(1):129–40.

[64] Dafaalla MM, Abass SE, Abdoun S, Hassan AWF, Idris OF. Effect of ethanol extract of *Moringa oleifera* seeds on fertility hormone and sperm quality of male Albino Rats. Int J Multidiscip Res Dev 2017;4(4):222–6.

[65] Akunna GG, Ogunmodede OS, Saalu CL, Ogunlade BA, Bello AJ, Salawu EO. Ameliorative effect of *Moringa oleifera* (drumstick) leaf extracts on chromium-induced testicular toxicity in rat testes. World J Life Sci Med Res 2012;2:20–6.

[66] Afolabi AO, Aderoju HA, Alagbonsi IA. Effects of methanolic extract of *Moringa oleifera* leaves on semen and biochemical parameters in cryptorchid rats. Afr J Tradit Complement Altern Med 2013;10(5):230–5.

[67] Cabacungan. Inquirer.net, Legarda pushes for malunggay, her beauty soup; 2008.

[68] Chapman J, Hall P. Dictionary of natural products on CD-ROM. Chapman & Hall/CRC; 2000.

[69] Henkel R, Fransman W, Hipler U-C, Wiegand C, Schreiber G, Menkveld R, et al. *Typha capensis* (Rohrb.) N.E.Br. (bulrush) extract scavenges free radicals, inhibits collagenase activity and affects human sperm motility and mitochondrial membrane potential in vitro: a pilot study. Andrologia 2012;44(Suppl. 1):287–94.

[70] Shode FO, Mahomed AS, Rogers CB. Typhaphthalide and typharin, two phenolic compounds from *Typha capensis*. Phytochemistry 2002;61(8):955–7.

[71] Hutchings A. Zulu medicinal plants: An inventory. University of Natal Press; 1996. 480 pp.

[72] Henkel R, Fransman W, Hipler U-C, Schreiber G, Weitz F. *Typha capensis* extracts decrease ros production and affect human sperm functions. Afr J Tradit Complement Altern Med 2009;6:438–9.

[73] Ilfergane A, Henkel RR. Effect of *Typha capensis* (Rohrb.) N.E.Br. rhizome extract F1 fraction on cell viability, apoptosis induction and testosterone production in TM3-Leydig cells. Andrologia 2018;50(2), e12854.

[74] Ogwo E, Osim E, Nwankwo A, Ijioma S. Semen quality in male albino rats fed with various concentrations of *Pausinystalia yohimbe* bark powder (Burantashi). J Med Dent Sci Res 2016;3:16–24.

[75] EFSA. Yohimbe (*P. yohimbe* (K. Schum) Pierre ex Beille) for use in food. European Food Safety Authority; 2013. [cited 2019 Oct 21]. Available from: https://www.efsa.europa.eu/en/efsajournal/pub/3302.

[76] Balon R. Fluoxetine-induced sexual dysfunction and yohimbine. J Clin Psychiatry 1993;54(4):161–2.

[77] Tyler V. The honest herbal. [cited 2019 Oct 21]. Available from: https://www.goodreads.com/work/best_book/2941167-the-honest-herbal-a-sensible-guide-to-the-use-of-herbs-and-related-reme; 1993.

[78] Goldberg MR, Robertson D. Yohimbine: a pharmacological probe for study of the alpha 2-adrenoreceptor. Pharmacol Rev 1983;35(3):143–80.

[79] Adeniyi AA, Brindley GS, Pryor JP, Ralph DJ. Yohimbine in the treatment of orgasmic dysfunction. Asian J Androl 2007;9(3):403–7.

[80] Ajayi AA, Newaz M, Hercule H, Saleh M, Bode CO, Oyekan AO. Endothelin-like action of *Pausinystalia yohimbe* aqueous extract on vascular and renal regional hemodynamics in Sprague Dawley rats. Methods Find Exp Clin Pharmacol 2003;25(10):817–22.

[81] Mohammadi F, Nikzad H, Taherian A, Amini Mahabadi J, Salehi M. Effects of herbal medicine on male infertility. Anat Sci J 2013;10(4):3–16.

[82] CHEMEXCIL. *Tribulus terrestris* Linn. (N.O.-Zygophyllaceae). In: Selected medicinal plants of India (A monograph of identity, safety and clinical usage). Bombay: Tata Press; 1992. p. 323–6.

[83] Gauthaman K, Ganesan AP. The hormonal effects of *Tribulus terrestris* and its role in the management of male erectile dysfunction—an evaluation using primates, rabbit and rat. Phytomedicine Int J Phytother Phytopharm 2008;15(1–2):44–54.

[84] Gauthaman K, Ganesan AP, Prasad RNV. Sexual effects of puncturevine (*Tribulus terrestris*) extract (protodioscin): an evaluation using a rat model. J Altern Complement Med 2003;9(2):257–65.

[85] Mohammed M, Shaddad S, Mudathir A, Elshari B, Algasem A. Effects of *Tribulus terrestris* ethanolic extract in male rats and cock's fertility. J Pharm Biomed Sci 2013;30(30):S13–8.

[86] Massoma Lembè D, Gasco M, Rubio J, Yucra S, Sock EN, Gonzales GF. Effect of the ethanolic extract from *Fagara tessmannii* on testicular function, sex reproductive organs and hormone level in adult male rats. Andrologia 2011;43(2):139–44.

[87] Ngandjui A, Ngaha N, Kenmogne H, Koloko B, Massoma L, Bend E, et al. Evaluation of the fertility activity of the aqueous leaves extract of *Zanthoxylum macrophylla* (Rutaceae) on male rats. J Phytopharm 2017;6:277–81.

Chapter 5.4.1

Herbal medicine used to treat andrological problems: Asia and Indian subcontinent: *Withania somnifera, Panax ginseng, Centella asiatica*

Pallav Sengupta[a], Damayanthi Durairajanayagam[b], and Ashok Agarwal[c]

[a]*Physiology, MAHSA University, Jenjarom, Selangor, Malaysia,* [b]*Physiology, Faculty of Medicine, Universiti Teknologi MARA (UiTM), Sungai Buloh, Selangor, Malaysia,* [c]*American Center for Reproductive Medicine, Cleveland Clinic, Cleveland, OH, United States*

1 Introduction

Herbal medicines have been trusted as medicinal therapy since thousands of years ago. In the present era of scientific revolution, it has evoked great research interests that are directed toward revealing the exact therapeutic target and mechanism of action in the etiopathology of various diseases, especially in Asia, South America, and Africa. Western countries are also becoming more oriented toward the use of herbal therapy [1]. As per the WHO estimation, primarily based on surveys from developing countries, 80% of the global population have placed their trust on herbal remedies [2].

Herbal resources have always elicited a keen research interest owing to its versatile usage and it being a source of novel drugs. Herbal medicine is steadily gaining more importance worldwide [3, 4]. In India, *Ayurveda* or the "science of life or longevity" refers to the traditional medicinal system that reportedly can supplement the more modern forms of medicine. This medicinal system claims to be comprehensive enough to rejuvenate the health and impart a long, healthy life to its practitioners [4]. These medicines have been found effective even in the treatment of conditions such as hypertension, diabetes, gastritis, and reproductive complications [1]. In the Middle East, the use of herbal medicines was reported to result in improvement in fertility status in infertile diabetic males [5, 6]. Chinese traditional medicine is also one of the ancient medicinal systems with various treatment modalities. These include acupuncture, and natural and herbal supplements for different diseases [7]. In the United States, alternative medicine or complementary therapy is gaining acceptability among the general population and medical community [8].

Male infertility is a condition whose mechanisms still remain elusive in most of the cases and the exact diagnosis and treatment are still under advanced research. The use of various herbal drugs has shown potential in improving male reproductive health. These herbs include *Eurycoma longifolia* (Tongkat Ali), *Tribulus terrestris* (Gokhru or land caltrops), *Allium sativum* (garlic), *Cannabis sativa* (marijuana), *Allium cepa* (onion), *Capsicum frutescens* (chili pepper), *Withania somnifera* (Ashwagandha or the "Indian ginseng"), *Panax ginseng*, *Centella asiatica*, and *Zingiber officinale* (ginger) [9–13]. They were tested and proved to be highly beneficial for the treatment of oligozoospermia, erectile dysfunction, reproductive endocrinological disruptions, and other male infertility issues. Thus, this chapter will concisely present the role of herbal medicines in male infertility, including detailed analyses of the effects of three potential herbs, *W. somnifera*, *P. ginseng*, and *C. asiatica* on male fertility parameters.

2 Herbal medicine and its use in andrology

Infertility is defined as the inability of a couple to conceive even after a year of regular and unprotected, well-timed vaginal intercourse. Globally, infertility affects about 8.5 million couples and male factors contribute to half of these cases [14]. Infertility treatment mainly involves the management of stress, hormonal therapy, other forms of expensive medications, and assisted reproductive technology (ART). Despite its high cost, the success rate of treating infertility is only about

Herbal Medicine in Andrology. https://doi.org/10.1016/B978-0-12-815565-3.00015-1

10%–30%. Thus, herbal therapies for male infertility are being tested for their efficacy, which promise cost-effectiveness and cure with minimum or no side effects [15].

Male infertility may stem from numerous causes including endocrine disruptions, varicocele, infections, and sexual dysfunctions, while almost half of the male infertility cases are idiopathic [16]. Oxidative stress (OS) may serve as a common pathway by which the various causatives may incur male infertility [17]. OS is induced by an imbalance between the antioxidant capacity and the generation of reactive oxygen species (ROS) in favor of the latter [18].

Diverse use of herbal medicines for the treatment and amelioration of male infertility have been reported, which include but is not limited to *Ayurveda*, Traditional Chinese Medicine, as well as Western Alternative Medicine [7]. *Sheng Jing*, an herbal mixture of 15 plants, was able to restore hormone levels and semen quality in oligozoospermic men [19]. Herbal therapy for primary health care and reproductive problems are also popular in South Africa [20]. A Southern African plant, *Typha capensis* (love reed) showed antioxidant capacity and increased testicular steroidogenesis [21, 22].

In *Ayurvedic* treatment, a mixture of different herbs is used as a cure for male infertility. These herbs commonly include *W. somnifera* (Indian ginseng), *Mucuna pruriens* (velvet bean), *T. terrestris* (land caltrops), *Glycyrrhiza glabra* (licorice), *Phyllanthus emblica* (Indian gooseberry or amla), *Terminalia arjuna* (Arjuna tree), *Z. officinale* (ginger), and *Piper longum* (Indian long pepper) [1]. Thus, the efficacy of these entrusted therapeutic combinations should be well researched and tested for their specific actions and mechanism.

Herbal components have also been recently used in ART, including several animal studies on cryopreservation and IVF [23, 24]. Semen preparation for ART essentially include separation of seminal plasma. Seminal plasma is the antioxidant and nutrient medium required for the survival of spermatozoa in the vagina and cervix. In case of ART, the sperm are devoid of their own antioxidative protection, and are thus at a high risk of OS [14, 23]. Spermatozoa can also be cryopreserved to preserve their capability to fertilize for a duration. However, cryopreservation is also associated with ROS generation, lipid peroxidation (LPO), and reduced sperm functions [14]. These issues have led to numerous experiments to determine whether plant-derived antioxidants could aid in improving sperm quality, and they included polyphenol-rich grape pomace extract (obtained from *Vitis vinifera*) and crocin (the main apocarotenoids of *Crocus sativus*) [23]. Bovine sperm incubated in grape seed extracts showed improved motility and viability, owing to its antioxidant properties and polyphenol content [23, 25]. Crocin also reportedly reduced ROS and LPO levels with increase in viability and motility in cryopreserved sperm [26]. The Chinese herbal mixture *Bushen Shengjing* decoction was administered in oligozoospermic and azoospermic men for a couple of months before ICSI. The treatment was shown to improve sperm viability, concentration, and motility with increased rates of fertilization and clinical pregnancy [24]. However, herbal supplements for ART are subject to more extensive studies.

3 *Withania somnifera*: As an herbal medicine in andrology

W. somnifera or *Ashwagandha* in Ayurvedic medicine is commonly referred to as Indian ginseng, winter cherry, or poison gooseberry. *Ashwagandha* is a small evergreen shrub with long tuberous roots, belonging to the plant family of *Solanaceae* (nightshade). *W. somnifera* (WS) is characterized by tiny greenish-yellow colored flowers, and smooth, round fruits containing several seeds. The *Ashwagandha* shrub grows in tropical and subtropical areas, including Middle East India and China as well as in South Africa [27]. It is grown as a medicinal crop in India and the entire shrub as well as its different components are utilized for its unique medicinal properties. The WS root has been reported to act as a diuretic, adaptogen, antioxidant, sedative, and aphrodisiac [28]. Other parts of this shrub, such as the leaves and fruits, also possess high medical significance as a pain reliever, antineoplastic agent, memory enhancer, and antimicrobial and antiinflammatory mediators [28].

Numerous phytochemical studies have reported the various chemical constituents of different WS components [29, 30]. Withanolides, which are triterpene lactones with C28 ergosterone-based structures, are the principal bioactive components of WS. As many as 40 withanolides have been isolated, along with 12 alkaloids and numerous sitoindosides [31]. The most essential compounds of WS comprise withaferin-A, withanolide-D, and withanone [32, 33]. Withaferin-A was first isolated from WS by Lavie et al. in 1965 [34]. Moreover, this shrub is also a proven source of various important metabolites including iron, aspartate, alanine, lactate, fructose, glutamine, etc. [35]. Clinical and toxicological research have confirmed that WS is nontoxic even at a wide range of doses, and there are no reports on any herb-drug or herb-herb in vivo interactions that involve WS [36–38]. Withanolides, the active constituent of WS, are shown to be absorbed through the intestinal epithelium following oral administration, with withaferin-A having the highest bioavailability [39].

3.1 *Withania somnifera* and male infertility

Studies, both in vivo and in vitro, have reached a consensus that the WS roots have antiinflammatory properties. In the rodent arthritic model, WS was shown to significantly reduce paw size and bone degenerations as compared to the control rats. Moreover, the WS-mediated improvements in arthritic inflammation were even statistically higher than those in the positive control group that received the standard reference drug, hydrocortisone [31, 40]. A reduced level of proinflammatory transcription factors and cytokines were evident with WS therapy [41]. Studies have also reported that WS roots have a modulatory impact on the central nervous system, such as regulation of acetylcholinesterase activity and modulation of GABA activities and the serotonin receptors [42]. WS may also act as an antineoplastic agent and its leaf extract is reportedly able to attenuate cancer cells via several mechanisms, which include the p53 signaling pathway, activation of apoptotic cascades, and death receptors signaling pathways [25]. Withaferin-A, the active component of WS, has been found to be a potent activator of tumor suppressor proteins (p53 and pRB) as well as tumor necrosis factors to prevent apoptosis [43].

WS has pharmacological relevance in innumerable ways. It is evident through various studies that WS has antioxidant activities and can inhibit LPO in spermatozoa [44], which may be a prime factor for the disruption of sperm functions and in idiopathic male infertility. WS reportedly could ameliorate and restore the levels of sex hormones in infertile men with psychological and/or physiological stress. This further confirms that WS possesses adaptogenic qualities [45]. WS is thus suited to attenuate several causative factors that lead to male factor infertility or subfertility.

Ahmad et al. (2010) reported that WS root extract mediated a significant increase ($P < .01$) in sperm concentration and sperm motility in male subjects diagnosed with normozoospermia, azoospermia, and oligozoospermia [46]. The treatment used the WS root extract as an oral dose of 5 g per day in a cup of milk for 3 months. Earlier reports by Mahdi et al. [45], with the same dose and treatment duration, showed WS-mediated improvement in overall semen quality in stress-induced male infertility. In Mahdi's study, subjects with normozoospermia (aged between 25–38 years) with unexplained infertility were selected and some of the subjects had reported a history of smoking or experiencing incidences that caused psychological stress. These infertile male subjects were treated for 3 months with WS root powder (single oral dose of 5 g per day with a cup of skimmed milk). The study demonstrated a reduction in levels of seminal markers for LPO, stress markers, serum cortisol levels, reduced ROS generation together with enhanced antioxidant capacity, increase in testosterone and LH levels, and improved sperm functions [45]. Ambiye and colleagues had claimed to have obtained as much as a 167% increase in sperm concentration in oligozoospermic subjects through 90 days of treatment with 675 mg/kg of WS root extract given thrice daily [47]. This treatment had accounted for improvements in sperm motility and semen volume by more than 50%, as well as increase in levels of testosterone and luteinizing hormone (LH) [47].

Several animal studies have also reported the positive impact of WS on semen quality. Sahin et al. (2016) had observed the efficacy of several herbal plants in the amelioration of semen quality in rats; they also showed a significant improvement in sperm count and sperm motility via treatment with WS, at a dose of 300 mg/kg for 8 weeks [48]. Kumar et al. (2015) and Bhargavan et al. (2015) had also found that WS root extract could reverse male reproductive potency in alcohol- and arsenic-induced testicular damage in rats [49, 50]. They have also reported a significant improvement in sperm count and motility after WS treatment was given orally for 30 days at a dose of 100 mg/kg or 28 days at a 200 mg/kg dose. WS (at a dose of 200 mg/kg for 28 days) also significantly reduced the abnormalities seen in sperm morphology [50]. Dhumal et al. (2013) [51] had demonstrated that Afrodet Plus, an herbal drug that contains WS along with other herbal components, could improve semen quality in rats when given at a dose of 100 mg of WS root extract for 21 days.

3.2 Mechanism of action of *Withania somnifera*

The mechanism of actions of WS on the male reproductive system and fertility can be discussed by dividing it into the oxidative and nonoxidative mechanisms. The oxidative mechanism include alterations in antioxidant activities, impact on antioxidant enzymes, and furnish co-factors needed for antioxidant enzymes activities [52]. The nonoxidative mechanisms focus on the WS effects on the hypothalamic-pituitary-testicular (HPT) axis and its stress reversing activities by acting on the hypothalamic-pituitary-adrenal (HPA) axis. After administration, the WS extract is metabolized to several different main components: withaferin-A, withanolide-D, withanone, and other derivatives [52]. The biochemical components impact either directly male reproductive cells, or indirectly endocrine homeostasis to ameliorate male fertility [52]. These observations lead to postulations of the general mechanism of WS actions, which are presented in Fig. 1.

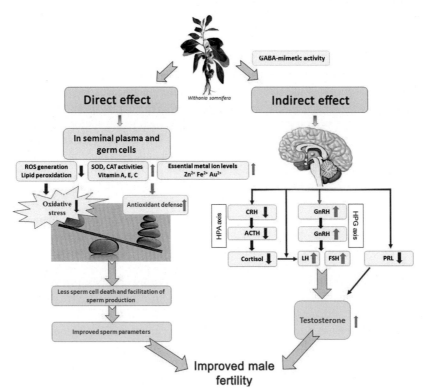

FIG. 1 Mechanism of action of *Withania somnifera* in the regulation of male fertility. Through direct and indirect mechanisms, this herb improves sperm parameters as well as the reproductive hormonal profile. Through the direct or oxidative mechanism, this herb improves seminal antioxidant status and decreases ROS generation to mitigate the effects of oxidative stress, whereas through the indirect or nonoxidative mechanism, it improves the reproductive hormonal profiles by directly acting on the HPG axis and by minimizing the endocrine-disrupting effects of the stress-induced HPA-HPG crosstalk as well by regulating the circulating prolactin levels in men.

3.2.1 Oxidative mechanisms

ROS are highly reactive molecules with one or several unpaired electrons in the outer orbit [53, 54] and have half-lives in the nano- to milliseconds range. Molecular oxygen exists in a diradical inert state. However, under certain physiological conditions, it may react with organic molecules to generate ROS. Mitochondria generates biological energy via oxidation of biological molecules, where the terminal electron acceptor is a molecular oxygen. The midpiece of sperm consists of a sperm-specific oxidoreductase, operated by nicotinamide adenine dinucleotide phosphate-oxidase (NOX) [55]. Electron leakage due to impaired electron transfer from Complex I or III in the mitochondrial electron transfer chain accounts mainly for the ROS generation [56]. Under aerobic conditions also, approximately 5% of the total consumed oxygen reacts to produce free radicals [57], which is an inevitable outcome of metabolism. Controlled concentration of ROS plays a vital role in maintaining normal sperm functions such as signal transduction for sperm capacitation, hyperactivation, and acrosome reaction [58]. Thus, a proper balance between ROS and antioxidant capacity must prevail to protect the testicular cells from oxidative damage. Since the sperm plasma membrane consists of high levels of polyunsaturated fatty acids, they are prone to LPO, impairments of subsequent cellular components, sperm DNA fragmentation, and loss of sperm functions [14].

Both endogenous and exogenous sources are responsible for the generation of ROS found in the seminal plasma. Endogenous sources mostly consist of immature spermatozoa, invasion of neutrophils, and macrophages [14]. Thus, oxidative stress-induced male infertility may be treated by inhibiting the excess ROS generation addressing the major sources of the same. A substantial number of studies have reported on the efficacy of different oral antioxidant supplements in improving male factor fertility [59]. Using solely antioxidants may not be effective, given the unknown cause of the problem. Moreover, as discussed earlier, the specific balance between oxidation and reduction is also vital for normal sperm physiology, and thus excess administration of antioxidants would result in the so-called "reductive stress," which is also detrimental for cells [60]. This paradoxical phenomenon is referred as the "antioxidant paradox," a term coined by Halliwell [61]. This is one of the crucial factors for the emergence of herbal supplements for male infertility management and treatment.

The daily administered daily of WS root powder at a dose of 5 g per day could decrease ROS generation in the seminal plasma and improved sperm count in infertile men with normozoospermia [44]. Several studies have conveyed the effects of WS on semen quality in infertile men and enzymatic antioxidant activities. It has been shown that WS could reduce the level of LPO as compared with the pretreatment group [44–46]. WS could act by donating electrons and inhibiting the consequent destructive chain reaction mediated by free radicals, thereby reducing the overall ROS burden [31].

Besides WS-mediated LPO reduction in infertile men, studies have also revealed that WS could alter the concentration of metal ions such as copper, zinc, iron, gold, and arsenic [49] in seminal plasma. Zinc in combination with copper act as a co-factor for superoxide dismutase (SOD), whereas the activation of glutathione peroxidase and catalase require selenium and iron, respectively [44]. Although gold does not have a direct role in the activities of antioxidant enzymes, its administration has been shown to improve spermatogenesis as well as steroidogenesis in immature Wistar rats [62]. It is evident that one of the mechanisms by which WS may combat oxidative damage and testicular cell death is via alterations in seminal levels of essential metals (copper, iron, zinc, and gold) in infertile men [44], which may function as co-factors for the proper functioning of antioxidant enzymes.

Thus, the ability of WS root extract to reduce levels of seminal ROS and testicular oxidative stress may be explained by two mechanisms: its high antioxidant activities in quenching excess ROS by itself, and its ability to induce antioxidant enzyme activities by supplementation of essential co-factors.

3.2.2 Nonoxidative mechanisms

Imbalance in the hormonal milieu present another set of causatives of male reproductive dysfunctions and male infertility. Studies have shown that stress-related hormones such as glucocorticoids adversely affect the hypothalamic-pituitary-gonadal (HPG) axis, thereby inhibiting steroidogenesis and spermatogenesis [63]. Hypothalamic gonadotrophin-releasing hormone (GnRH) stimulates the release of anterior pituitary trophic hormones, follicle-stimulating hormone (FSH), and luteinizing hormone (LH). These trophic hormones act on the testicular cells, i.e., LH on the Leydig cells and FSH on the Sertoli cells to mediate steroidogenesis and spermatogenesis. Therefore, disruption of the HPG axis by crosstalk with other hormones such as the adipose tissue-derived hormones, gonadotrophin-inhibiting hormone, and cortisol immensely affect male reproductive functions [64].

As WS root extract is claimed to act as an adaptogen, it can bring about physiological homeostasis by attenuating the stress response and cortisol levels, thus leading to improved reproductive functions to a certain extent. It has been shown that WS treatment (at the dose of 5 g per day for 3 months) in infertile normozoospermic men under either psychological or environmental stress or with idiopathic infertility of unknown cause could significantly reduce their cortisol levels and increase their testosterone and LH levels [45]. Moreover, WS treatment was demonstrated to have increased fertility rates by about 14% among couples with prior male factor subfertility or infertility [46]. Thus, WS can modulate the levels of serum sex hormones and improve testicular functions by regulating the HPG axis.

WS may stabilize the normal regulations of the HPA and HPG axes on male reproduction by acting at various regulatory levels, i.e., at the testicular, adrenal cortex, pituitary, or hypothalamic levels. There are studies that support the action of the WS root powder on hypothalamic secretions [27, 65]. Also, the aqueous extract of WS leaves could stimulate hypothalamic GnRH activities via its GABA-mimetic activity [65]. Since WS is able to stimulate GnRH, it may induce the secretion and release of the downstream pituitary hormones, LH, and FSH, followed by an increased production of testicular testosterone. The major bioactive compounds in WS that are mostly responsible for these physiological actions are Withaferin A [66] and Withanone [32].

Seminal plasma composition is a major determinant of vitality and functionality of spermatozoa [67]. Gupta et al. (2013) studied the efficacy of WS in improving the levels of seminal plasma metabolites in infertile men. They demonstrated that WS root extract powder at a dose of 5 g per day for 4 months could enhance the seminal constituents almost to the levels of that in fertile men [68]. The parameters investigated in the study included those for spermatozoa quality, such as sperm count, motility, lipid peroxide levels, concentration of hormones, and seminal concentrations of glutamine, citrate, lactate, lysine, alanine, glutamate, glycerophosphocholine, choline, glycine, tyrosine, phenylalanine, histidine, and uridine. These results suggest that WS can be a potential substance for empirical treatment of male infertility. Several other studies have supported this suggestion, which also showed that WS root comprises a substantial amount of lactate and lactate dehydrogenase, which could lead to an improvement in the seminal plasma lactate content [35]. Lactate is the product of an LDH-controlled reaction. It is known that a reduction in lactate dehydrogenase activities is associated with reduced sperm motility and viability [69].

WS treatment have also been shown to elevate the concentrations of several essential metals (zinc, copper, iron, and gold) that act to maintain robust testicular functions, by ameliorating both steroidogenesis and spermatogenesis [44].

Since WS can improve seminal plasma concentrations of citrate, lactate, histidine, alanine, and phenylalanine, this may lead to an overall improvement in spermatozoa metabolism and spermatogenesis.

4 *Panax ginseng*: As an herbal medicine in andrology

4.1 *Panax ginseng* and male infertility

Ginseng, often considered as "the king of herbs," is a well-known agent for its characteristics to improve an individual's general well-being, including the cardiovascular, neuronal, and immune systems. It also acts as a promising aphrodisiac and has been shown to have immense application in the treatment of sexual dysfunction and in amelioration of sexual behavior, mostly in the traditional Chinese medical practices. The term, "Panax," Greek meaning "all-healing," was added to ginseng by the Russian Botanist, Carl A Meyer in 1843. Conventionally, *P. ginseng* (PG) refers to the Asian ginseng [70, 71].

PG can improve sexual performance and satisfaction as evidenced by data from various studies in animals and humans, which have demonstrated that PG treatment has positive effects on libido and copulatory performances. It also enhances sperm quality and sperm count in healthy individuals as well as in infertile patients. These effects of PG are mostly attributed to its main pharmacological active component, ginsenosides [70].

4.2 *Panax ginseng* and penile erection

PG is a traditional Chinese medicine that may be taken with an herbal formulation or by itself to improve sexual performance [70, 72]. Meta-analyses of randomized clinical trials with ginseng treatment have supported the beneficial effects of PG on male reproductive functions. A double-blind, placebo-controlled study showed ginseng mediated increase in scores on erectile function and sexual satisfaction in 45 male subjects, who had presented with moderate to severe erectile dysfunction [73]. Another study comprising 60 men with erectile dysfunction also showed substantially improved erectile functions such as penile rigidity, penetration, and sustenance of erection, following 12 weeks of ginseng treatment [74]. Animal studies have also demonstrated ginseng-mediated relaxation of the smooth muscles of precontracted penile corpus cavernosum of rabbits in vitro, and enhanced intracavernosal pressure in rats in vivo [75, 76]. Available reports suggest that these ginseng actions are nitric oxide (NO) dependent. Ginsenosides, the major active components of ginseng, have been shown to induce synthesis of NO in perivascular nerves and endothelial cells, thereby increasing the sensitivity of vascular smooth muscle cell to NO [19, 77]. The release of NO leads to smooth muscle relaxation thereby causing greater volume of blood to flow to the erectile bodies known as corpus cavernosum, leading to an erection [78]. The ginsenoside found in PG is the ginsenoside Rg1 that acts via glucocorticoid receptor-dependent, nongenomic mechanisms to trigger NO synthesis in endothelial cells [79]. It has been shown that Rg1 administration at a dose of 10 mg/kg significantly upregulates NO release and intracellular cyclic GMP (cGMP) concentration in the corpus cavernosum of mice [80].

4.3 *Panax ginseng* and libido

Experiments using rodent models have revealed that Asian ginseng or PG [81] can facilitate sexual behavior. PG treatment at doses of 25–100 mg/kg or ginsenoside Rg1 (2.5–10 mg/kg) have shown dose-dependent enhancement in copulatory behavior patterns like mounting, penile licking, and intromission in mice exposed to estrous females [82].

In higher mammals, sex drive is coordinated by complex crosstalk among the hormonal and neuronal components. Testosterone, the male sex steroid, is produced by the Leydig cell as per regulation by the anterior pituitary hormone, luteinizing hormone (LH) [83]. Testosterone levels are a major determinant of a robust libido and sex drive [84]. Interestingly, a 5% PG dose given to rats with their regular diet for 60 days resulted in increased levels of testosterone in blood, while a 1% PG dose did not show similar results [85]. The active component of PG, ginsenoside Rg1 at a dose of 10 mg/kg could increase serum testosterone levels and significantly improve copulatory behavior [80]. Various ginseng species have also been shown to increase LH secretion by its direct effects on the anterior pituitary gland [86]. A clinical study with 66 subjects showed that PG treatment significantly increased the plasma levels of total and free testosterone, as well as increased follicle stimulating hormone (FSH) and LH levels [87].

Libido is influenced by several neurotransmitters, such as dopamine (DA) which implicates desire, acetylcholine (ACh) which mediates arousal, and γ-aminobutyric acid (GABA) that is needed to attain an orgasm. Receptor-ligand binding assays have shown that various ginsenosides including the PG specific Rg1 are agonists of the GABA(A) receptor [88]. These findings indicate that PG may have direct effects on the hypothalamic-pituitary-testicular (HPT) axis for both hormonal and neuronal regulation over male reproduction.

4.4 *Panax ginseng* on sperm count and motility

The pioneer report on the positive effects of ginseng on spermatogenesis was published in 1977 [89]. The study had demonstrated that ginseng extracts could stimulate rat testicular DNA and protein syntheses [89]. With advances in research, various studies on humans and rodents have reported that ginseng has positive effects on sperm count. Ginseng treatment in rats have been shown to increase the spermatogenic rate by inducing expression of glial cell-derived neurotrophic factor (GDNF) in the Sertoli cells [90] and activating the cAMP-responsive element modulator (CREM) in the testis [91]. GDNF acts as a possible regulator of the spermatogonial survival and differentiation [92] and is vital for spermatid maturation [93]. Little or absence of expression in CREM protein or mRNA have been shown to result in particular arrest of maturation of round spermatids, possibly causing male infertility [94]. PG use has been reported to have a positive impact over sperm density and motility in oligoasthenozoospermic patients as compared to that of healthy, age-matched controls [87]. PG has also been shown to improve progressive sperm motility in asthenozoospermia patients [95]. Specifically, the polysaccharide, aqueous, and organic fractions of PG correlate positively with increased directional sperm motility within 60–120 minutes in humans [96]. These functions may be mediated via activating the nitric oxide synthase (NOS) and generation of NO [97], which plays a major role in sperm physiology, enhancing capacitation as well as the acrosome reaction [98].

4.5 *Panax ginseng* and sperm preservation

Various ginseng species have been found to have immense applicability in the preservation of ejaculated sperms. There are evidences suggesting that incubation of ejaculated sperms with ginseng extracts significantly increases the sperm count as compared to that of vehicle-treated controls [99]. The active component in PG, ginsenoside Rg1, at a dose of 50 μg/mL has been reported to highly enhance sperm motility and integrity of sperm membrane of postthawed sperm when compared to that of untreated freshly thawed sperm [100]. Thus, PG may serve as a potent herbal agent that can ameliorate the quality of cryogen for sperm storage, thereby improving ART outcomes.

4.6 Mechanism of action of *Panax ginseng*

The active constituent of the ginseng ginsenosides are chemically triterpenoid saponins whose structure resembles that of steroid hormones. Male sexual behavior, gonadal development, and testicular functions such as steroidogenesis and spermatogenesis are largely regulated by androgens. The structural resemblance of ginsenosides to steroid hormones may suggest that it can activate steroid hormone receptors in the reproductive tissues regulating gametogenesis, steroidogenesis, and other gonadal functions. Expression of androgen receptor (AR) is high in male gonadal tissues as well as in spermatozoa [101], while in infertile men, these expressions become significantly reduced [102]. Ginsenosides may act as AR agonists to activate NOS and induce intracellular NO production. This increase in intracellular NO levels in spermatozoa is perhaps the key mechanism by which ginseng improves overall sperm functions, notably sperm capacitation and the acrosome reaction [98, 103, 104]. Ginseng-induced increase in NO production has also been shown to improve erectile dysfunction in a rodent model [76].

5 *Centella asiatica*: As an herbal medicine in andrology

C. asiatica L. (Urban), also known as the "Indian pennywort," "Asiatic pennywort," or "gotu kola," is renowned for its high medicinal value. This perennial herb from the Apiaceae family has been used for centuries for its multifunctional properties in Indian Ayurvedic medicine, as well as in herbal medicine in Malaysia, China, and other Asian regions [105]. *C. asiatica* (CA) has been traditionally used in the ancient medicinal systems throughout the world as a remedy for a wide range of disorders (reviewed in Ref. [106]). It is most popularly used for its neuroprotective activities and in the treatment of disorders concerning the central nervous system, such as for the treatment of mental fatigue and anxiety as well as memory enhancement (reviewed in Ref. [107]). Additionally, it is also known for its antiinflammatory [108] and antioxidant [109] properties among numerous others.

Bioactive compounds that have been isolated from CA include triterpene acids, polyphenolic compounds, glycosides, volatiles, fatty acids, and alkaloids [106]. Of these, the most biologically active constituents of CA are pentacyclic triterpenes such as asiatic acid, asiaticoside, madecassic acid, and madecassoside [110]. These compounds are potent antioxidants and are present in high amounts in the CA plant, contributing to its antioxidant properties. Other terpenoids found in CA include centelloside and brahmoside.

CA is also a rich source of phenols such as quercetin, kaempferol, and luteolin. The high concentration of phenolic compounds found in CA also serve as key contributors to the antioxidant activities of CA [111]. Besides these, carbohydrates (such as glucose and centellose) and amino acids (such as glutamate and aspartate) can be found in CA [106]. It is also a source of micronutrients such as sodium, iron, phosphorus, carotene, vitamins A, B, and C, and dietary fibers [112].

5.1 *Centella asiatica* and male contraception

Extracts of the CA leaves have been reported to be traditionally used as a male contraceptive in India and Eastern Asia [113]. Heidari and coworkers [113] studied the effects of CA on testicular tissue and spermatogenesis by administering the aqueous (crude) extract of CA leaves (at doses of 10, 50, 80, and 100 mg/kg) daily for 60 days in Wistar albino rats. They found that body weight was significantly higher, while testicular weight was significantly lower in CA-treated rats compared to that of the control group. In addition, these authors have reported a significant decrease in the number of epididymal sperm, sperm motility, and viability in rats given CA. Serum levels of testosterone, FSH, and LH in CA-treated rats were significantly reduced compared to the control group [113].

Moreover, the number of spermatogenic cells in the seminiferous tubules were significantly lower in CA-treated rats [113]. Degeneration of the Leydig cells and seminiferous tubules along with a decline in sperm density was also observed in the CA groups. Spermatogonia and spermatocytes of CA-treated rats showed signs of apoptosis compared to those in control rats. Thus, it was apparent that the crude extract of CA leaves (100 mg/kg) caused significant adverse effects on the reproductive system of male rats [113]. The negative effects of CA on spermatogenesis was also evident when oral administration of the ethanolic extract of CA leaves (125 mg/kg) for 30 days significantly lowered the number of spermatogonia, primary spermatocytes, and spermatids in fertile mice [114].

Yunianto's group demonstrated the dose-dependent effect (100, 200, and 300 mg/kg) of CA on sperm parameters and testicular tissue [115]. They showed that oral administration of ethanolic extract of CA at doses of 200 and 300 mg/kg for 42 consecutive days resulted in decreased sperm count and sperm motility, with the higher dose of 300 mg/kg giving a more pronounced effect. Serum testosterone levels were also decreased in CA-treated groups compared to controls in a dose-dependent manner. These changes in sperm parameters and testosterone level were accompanied by abnormalities of the seminiferous tubules and interstitial cells, particularly in the 300 mg/kg CA-treated group [115].

In a subsequent study, Yunianto and colleagues performed a proteomic analysis on sperm from proven fertile male rats given daily oral administration of CA (ethanol extract 300 mg/kg) for 42 consecutive days [116]. The percentage of infertile male rats was higher among the CA-treated rats (43.75%) compared to the control animals (18.75%). This was because the CA-treated rats had lower sperm count and fewer number of implantation sites in their female partner compared to the controls. In addition, sperms with abnormal morphology (e.g., flattened head and bent tail) were observed in CA-treated rats while those in the controls exhibited normal morphology (hook-shaped head and long straight tail) [116].

The researchers also identified 15 proteins of which 5 were differentially expressed in the CA-treated group [116]. Of the five proteins, α-enolase and aldolase A were upregulated and downregulated, respectively, in CA-treated rats. However, sorbitol dehydrogenase, glutamine synthetase, and lipocalin were absent in the sperm proteome of CA-treated rats. Both lipocalin and sorbitol dehydrogenase play important roles in spermatogenesis, with the former being involved in epididymal function and sperm maturation, while the latter is involved in sperm motility [116]. These animal studies suggest that CA exerts antispermatogenic and antifertility effects on the male reproductive system. Therefore, CA could potentially serve as a useful natural contraceptive agent in males.

The antifertility effects of CA on the reproductive system have also been observed in females. The CA leaf extracts (125, 200, 275, and 300 mg/kg) were shown to reduce the number of follicles (primary, secondary, and tertiary) and corpus luteum, theca cell thickness, and ovarian weight in mice [117]. In an earlier study, Fitriyah (2009) had reported that lower doses of CA extract (25 and 75 mg/kg) increased the number of primary, secondary, and tertiary follicles, while higher doses of CA (100 and 125 mg/kg) decreased the number of these follicles in the mice ovary [118].

5.2 Mechanism of action of *Centella asiatica*

Some studies suggest that CA may be useful as a natural contraceptive agent due to its antispermatogenesis and antifertility properties [113, 114, 116]. The primary constituents responsible for the pharmacological properties of CA are its active compounds: asiatic and madecassic acids, asiaticoside, and madecassoside. Higher doses of CA would contain a higher amount of these active ingredients. CA is also a rich source of flavonoids and terpenoids [119] and pentacyclic triterpenoid saponins (centelloids) [120].

Terpenoids such as asiaticoside, madecassoside, asiatic acid, madecassic acid, and brahmic acid are chemically triterpenoid saponins with structures that resemble that of steroid hormones. The total saponoside fraction of CA containing brahmic acid and its derivatives has been reported to negatively impact human and rat sperm leading to infertility [121]. Triterpenoid glycosides could exert adverse effects on the reproductive system by dysregulating the hypothalamus-pituitary-gonadal axis or via a direct cytotoxic effect on the testes, leading to impaired spermatogenesis [114, 122].

Aqueous extract of CA was shown to induce the apoptosis of spermatogenic cells (mainly spermatogonia and spermatocytes) thereby reducing fertility in male rats [113]. It was proposed that these CA-induced effects were due to a direct effect on the seminiferous tubules, causing degeneration of Leydig and Sertoli cells. Consequently, testosterone production and the spermatogenesis process are disrupted. It was also proposed that CA administration leads to an increase in the generation of peroxide radicals in the testes leading to germ cell apoptosis [113]. Germ cell death by apoptosis occurs during normal spermatogenesis to maintain normal germ cell development and sperm output [123]. CA treatment could lead to the activation of caspases [113], either through the intrinsic mitochondrial pathway or the extrinsic death receptor pathway, resulting in apoptosis.

Several experimental studies have examined the antioxidant properties of CA extracts. Concurrent treatment of CA aqueous extract in lead-exposed rats increased epididymal sperm count, sperm motility, and viability compared to that of the controls [124]. They also found that co-treatment with CA significantly decreased lipid peroxidation levels and increased SOD and catalase activities in the testes of lead-exposed rats compared to rats exposed only to lead. These results suggest that CA prevents the adverse effects of lead-induced oxidative stress on sperm parameters and testicular steroidogenic enzyme activities [124]. An earlier study reported that the ethanolic extract of CA whole plant has significantly higher antioxidative activity than the water extract [109]. The leaves and roots of CA have also been demonstrated to have high antioxidative activity that were comparable to that of alpha tocopherol. These effects were attributed to the phenolic content of CA [111].

Hussin et al. have evaluated the ability of CA extract and powder in reducing oxidative stress in the red blood cells of Sprague-Dawley rats. CA treatment for 25 weeks decreased ROS generation and H_2O_2 induced-oxidative stress in these rats, accompanied by an increase in catalase levels and a decrease in SOD levels. These effects may be due to the presence of antioxidant compounds in CA, particularly flavonoids such as quercetin, catechin, and rutin, which are known potent antioxidants [125]. The cardioprotective effect of CA (freeze-dried whole plant water extract) on myocardial markers and antioxidant enzymes have been reported in a cardiomyopathy animal model [126]. The whole plant powder of CA was reported to be effective in reducing lipid peroxidation and protein carbonyl levels, in addition to increasing the antioxidant status in regions of the brain [127].

When given crude methanol extract of CA whole plant for 14 days, the activities of antioxidant enzymes (glutathione peroxidase, SOD, catalase) and levels of antioxidants (glutathione, ascorbic acid) were significantly increased in both the liver and kidney of lymphoma-bearing mice [128]. The ethanolic extract of CA has also been found to enhance SOD activity in hepatocytes [129]. Treatment of diabetic male Sprague-Dawley rats with CA (500 mg/kg) for 14 days decreased hepatic malondialdehyde levels and increased the levels of reduced glutathione, along with the activities of glutathione S-transferase and glutathione peroxidase [130].

CA leaves were reported to possess higher antioxidant activity compared to other parts of the plants [111]. The phenolic compounds in CA could be a major contributor to its antioxidative activity, although the exact compounds are yet to be elucidated [124]. The antioxidant properties of CA could perhaps be attributed to one of its main active compounds, asiaticoside. Topical application of asiaticoside was found to cause a significant increase in the levels of both enzymatic antioxidants (catalase, glutathione peroxidase, SOD) and nonenzymatic antioxidants (vitamin E, ascorbic acid) in excision-type cutaneous wounds in rats, particularly at the initial stage of healing. These increases in antioxidant activity was accompanied by a reduction in lipid peroxidation [131]. Asiaticoside derivatives were also shown to reduce H_2O_2-induced cell death and intracellular concentrations of free radicals [132]. Asiaticoside is hydrolyzed in vivo into another major bioactive compound of CA, asiatic acid. Asiatic acid has also been reported to cause attenuation of oxidative stress [133].

6 Future perspectives

Over the years, a diverse array of natural products and herbal remedies have been used around the world to treat subfertility and disorders of the male reproductive system. In order to make these herbal medicines more widely accepted, particularly in the current modern medicine practices, evidence-based methods must to be applied to studies examining the safety and efficacy of herbal treatment. Pharmacokinetic, pharmacological, and clinical data are still lacking on most herbal medicinal products despite them having been used for centuries. The active compounds and standard doses of these herbs need to be clearly established to regulate its pharmacodynamics [134]. Large-scale, multicenter randomized controlled trials will be required for these herbal medicines to gain wider acceptance alongside the standard modern medicine. Investigations should also aim to elucidate the therapeutic mechanisms of herbal medicines in male infertility at a molecular and cellular level to better understand its drug efficacy [135].

The possibility of developing drugs that utilize the synergism either between herbal medicines or between herbal medicines and synthetic compounds deserves to be explored in the treatment of infertility. Synergistic effects may be result due to the ability of the bioactive constituents with different polarities to solubilize concurrently or to act on multiple different targets such as receptors, transport proteins, enzymes, and ion channels, thereby improving bioavailability [136]. The omics technologies may be utilized to further understand the underlying synergistic mechanisms and to establish combination therapies of herbal medicines and synthetic drugs that could improve treatment efficacy and reduce adverse reactions [137]. Further studies are also required to examine the efficacy of herbal medicines in the treatment of disorders related to male infertility with emphasis on its use either alone or as an adjuvant/concurrent therapy for male partners of couples seeking ART treatment.

7 Conclusion

Herbal medicines have been entrusted for use in the treatment of male infertility since ancient times, and in recent decades it is regaining its popularity. However, research regarding the efficacy of herbal medicine seems to be a rediscovery of ancient traditional medicines. This chapter has discussed numerous evidences that showed the various pharmacological effects of *W. somnifera*, *P. ginseng*, and *C. asiatica* on semen quality and also on sex hormones. The molecular mechanisms of actions of these herbs have also been presented for better understanding of their effects on male reproduction. It may be recommended that future studies should emphasize more on the synergistic effects of these herbal extracts with standard medicines in the treatment of male fertility. Moreover, further studies on the use of herbal components in ART would be beneficial. Advances in research, combination of standard medical therapy with herbal therapy, along with lifestyle modifications, may maximize the treatment efficacy in male infertility.

References

[1] Samy RP, Pushparaj PN, Gopalakrishnakone P. A compilation of bioactive compounds from Ayurveda. Bioinformation 2008;3(3):100.

[2] Gurib-Fakim A. Medicinal plants: traditions of yesterday and drugs of tomorrow. Mol Aspects Med 2006;27(1):1–93.

[3] Kuo Y-T, Liao H-H, Chiang J-H, Wu M-Y, Chen B-C, Chang C-M, et al. Complementary Chinese herbal medicine therapy improves survival of patients with pancreatic cancer in Taiwan: a nationwide population-based cohort study. Integr Cancer Ther 2018;17(2):411–22.

[4] Pandey MM, Rastogi S, Rawat AK. Indian traditional ayurvedic system of medicine and nutritional supplementation. Evid Based Complement Alternat Med 2013;2013:376327. https://doi.org/10.1155/2013/376327.

[5] Khaki A, Ainehchi N. Herbal medicine and sexual behavior in diabetic patients. Int J Womens Health Reprod Sci 2017;5:1–2.

[6] Ouladsahebmadarek E, Giasi GS, Khaki A, Ahmadi Y, Farzadi L, Ghasemzadeh A, et al. The effect of compound herbal remedy used in male infertility on spermatogenesis and pregnancy rate. Int J Womens Health Reprod Sci 2016;4(4):185–8.

[7] Crimmel AS, Conner CS, Monga M. Withered Yang: a review of traditional Chinese medical treatment of male infertility and erectile dysfunction. J Androl 2001;22(2):173–82.

[8] Clarke TC, Black LI, Stussman BJ, Barnes PM, Nahin RL. Trends in the use of complementary health approaches among adults: United States, 2002–2012. Natl Health Stat Rep 2015;79:1.

[9] Tambi M, Imran M, Henkel R. Standardised water-soluble extract of *Eurycoma longifolia*, Tongkat ali, as testosterone booster for managing men with late-onset hypogonadism? Andrologia 2012;44:226–30.

[10] Henkel RR, Wang R, Bassett SH, Chen T, Liu N, Zhu Y, et al. Tongkat Ali as a potential herbal supplement for physically active male and female seniors—a pilot study. Phytother Res 2014;28(4):544–50.

[11] Mansouri E, Keshtkar A, Khaki AA, Khaki A. Antioxidant effects of *Allium cepa* and cinnamon on sex hormones and serum antioxidant capacity in female rats exposed to power frequency electric and magnetic fields. Int J Womens Health Reprod Sci 2016;4:141–5.

[12] Lohiya N, Balasubramanian K, Ansari A. Indian folklore medicine in managing men's health and wellness. Andrologia 2016;48(8):894–907.

[13] Malviya N, Malviya S, Jain S, Vyas S. A review of the potential of medicinal plants in the management and treatment of male sexual dysfunction. Andrologia 2016;48(8):880–93.

[14] Agarwal A, Durairajanayagam D, Virk G, Du Plessis SS. Strategies to ameliorate oxidative stress during assisted reproduction. Springer; 2014.

[15] Dabaja AA, Schlegel PN. Medical treatment of male infertility. Transl Androl Urol 2014;3(1):9.

[16] Chachamovich J, Chachamovich E, Fleck M, Cordova FP, Knauth D, Passos E. Congruence of quality of life among infertile men and women: findings from a couple-based study. Hum Reprod 2009;24(9):2151–7.

[17] Agarwal A, Prabakaran S, Allamaneni SS. Relationship between oxidative stress, varicocele and infertility: a meta-analysis. Reprod Biomed Online 2006;12(5):630–3.

[18] Hall J. Infertility and contraception. In: Kasper D, Fauci A, Hauser S, Longo D, Jameson JL, Loscalzo J, editors. Harrison's principles of internal medicine. 19th ed; 2015. p. 2387–91.

[19] Chen X, Lee TJF. Ginsenosides-induced nitric oxide-mediated relaxation of the rabbit corpus cavernosum. Br J Pharmacol 1995;115(1):15–8.

[20] Abdillahi H, Van Staden J. South African plants and male reproductive healthcare: conception and contraception. J Ethnopharmacol 2012;143(2):475–80.

[21] Henkel R, Fransman W, Hipler UC, Wiegand C, Schreiber G, Menkveld R, et al. *Typha capensis* (Rohrb.) NE Br.(bulrush) extract scavenges free radicals, inhibits collagenase activity and affects human sperm motility and mitochondrial membrane potential in vitro: a pilot study. Andrologia 2012;44:287–94.

[22] Ilfergane A, Henkel R. Effect of *Typha capensis* (Rohrb.) NE Br. rhizome extract F1 fraction on cell viability, apoptosis induction and testosterone production in TM 3-Leydig cells. Andrologia 2018;50(2):e12854.

[23] Sapanidou VG, Margaritis I, Siahos N, Arsenopoulos K, Dragatidou E, Taitzoglou IA, et al. Antioxidant effect of a polyphenol-rich grape pomace extract on motility, viability and lipid peroxidation of thawed bovine spermatozoa. J Biol Res Thessaloniki 2014;21(1):19.

[24] Zhang H, Zhao H, Zhang A. Male infertility with severe oligospermatism and azoospermia treated by Bushen Shengjing Decoction combined with intracytoplasmic sperm injection. Zhongguo Zhong xi yi jie he za zhi Zhongguo Zhongxiyi jiehe zazhi = Chin J Integr Tradit West Med 2007;27(11):972–5.

[25] Belviranli M, Gökbel H, Okudan N, Büyükbaş S. Effects of grape seed extract on oxidative stress and antioxidant defensemarkers in streptozotocin-induced diabetic rats. Turk J Med Sci 2015;45(3):489–95.

[26] Maleki EM, Eimani H, Bigdeli MR, Ebrahimi B, Shahverdi AH, Narenji AG, et al. A comparative study of saffron aqueous extract and its active ingredient, crocin on the in vitro maturation, in vitro fertilization, and in vitro culture of mouse oocytes. Taiwan J Obstet Gynecol 2014;53(1):21–5.

[27] Dar NJ, Hamid A, Ahmad M. Pharmacologic overview of *Withania somnifera*, the Indian ginseng. Cell Mol Life Sci 2015;72(23):4445–60.

[28] Narinderpal K, Junaid N, Raman B. A review on pharmacological profile of *Withania somnifera* (Ashwagandha). Res Rev J Bot Sci 2013;2:6–14.

[29] Kuboyama T, Tohda C, Komatsu K. Effects of Ashwagandha (roots of *Withania somnifera*) on neurodegenerative diseases. Biol Pharm Bull 2014;37(6):892–7.

[30] RajaSankar S, Manivasagam T, Sankar V, Prakash S, Muthusamy R, Krishnamurti A, et al. *Withania somnifera* root extract improves catecholamines and physiological abnormalities seen in a Parkinson's disease model mouse. J Ethnopharmacol 2009;125(3):369–73.

[31] Mishra L-C, Singh BB, Dagenais S. Scientific basis for the therapeutic use of *Withania somnifera* (ashwagandha): a review. Altern Med Rev 2000;5(4):334–46.

[32] Dar NJ, Bhat JA, Satti NK, Sharma PR, Hamid A, Ahmad M. Withanone, an active constituent from *Withania somnifera*, affords protection against NMDA-induced excitotoxicity in neuron-like cells. Mol Neurobiol 2017;54(7):5061–73.

[33] Mirjalili M, Moyano E, Bonfill M, Cusido R, Palazón J. Steroidal lactones from *Withania somnifera*, an ancient plant for novel medicine. Molecules 2009;14(7):2373–93.

[34] Lavie D, Glotter E, Shvo Y. Constituents of *Withania somnifera* Dun. III. The side chain of withaferin A*, 1. J Org Chem 1965;30(6):1774–8.

[35] Chatterjee S, Srivastava S, Khalid A, Singh N, Sangwan RS, Sidhu OP, et al. Comprehensive metabolic fingerprinting of *Withania somnifera* leaf and root extracts. Phytochemistry 2010;71(10):1085–94.

[36] Kulkarni S, Dhir A. *Withania somnifera*: an Indian ginseng. Prog Neuro-Psychopharmacol Biol Psychiatry 2008;32(5):1093–105.

[37] Patel SB, Rao NJ, Hingorani LL. Safety assessment of *Withania somnifera* extract standardized for Withaferin a: acute and sub-acute toxicity study. J Ayurveda Integr Med 2016;7(1):30–7.

[38] Prabu P, Panchapakesan S, Raj CD. Acute and sub-acute oral toxicity assessment of the hydroalcoholic extract of *Withania somnifera* roots in Wistar rats. Phytother Res 2013;27(8):1169–78.

[39] Devkar ST, Kandhare AD, Sloley BD, Jagtap SD, Lin J, Tam YK, et al. Evaluation of the bioavailability of major withanolides of *Withania somnifera* using an in vitro absorption model system. J Adv Pharm Technol Res 2015;6(4):159.

[40] Begum VH, Sadique J. Long term effect of herbal drug *Withania somnifera* on adjuvant induced arthritis in rats. Indian J Exp Biol 1988;26(11):877–82.

[41] Kaileh M, Berghe WV, Heyerick A, Horion J, Piette J, Libert C, et al. Withaferin A strongly elicits IκB kinase β hyperphosphorylation concomitant with potent inhibition of its kinase activity. J Biol Chem 2007;282(7):4253–64.[42]Ashwagandha: Natural Product Database (NPD). Lexi-Comp. Inc. Available from: http://naturaldatabase.therapeuticresearch.com/nd/Search.aspx?cs=&s=ND&pt=9&Product=Ashwaganda&btnSearch.x=0&btnSearch.y=0.Ashwagandha: Natural Product Database (NPD). Lexi-Comp. Inc. Available from: http://naturaldatabase.therapeuticresearch.com/nd/Search.aspx?cs=&s=ND&pt=9&Product=Ashwaganda&btnSearch.x=0&btnSearch.y=0.

[43] Wadhwa R, Singh R, Gao R, Shah N, Widodo N, Nakamoto T, et al. Water extract of Ashwagandha leaves has anticancer activity: identification of an active component and its mechanism of action. PLoS One 2013;8(10):e77189.

[44] Shukla KK, Mahdi AA, Mishra V, Rajender S, Sankhwar SN, Patel D, et al. *Withania somnifera* improves semen quality by combating oxidative stress and cell death and improving essential metal concentrations. Reprod Biomed Online 2011;22(5):421–7.

[45] Mahdi AA, Shukla KK, Ahmad MK, Rajender S, Shankhwar SN, Singh V, Dalela D. *Withania somnifera* improves semen quality in stress-related male fertility. Evid Based Complement Alternat Med 2009;2011:576962. https://doi.org/10.1093/ecam/nep138.

[46] Ahmad MK, Mahdi AA, Shukla KK, Islam N, Rajender S, Madhukar D, et al. *Withania somnifera* improves semen quality by regulating reproductive hormone levels and oxidative stress in seminal plasma of infertile males. Fertil Steril 2010;94(3):989–96.

[47] Ambiye VR, Langade D, Dongre S, Aptikar P, Kulkarni M, Dongre A. Clinical evaluation of the spermatogenic activity of the root extract of Ashwagandha (*Withania somnifera*) in oligospermic males: a pilot study. Evid Based Complement Alternat Med 2013;2013:571420. https://doi.org/10.1155/2013/571420.

[48] Sahin K, Orhan C, Akdemir F, Tuzcu M, Gencoglu H, Sahin N, et al. Comparative evaluation of the sexual functions and NF-κB and Nrf2 pathways of some aphrodisiac herbal extracts in male rats. BMC Complement Altern Med 2016;16(1):318.

[49] Kumar A, Kumar R, Rahman MS, Iqubal MA, Anand G, Niraj PK, et al. Phytoremedial effect of *Withania somnifera* against arsenic-induced testicular toxicity in Charles Foster rats. Avicenna J Phytomedicine 2015;5(4):355.

[50] Bhargavan D, Deepa B, Shetty H, Krishna A. The protective effect of *Withania somnifera* against oxidative damage caused by ethanol in the testes of adult male rats. Int J Basic Clin Pharmacol 2015;4(6):1104–8.

[51] Dhumal R, Vijaykumar T, Dighe V, Selkar N, Chawda M, Vahlia M, et al. Efficacy and safety of a herbo-mineral ayurvedic formulation 'Afrodet Plus®' in male rats. J Ayurveda Integr Med 2013;4(3):158.

[52] Sengupta P, Agarwal A, Pogrebetskaya M, Roychoudhury S, Durairajanayagam D, Henkel R. Role of *Withania somnifera* (Ashwagandha) in the management of male infertility. Reprod Biomed Online 2018;36(3):311–26.

[53] Griveau J, Lannou DL. Reactive oxygen species and human spermatozoa: physiology and pathology. Int J Androl 1997;20(2):61–9.

[54] Sharma RK, Agarwal A. Role of reactive oxygen species in male infertility. Urology 1996;48(6):835–50.

[55] Gavella M, Lipovac V. NADH-dependent oxidoreductase (diaphorase) activity and isozyme pattern of sperm in infertile men. Arch Androl 1992;28(2):135–41.

[56] Finkel T, Holbrook NJ. Oxidants, oxidative stress and the biology of ageing. Nature 2000;408(6809):239.

[57] Chance B, Sies H, Boveris A. Hydroperoxide metabolism in mammalian organs. Physiol Rev 1979;59(3):527–605.

[58] de Lamirande E, Jiang H, Zini A, Kodama H, Gagnon C. Reactive oxygen species and sperm physiology. Rev Reprod 1997;2(1):48–54.

[59] Gharagozloo P, Aitken RJ. The role of sperm oxidative stress in male infertility and the significance of oral antioxidant therapy. Hum Reprod 2011;26(7):1628–40.

[60] Henkel R, Sandhu IS, Agarwal A. The excessive use of antioxidant therapy: a possible cause of male infertility? Andrologia 2019;51(1):e13162.

[61] Halliwell B. The antioxidant paradox. Lancet 2000;355(9210):1179–80.

[62] Biswas N, Chattopadhyay A, Sarkar M. Effects of gold on testicular steroidogenic and gametogenic functions in immature male albino rats. Life Sci 2004;76(6):629–36.

[63] Chandra AK, Sengupta P, Goswami H, Sarkar M. Excessive dietary calcium in the disruption of structural and functional status of adult male reproductive system in rat with possible mechanism. Mol Cell Biochem 2012;364(1–2):181–91.

[64] Nargund VH. Effects of psychological stress on male fertility. Nat Rev Urol 2015;12(7):373.

[65] Kataria H, Gupta M, Lakhman S, Kaur G. *Withania somnifera* aqueous extract facilitates the expression and release of GnRH: in vitro and in vivo study. Neurochem Int 2015;89:111–9.

[66] Ray S, Jha S. Production of withaferin A in shoot cultures of *Withania somnifera*. Planta Med 2001;67(05):432–6.

[67] López Rodríguez A, Rijsselaere T, Beek J, Vyt P, Van Soom A, Maes D. Boar seminal plasma components and their relation with semen quality. Syst Biol Reprod Med 2013;59(1):5–12.

[68] Gupta A, Mahdi AA, Shukla KK, Ahmad MK, Bansal N, Sankhwar P, et al. Efficacy of *Withania somnifera* on seminal plasma metabolites of infertile males: a proton NMR study at 800 MHz. J Ethnopharmacol 2013;149(1):208–14.

[69] Gershbein LL, Thielen DR. Enzymatic and electrolytic profiles of human semen. Prostate 1988;12(3):263–9.

[70] Leung KW, Wong AS. Ginseng and male reproductive function. Spermatogenesis 2013;3(3):e26391.

[71] Yun TK. Brief introduction of *Panax ginseng* CA Meyer. J Korean Med Sci 2001;16(Suppl):S3.

[72] Dehkordi RZ, Asadi E, Najafi A. Ginseng and male reproductive function. Int J Fertil Steril 2015;9:102.

[73] Hong B, Ji YH, Hong JH, Nam KY, Ahn TY. A double-blind crossover study evaluating the efficacy of Korean red ginseng in patients with erectile dysfunction: a preliminary report. J Urol 2002;168(5):2070–3.

[74] De Andrade E, De Mesquita AA, de Almeida CJ, De Andrade PM, Ortiz V, Paranhos M, et al. Study of the efficacy of Korean Red Ginseng in the treatment of erectile dysfunction. Asian J Androl 2007;9(2):241–4.

[75] Choi YD, Rha KH, Choi HK. In vitro and in vivo experimental effect of Korean red ginseng on erection. J Urol 1999;162(4):1508–11.

[76] Cho KS, Park CW, Kim C-K, Jeon HY, Kim WG, Lee SJ, et al. Effects of Korean ginseng berry extract (GB0710) on penile erection: evidence from in vitro and in vivo studies. Asian J Androl 2013;15(4):503.

[77] Murphy LL, LEE TJF. Ginseng, sex behavior, and nitric oxide. Ann N Y Acad Sci 2002;962(1):372–7.

[78] Toda N, Ayajiki K, Okamura T. Nitric oxide and penile erectile function. Pharmacol Ther 2005;106(2):233–66.

[79] Leung KW, Cheng Y-K, Mak NK, Chan KK, David Fan T, Wong RN. Signaling pathway of ginsenoside-Rg1 leading to nitric oxide production in endothelial cells. FEBS Lett 2006;580(13):3211–6.

[80] Wang X, Chu S, Qian T, Chen J, Zhang J. Ginsenoside Rg1 improves male copulatory behavior via nitric oxide/cyclic guanosine monophosphate pathway. J Sex Med 2010;7(2):743–50.

[81] Kim C, Choi H, Kim CC, Kim JK, Kim MS, Ahn BT, et al. Influence of ginseng on mating behavior of male rats. Am J Chin Med 1976;4(02):163–8.

[82] Yoshimura H, Kimura N, Sugiura K. Preventive effects of various ginseng saponins on the development of copulatory disorder induced by prolonged individual housing in male mice. Methods Find Exp Clin Pharmacol 1998;20:59–64.

[83] Nelson WO. The male sex hormone: Some factors controlling its production and some of its effects on the reproductive organs; 1937.

[84] Seftel AD, Mack RJ, Secrest AR, Smith TM. Restorative increases in serum testosterone levels are significantly correlated to improvements in sexual functioning. J Androl 2004;25(6):963–72.

[85] Fahim M, Fahim Z, Harman J, Clevenger T, Mullins W, Hafez E. Effect of *Panax ginseng* on testosterone level and prostate in male rats. Arch Androl 1982;8(4):261–3.

[86] Tsai S-C, Chiao Y-C, Lu C-C, Wang PS. Stimulation of the secretion of luteinizing hormone by ginsenoside-Rb1 in male rats. Chin J Physiol 2003;46(1):1–8.

[87] Salvati G, Genovesi G, Marcellini L, Paolini P, De IN, Pepe M, et al. Effects of *Panax ginseng* CA Meyer saponins on male fertility. Panminerva Med 1996;38(4):249–54.

[88] Kimura T, Saunders P, Kim H, Rheu H, Oh K, Ho I. Interactions of ginsenosides with ligand-bindings of GABA (A) and GABA (B) receptors. Gen Pharmacol 1994;25(1):193–9.

[89] Yamamoto M, Kumagai A, Yamamura Y. Stimulatory effect of *Panax ginseng* principles on DNA and protein synthesis in rat testes. Arzneimittelforschung 1977;27(7):1404–5.

[90] Yang WM, Park SY, Kim HM, Park EH, Park SK, Chang MS. Effects of *Panax ginseng* on glial cell-derived neurotrophic factor (GDNF) expression and spermatogenesis in rats. Phytother Res 2011;25(2):308–11.

[91] Park WS, Shin DY, Yang WM, Chang MS, Park SK. Korean ginseng induces spermatogenesis in rats through the activation of cAMP-responsive element modulator (CREM). Fertil Steril 2007;88(4):1000–2.

[92] Meng X, Lindahl M, Hyvönen ME, Parvinen M, de Rooij DG, Hess MW, et al. Regulation of cell fate decision of undifferentiated spermatogonia by GDNF. Science 2000;287(5457):1489–93.

[93] Behr R, Weinbauer G. cAMP response element modulator (CREM): an essential factor for spermatogenesis in primates? Int J Androl 2001;24(3):126–35.

[94] Steger K, Behr R, Kleiner I, Weinbauer GF, Bergmann M. Expression of activator of CREM in the testis (ACT) during normal and impaired spermatogenesis: correlation with CREM expression. Mol Hum Reprod 2004;10(2):129–35.

[95] Morgante G, Scolaro V, Tosti C, Di AS, Piomboni P, De VL. Treatment with carnitine, acetyl carnitine, L-arginine and ginseng improves sperm motility and sexual health in men with asthenopermia. Minerva Urol Nefrol = Ital J Urol Nephrol 2010;62(3):213–8.

[96] Chen J-C, Xu M-X, Chen L-D, Chen Y-N, Chiu TH. Effect of Panax notoginseng extracts on inferior sperm motility in vitro. Am J Chin Med 1999;27(01):123–8.

[97] Zhang H, Zhou Q-M, Li X-D, Xie Y, Duan X, Min F-L, et al. Ginsenoside Re increases fertile and asthenozoospermic infertile human sperm motility by induction of nitric oxide synthase. Arch Pharm Res 2006;29(2):145–51.

[98] Zhang H, Zhou Q, Li X, Zhao W, Wang Y, Liu H, et al. Ginsenoside Re promotes human sperm capacitation through nitric oxide-dependent pathway. Mol Reprod Dev Inc Gamete Res 2007;74(4):497–501.

[99] Wiwanitkit V. In vitro effect of ginseng extract on sperm count. Sex Disabil 2005;23(4):241–3.

[100] Kim DY, Hwang YJ. Effects of ginsenoside-Rg1 on post-thawed miniature pig sperm motility, mitochondria activity, and membrane integrity. J Embryo Transfer 2013;28:63–71.

[101] Solakidi S, Psarra AG, Nikolaropoulos S, Sekeris CE. Estrogen receptors α and β (ERα and ERβ) and androgen receptor (AR) in human sperm: localization of ERβ and AR in mitochondria of the midpiece. Hum Reprod 2005;20(12):3481–7.

[102] Zalata AA, Mokhtar N, Badawy AE-N, Othman G, Alghobary M, Mostafa T. Androgen receptor expression relationship with semen variables in infertile men with varicocele. J Urol 2013;189(6):2243–7.

[103] Furukawa T, Bai C-X, Kaihara A, Ozaki E, Kawano T, Nakaya Y, et al. Ginsenoside Re, a main phytosterol of *Panax ginseng*, activates cardiac potassium channels via a nongenomic pathway of sex hormones. Mol Pharmacol 2006;70(6):1916–24.

[104] Yu J, Eto M, Akishita M, Kaneko A, Ouchi Y, Okabe T. Signaling pathway of nitric oxide production induced by ginsenoside Rb1 in human aortic endothelial cells: a possible involvement of androgen receptor. Biochem Biophys Res Commun 2007;353(3):764–9.

[105] Brinkhaus B, Lindner M, Schuppan D, Hahn EG. Chemical, pharmacological and clinical profile of the East Asian medical plant *Centella asiatica*. Phytomedicine 2000;7(5):427–48.

[106] Belwal T, Andola HC, Atanassova MS, Joshi B, Suyal R, Thakur S, et al. Gotu Kola (*Centella asiatica*). In: Nabavi S, Silva AS, editors. Nonvitamin and nonmineral nutritional supplements. 1st ed. Elsevier; 2019. p. 265–75.

[107] Kant R, Srivastav PP, Datta AK. The medicinal role of *Centella asiatica* and its applications in the Dahi: a research review. J Pharm Res Int 2019;28(6):1–9.

[108] Somchit M, Sulaiman M, Zuraini A, Samsuddin L, Somchit N, Israf D, et al. Antinociceptive and antiinflammatory effects of *Centella asiatica*. Indian J Pharmacol 2004;36(6):377–80.

[109] Hamid AA, Md. Shah Z, Muse R, Mohamed S. Characterisation of antioxidative activities of various extracts of *Centella asiatica* (L) Urban. J Food Chem 2002;77:465–9.

[110] Inamdar PK, Yeole RD, Srivastava MM, De Souza NJ. Stability study of the active constituents in the *Centella asiatica* extract formulations. Drug Dev Ind Pharm 1996;22(3):211–6.

[111] Zainol MK, Hamid AA, Yusof S, Muse S. Antioxidant activity and total phenolic compounds of leaf, root and petiole of four accessions of *Centella asiatica* (L.) urban. Food Chem 2003;67:456–66.

[112] Hashim P, Sidek H, Helan MH, Sabery A, Palanisamy UD, Ilham M. Triterpene composition and bioactivities of *Centella asiatica*. Molecules 2011;16(2):1310–22.

[113] Heidari M, Heidari-Vala H, Sadeghi MR, Akhondi MM. The inductive effects of *Centella asiatica* on rat spermatogenic cell apoptosis in vivo. J Nat Med 2012;66(2):271–8.

[114] Hasaaanah IW. Pengaruh ekstrak daun pegagan (*Centella asiatica*) terhadap spermatogenesis mencit (*Mus musculus*). Indonesia: Universitas Islam Negeri Maulana Malik Ibrahim Malang; 2009.

[115] Yunianto I, Das S, Mat NM. Antispermatogenic and antifertility effect of Pegaga (*Centella asiatica* L) on the testis of male Sprague-Dawley rats. Clin Ter 2010;161(3):235–9.

[116] Yunianto I, Bashah NAK, Noor MM. Antifertility properties of *Centella asiatica* ethanolic extract as a contraceptive agent: preliminary study of sperm proteomic. Asian Pacific J Reprod 2017;6(5):212–6.

[117] Muchtaromah B, Romaidi, Griani TP, Hasfita Y. Potential antifertilty of *Centella asiatica* leaf extract. Aust J Basic Appl Sci 2015;9(7):102–5.

[118] Fitriyah. Pengaruh Pemberian Ekstrak Pegagan (*Centella asiatica* (L.) Urban) Terhadap Perkembangan Folikel Ovarium Mencit (*Mus musculus*) Betina. Indonesia: Universitas Islam Negeri Maulana Malik Ibrahim Malang; 2009.

[119] Roy D, Barman S, Shaik M. Current updates on *Centella asiatica*: phytochemistry, pharmacology and traditional uses. Med Plant Res 2013;3(4):70–7.

[120] James JT, Dubery IA. Pentacyclic triterpenoids from the medicinal herb, *Centella asiatica* (L.) urban. Molecules 2009;14(10):3922–41.

[121] Singh B, Rastogi R. Chemical examination of *Centella asiatica* linn-III. Constitution of brahmic acid. Phytochemistry 1968;7(8):1385–93.

[122] Amilah S, Sukarjati S, Rachmatin DP, Masruroh M. Leaf and petiole extract of *Centella asiatica* are potential for antifertility and antimicrobial material. Folia Medica Indonesiana 2019;55(3):188–97.

[123] Sinha Hikim AP, Swerdloff RS. Hormonal and genetic control of germ cell apoptosis in the testis. Rev Reprod 1999;4(1):38–47.

[124] Sainath SB, Meena R, Supriya C, Reddy KP, Reddy PS. Protective role of *Centella asiatica* on lead-induced oxidative stress and suppressed reproductive health in male rats. Environ Toxicol Pharmacol 2011;32(2):146–54.

[125] Hussin M, Abdul-Hamid A, Mohamad S, Saari N, Ismail M, Bejo M. Protective effect of *Centella asiatica* extract and powder on oxidative stress in rats. Food Chem 2007;100(2):535–41.

[126] Gnanapragasam A, Ebenezar KK, Sathish V, Govindaraju P, Devaki T. Protective effect of *Centella asiatica* on antioxidant tissue defense system against adriamycin induced cardiomyopathy in rats. Life Sci 2004;76(5):585–97.

[127] Subathra M, Shila S, Devi MA, Panneerselvam C. Emerging role of *Centella asiatica* in improving age-related neurological antioxidant status. Exp Gerontol 2005;40(8–9):707–15.

[128] Jayashree G, Kurup Muraleedhara G, Sudarslal S, Jacob VB. Anti-oxidant activity of *Centella asiatica* on lymphoma-bearing mice. Fitoterapia 2003;74(5):431–4.

[129] Jatayu D, Nursyam H, Hertika A. Antioxidant effect of *Centella asiatica* ethanolic extract to superoxide dismutase (SOD) level on *Cyprinus carpio* liver. Res J Life Sci 2018;5(3):163–72.

[130] Oyenihi AB, Chegou NN, Oguntibeju OO, Masola B. *Centella asiatica* enhances hepatic antioxidant status and regulates hepatic inflammatory cytokines in type 2 diabetic rats. Pharm Biol 2017;55(1):1671–8.

[131] Shukla A, Rasik AM, Dhawan BN. Asiaticoside-induced elevation of antioxidant levels in healing wounds. Phytother Res 1999;13(1):50–4.

[132] Mook-Jung I, Shin JE, Yun SH, Huh K, Koh JY, Park HK, et al. Protective effects of asiaticoside derivatives against beta-amyloid neurotoxicity. J Neurosci Res 1999;58(3):417–25.

[133] Lv J, Sharma A, Zhang T, Wu Y, Ding X. Pharmacological review on asiatic acid and its derivatives: a potential compound. SLAS Technol 2018;23(2):111–27.

[134] Parveen A, Parveen B, Parveen R, Ahmad S. Challenges and guidelines for clinical trial of herbal drugs. J Pharm Bioallied Sci 2015;7(4):329–33.

[135] Zhou SH, Deng YF, Weng ZW, Weng HW, Liu ZD. Traditional Chinese medicine as a remedy for male infertility: a review. World J Mens Health 2019;37(2):175–85.

[136] Wagner H, Ulrich-Merzenich G. Synergy research: approaching a new generation of phytopharmaceuticals. Phytomedicine 2009;16(2–3):97–110.

[137] Ulrich-Merzenich G, Panek D, Zeitler H, Wagner H, Vetter H. New perspectives for synergy research with the "omic"-technologies. Phytomedicine 2009;16(6–7):495–508.

Chapter 5.4.2

Herbal medicine used to treat andrological problems: Asia and Indian subcontinent: Tongkat Ali (*Eurycoma longifolia* jack)

Ismail Tambi

Men Wellness Clinic, Damai Service Hospital, Kuala Lumpur, Malaysia

Herbal medicines originated since the dawn of mankind. Plants provide basic necessities in the form of roof, food, warmth, clothing, and wellness. In the context of wellness, specific plants are used for the treatment of specific diseases. Traditional healers chopped tree barks and dug up roots and decoction of these were given to the tribes to treat their ailments. Enhancement of wellness and strength had placed these discoveries as miracle or "magic potion" and were revered forever. Tongkat Ali (T. Ali) was one of such discoveries.

Men who consume decoction of the dried roots of Tongkat Ali found energized, virile, fertile, and never tied out. This "magical secrets" were handed down from generation to generation but were eventually found out by the British Colonists who were ethnobotanists, looking for plants with medicinal properties in the new land. The discovery of the Malay traditional medicine manuscript published in 1930 by Garden Bulletin as "The Medical Book of Malayan Medicine" edited by Dr. J. D. Gimlett and I. H. Burkill glorified Malayan plants among which is the Simaroubaceae species, *Eurycoma longifolia* jack, the fabulous T. Ali [1] was the beginning of the journey of the elixir for men.

T. Ali or *E. longifolia* jack, as it is scientifically known, from Malaysia has come a long way from just a common rainforest jungle herb to a world class herbal supplement. The herbal shrub is also native to Indonesia, Vietnam, Cambodia, Myanmar, Laos, and Thailand. However, the phytocompounds found in these plants are unique for each of these Asian countries [2, 3]. *E. longifolia* is a folk medicine well known for its aphrodisiac effects as well as is used to treat sexual dysfunction, aging, malaria, cancer, diabetes, anxiety, aches, constipation, exercise recovery, fever, increase energy, increase strength, leukemia, osteoporosis, stress, syphilis, and glandular swelling, and intermittent fever (malaria) in Asia [4]. Traditionally, the water decoction of the *E. longifolia* root is consumed. Nowadays, more convenient formulations are available, primarily additives mixed with teas and coffees, and over 200 products are available either in the form of raw crude root powder or as capsules mixed with other herbs in the health-food market [5].

T. Ali, which literally means "Ali's walking stick," refers to its aphrodisiac property, strength, and energy and probably that is the reason it is named after a famous ancient Islamic Warrior, the son-in-law of Prophet Mohammad, "Ali." It has made an impact in the international market and is one of the sought after herbal ingredients.

T. Ali is an evergreen [5], tall, slender, shrubby tree, which grows in sandy soil. Besides *E. longifolia* jack, being locally known as Ali's cane, there are three other plant species, namely *Entomophthora apiculata*, *Polyalthia bullata*, and *Goniothalamus* sp. [4]. However, *E. longifolia* jack is the only species that have been much studied. It belongs to the Simaroubaceae family and has compound leaves on branches that can grow up to 1 m long. The shrubs grow slowly and reach up to 15–18 m in height on jungle slopes where they receive adequate shade and water [5]. The tree starts bearing fruits after 2–3 years, yet complete maturation takes up to 25 years. Its long, twisted roots are harvested, and aqueous concoctions are used by the local people to restore energy and vitality [5] or for its aphrodisiac properties [6]. Particularly, the roots of *E. longifolia* contain a wide variety of chemical compounds including alkaloids, quassinoids, quassinoid diterpenoids, eurycomaoside, euycolactone, laurycolactone or eurycomalactona [7–9]. Recently, liquid chromatography-tandem mass spectrometry method for the simultaneous determination of six major quassinoids of *E. longifolia*, i.e., eurycomanone, 13α (21)-epoxyeurycomanone, 13, 21-dihydroeurycomanone, 14,15β-dihydroxyklaineanone, longilactone, and eurycomalactone was developed. By using the liquid chromatography-mass spectrometry (LC-MS) method, the content of these quassinoids was measured in dietary supplement tablets and capsules to confirm the purity of *E. longifolia* in commercial products [10].

Herbal Medicine in Andrology. https://doi.org/10.1016/B978-0-12-815565-3.00016-3

A patented, standardized water-soluble extract of *E. longifolia* has undergone numerous clinical trials and evaluations locally and internationally and has been found to be a specifically beneficial botanical optimizing men's sexual and reproductive health as well as for general wellness. The standardized water-soluble extract contains phenolic compounds, tannins, high molecular weight polysaccharides, polypeptides with 30–39 amino acids and 4300 Da (labeled as eurypeptides), glycoprotein and mucopolysaccharides [11]. The eurypeptides and glycoprotein complex exert antioxidant and antinitrogen effects that promote cellular energizer, anticancer, pro-fertility, aphrodisiacs, antiaging and many more properties. Although *E. longifolia* has been used in traditional medicine for generations in Malaysia, it was only in the late 1990s that researchers started to pay more attention to its safe dosage and toxicity profile. Safety studies carried out thus far show that *E. longifolia* concentrations used therapeutically (2.5 μg/mL) appear not to have any detrimental effects on human spermatozoa in vitro [2]. However, at concentrations higher than 100 μg/mL, cytotoxic effects might occur [12, 13], supporting in vivo data by Tambi and Kadir that the extract is not toxic [14]. The water-based fraction of *E. longifolia* is considered the safest among others, as its LD50 value is comparatively higher (>3000 mg/kg) than other fractions, therefore this needs attention when using different fractions of *E. longifolia* and proper reference of the corresponding range of LD50 [15]. Numerous studies have shown that the extract is nontoxic to the vital bodily functions even at a high dose of 600 mg. The standardized water-soluble extract has been patented in the United States (US patent no. 7132117) after having gone through extensive animal and human clinical evaluation [16]. Extended studies on the same extract have proven the herb to be an energizer, an aphrodisiac, and an ergogenic botanical which also facilitate muscle fatigue recovery and antistress. Henkel et al. investigated the ergogenic effect of *E. longifolia* in elderly people and found that it is a potential herbal supplement for physically active aged male and female (age 57–72 years). Treatment resulted in significant increases in total and free testosterone concentrations and muscular force in men and women when *E. longifolia* extract 400 mg/day was used for 5 weeks [17]. It is a potent adaptogen as well [18–20].

The overall effects of *E. longifolia* on various hormones are also positive. It enhanced total testosterone and DHEA (dehydroepiandrosterone) which also modulate testosterone level, ensuring enough free testosterone for the body's need. Its other adaptogenic effects include positive effect on body cortisol levels as well as on growth hormone as it modulates the release of IGF-1 [20–22]. The water-soluble extract of *E. longifolia* extracts was reported to be able to enhance male fertility (with regard to higher semen volumes, spermatozoa count, and motility) in rodents [23, 24] and in human trials [25–28]. With regard to male infertility as seen by low semen volume, low sperm concentration, low sperm motility, and low percentage of spermatozoa with normal morphology, the consumption of the standardized water-soluble extract of T. Ali has been found to improve these parameters significantly. A randomized, double-blind, placebo-controlled, parallel group study was conducted to investigate the aphrodisiac clinical evidence of *E. longifolia* extract in men. The 12-week study in 109 men between 30 and 55 years of age is divided into a group of 300 mg of water extract of *E. longifolia* treated and placebo. The *E. longifolia* group showed higher scores in the overall erectile function domain (IIEF, $P < .001$), the sexual libido (14% by week 12), seminal fluid analysis (SFA) with sperm motility at 44.4%, and semen volume at 18.2% after treatment [26]. Yet another study showed that men with idiopathic normo-gonadotropic infertility were able to sire pregnancies through their wives after the consumption of T. Ali in as little as 3 months [27]. In another study conducted to demonstrate the effect of *E. longifolia* on spermatozoa, Erasmus et al. treated semen samples with *E. longifolia* extract (in vitro condition), and found a significant dose-dependent trends for vitality, total motility, acrosome reaction, and reactive oxygen species-positive spermatozoa without deleterious effects on sperm functions at therapeutically used concentrations (<2.5) [28].

A randomized controlled trial investigating *E. longifolia* compared to placebo by Kotirum et al. postulated that *E. longifolia* root extract may have a clinical benefit on improving erectile dysfunction experience by men. Based on current evidence, the standardized extract of *E. longifolia* may have clinical effect on erectile dysfunction; however this needs further clinical evidence of efficacy trials to make any firm recommendation [29]. A recent study by Udani et al. on the effect of T. Ali on sexual performance and well-being, a randomized, double-blind, and placebo-controlled study on 14 healthy males with mild ED, showed that T. Ali significantly improves sexual performance and satisfaction compared to the placebo group [30]. He highlighted the uniqueness of T. Ali in improving penile erection, penile hardness, and other important parameters of male sexual health, substantiating the therapeutic feasibility of T. Ali in the management of ED. Udani and coworkers proposed that daily intake of T. Ali can improve physical health, erectile performance, sexual desire and satisfaction, and the meaningful improvement in overall male sexual activities, compared to placebo groups [30]. In yet another recent study T. Ali extract enriched cream when gently rubbed to the glans penis in men with mild ED created confidence and ability to keep erection for penetrative sex [31]. It has been established that the mechanism of erection is through the relaxation of the smooth muscle of the corpus cavernosum of the penis and the relaxation of the penile arteries is contributed by the Rho-kinase potential of T. Ali [32].

Male senesce as menopause in women is a recognized condition. In a pilot study, Henkel et al. investigated the ergogenic effect of *E. longifolia* in elderly people and found that it is a potential herbal supplement for physically active aged male and female (age 57–72 years). Treatment resulted in significant increases in total and free testosterone concentrations and muscular force in men and women, when *E. longifolia* extract 400 mg/day was used for 5 weeks [17].

In a study, men with late-onset hypogonadism with typical symptoms of lethargy, generalized debility, and poor libido and low testosterone with poor score of the AMS (Aging Male Score) did well with testosterone replacement therapy [33]. Tambi et al. treated a group of patients suffering from late-onset hypogonadism (LOH) with T. Ali extract, which showed significantly ($P < .0001$) improved the AMS score as well as the serum testosterone concentration. Thus, T. Ali extract appears to be useful as a supplement in overcoming the symptoms of LOH and for the management of hypogonadism [34]. The testosterone deficiency syndrome (TDS) can be characterized by numerous symptoms, including low libido, fatigue, increased fat mass, osteoporosis, or erectile dysfunction, and up to 80% of men have experienced some sort of AMS [33]. Conventionally, TDS is treated with testosterone replacement therapy (TRT). With the beneficial effects of this therapy, significant adverse effects have been indicated, including prostate cancer [33]. *E. longifolia* is the herbal alternative to TRT, which has been shown to successfully restore serum testosterone levels, and significantly improve the physical condition and sexual health of patients [33]. Therefore, *E. longifolia* might be considered a safe alternative to TRT [33]. Supplementation with water-soluble extract of T. Ali has been found to improve the LOH symptoms tremendously [34] by the phytoandrogenic properties of T. Ali through its functions as a natural alternative to testosterone replacement therapy [33]. Knowing that aging has some element of stress and general debility, Talbott et al. studied and inferred that T. Ali root extract improves stress hormone profile (lower cortisol; higher testosterone) and certain mood state parameters (lower tension, anger, and confusion) [35]. These findings are in agreement with several recent supplementation trials in humans, suggesting that T. Ali may be an effective approach to shielding the body from the detrimental effects of chronic stress from daily stressors, dieting for weight loss, sleep deprivation, and intense exercise training [35].

Osteoporosis in men is receiving attention in men's health issue as it is becoming one of the main causes of morbidity and mortality in older men [36]. Approximately 2 million men in the United States suffer from osteoporosis [36]. Worldwide, one in three women over the age of 50 years will experience osteoporotic fractures, as will one in five men [36–38]. *E. longifolia* may well be the best herbal supplement that can be a perfect remedy for this condition. The possible reasons for this are discussed. According to Tambi and Kamarul, *E. longifolia* contains high concentrations of superoxide dismutase (SOD), an antioxidant that plays an important role in counteracting oxidative stress [27]. Other components of *E. longifolia*, such as alkaloids and triterpenes, can also act as antioxidants that may reduce bone loss and maintain the bone formation rate [39]. Recently, it was established that *E. longifolia* may be used in the prevention and treatment of osteoporosis, or more specifically, male osteoporosis. Shuid et al. showed that both testosterone replacement and *E. longifolia* supplementation to orchidectomized rats were able to maintain the bone calcium levels, with the former showing better effects. Hence *E. longifolia* prevented bone calcium loss in orchidectomized rats and thus has the potential to be used as an alternative treatment for androgen-deficient osteoporosis [40]. The bioactive complex polypeptides from the *E. longifolia* root extract, labeled as eurypeptides, can exert and enhance their effects on the biosynthesis of various androgens [41]. Eurypeptides acts by stimulating dehydroepiandrosterone (DHEA) [34]. DHEA in turn will act on androgen receptors to initiate the conversion of androstenedione and androstenediol to testosterone and estrogen, respectively [33]. These eurypeptides may also alleviate sex hormone binding globulin (SHBG) levels and subsequently increase the free testosterone level [42]. Due to these proandrogen properties of *E. longifolia*, they are able to stimulate osteoblast proliferation and differentiation, resulting in increased bone formation rate. High levels of testosterone and estrogen may also exert proapoptotic effects on osteoclasts, reducing the bone resorptive activity. As testosterone levels decrease with age, it has been suggested that men can consume *E. longifolia* (at suitable dosages) as a supplement [34]. Male osteoporosis can also be explained in terms of an oxidative stress mechanism. Free radicals, mainly reactive oxygen species (ROS), are efficiently scavenged in the body. However, oxidative stress will occur when there is an imbalance between increased ROS levels and inadequate antioxidant activity [43]. Orchiectomy (a model of androgen-deficient osteoporosis) can promote upregulation of ROS, which leads to oxidative stress. Oxidative stress plays a role in osteoblast apoptosis and osteoclast differentiation [44]. There are several mechanisms proposed for its antiosteoporotic effects. The main mechanism is via its testosterone-enhancing effects for the prevention and treatment of androgen-deficient osteoporosis [4, 39]. Other mechanisms involved are its nitric oxide generation and antioxidative properties. Androgen-deficient osteoporosis in men is treated with testosterone therapy, which is associated with many side effects. *E. longifolia* exerts proandrogenic effects that enhance the testosterone level, as well as stimulate osteoblast proliferation and osteoclast apoptosis. This will maintain bone remodeling activity and reduce bone loss. Phytochemical components of *E. longifolia* may also prevent osteoporosis via its antioxidative property. Hence, *E. longifolia* has the potential as a complementary treatment for male osteoporosis [39].

Androgens such as testosterone and 5α-dihydrotestosterone (DHT) are important for the development, maturation, and function of the prostate gland. Nevertheless, deregulation of the androgen receptor (AR) pathway has been implicated in benign and malignant prostate disorders, such as benign prostatic hypertrophy (BPH) and prostate cancer [45, 46]. Since an elevation of testosterone has been associated with an increased risk for prostate carcinogenesis, it would be pertinent to evaluate if *E. longifolia* extract would trigger this if consumed for a long time. Tong et al. investigated the in vitro and in vivo anticancer activities of a standardized quassinoid mixture (SQ40) from *E. longifolia* on LNCaP human prostate cancer cells, and showed that it induced selective cytotoxicity on human prostate cancer cells and inhibited the growth of LNCaP cells. SQ40 also inhibited androgen receptor translocation to nucleus which is important for the transactivation of its target gene, prostate-specific antigen (PSA), and resulted in a significant reduction in PSA secretion after the treatment [47]. The antitumorigenic activity of SQ40 was successfully demonstrated in the mouse xenograft model [47]. Thus *E. longifolia* has the potential of being a prostate cancer protective if taken as a health supplement.

Chronic hyperglycemia in diabetes affects glucose metabolism and an array of heath conditions including low testosterone, peripheral neuropathy, and erectile dysfunction in men. An herbal health supplement that can modulate glucose as well as a host of other properties like boost testosterone production and function as a pro-erectile herbal supplement would be of value to men. *E. longifolia* extract has been investigated to explore its hypoglycemia properties. In a study using streptozotocin-induced hyperglycemic adult rats, treated with 150 mg/kg body weight using aqueous extracts of *E. longifolia*, blood glucose levels decreased by 38% ($P<.05$) and 47% ($P<.001$) for two different *E. longifolia* extracts. However, in normo-glycemic rats, no significant reduction was noted when the same extracts were used [48]. *E. longifolia* root extract increased insulin sensitivity through the enhancement of glucose uptake by more than 200% at 50 g/mL and suppressed lipid accumulation in a concentration-dependent manner, inferring that the ability of *E. longifolia* to suppress lipid production would provide additional benefits in the treatment of diabetes [49].

1 Conclusion

With all these ample scientific and clinical findings, standardized patented water-soluble extract of T. Ali has emerged as a potent botanical supplement in men's health and a most sought-after herbal ingredient for supplementary product and supplement formulary for men's health.

This Malaysian herbal extract is on the shelves of many pharmacies in the United States, Japan, Eastern Europe, the Middle East, Hong Kong, and the Far East as an herbal medicine in the mainstream health care in managing men's health.

References

[1] Burkill IH, Hanif M. Malay village medicine, prescriptions collected. Gardens Bull Strait Settlements 1930;6:176–7.
[2] Hussein S, Ibrahim R, LingPick K. A summary of reported chemical constituents and medicinal uses of *Eurycoma longifolia*. J Trop Med Plants 2007;8:103–10.
[3] Chua LS, Amin NAM, Neo JCH, Lee TH, Lee CT, Sarmidi MR, Aziz RA. LC-MS/MS-based metabolites of *Eurycoma longifolia* (Tongkat Ali) in Malaysia (Perak and Pahang). J Chromatogr B 2011;879:3909–19.
[4] Rehman SU, Choe K, Yoo HH. Review on a traditional herbal medicine, *Eurycoma longifolia* Jack (Tongkat Ali): its traditional uses, chemistry, evidence-based pharmacology and toxicology. Molecules 2016;21(3):331.
[5] Bhat R, Karim AA. Tongkat Ali (*Eurycoma longifolia* Jack): a review on its ethnobotany and pharmacological importance. Fitoterapia 2010;10:1–11.
[6] Zanoli P, Zavatti M, Montanari C, Baraldi M. Influence of *Eurycoma longifolia* on the copulatory activity of sexually sluggish and impotent male rats. J Ethnopharmacol 2009;126:308–13.
[7] Morita H, Kishi E, Takeya K, Itokawa H, Iitaka Y. Squalene derivatives from *Eurycoma longifolia*. Phytochemistry 1993;4:765–71.
[8] Ang HH, Hitotsuyanagi Y, Fukuya H, Takeya K. Quassinoids from *Eurycoma longifolia*. Phytochemistry 2002;59:833–7.
[9] Bedir E, Abou-Gazar H, Ngwendson JN, Khan IA. Eurycomaoiside: a new quassinoid-type glycoside from the root of *Eurycoma longifolia*. Chem Pharm Bull (Tokyo) 2003;51:1301–3.
[10] Han YM, Jang M, Kim IS, Kim SH, Yoo HH. Simultaneous quantitation of six major quassinoids in Tongkat Ali dietary supplements by liquid chromatography with tandem mass spectrometry. J Sep Sci 2015;38:2260–6.
[11] Asiah O, Nurhanan MY, Ilham MA. Determination of bioactive peptide (4.3 kDa) as an aphrodisiac marker in six Malaysia plants. J Trop For Sci 2007;19:61–3.
[12] Kuo PC, Damu AG, Lee KH, Wu TS. Cytotoxic and antimalarial constituents from the roots of *Eurycoma longifolia*. Biorg Med Chem 2004;12:537–44.
[13] Nurhanan M, Hawariah L, Ilham AM, Shukri M. Cytotoxic effects of the root extracts of *Eurycoma longifolia* Jack. Phytother Res 2005;19:994–6.
[14] Sulaiman B, Jaafar A, Mansor M. Some medicinal plants from Sungai Kinchin, Pahang, Malaysia. Malay Nat J 1990;43:267.
[15] Shuid A, Siang L, Chin T, Muhammad N, Mohamed N, Soelaiman I. Acute and subacute toxicity studies of *Eurycoma longifolia* in male rats. Int J Pharm 2011;7:641–6.
[16] Sambandan TG, Rha C, Kadir AA, Aminudim N, Saad JM. Bioactive fraction of *Eurycoma longifolia*. US Patent: US7, 132, 117; 2006.
[17] Henkel RR, Wang R, Bassett SH, Chen T, Liu N, Zhu Y, Tambi MI. Tongkat Ali as a potential herbal supplement for physically active male and female seniors—a pilot study. Phytother Res 2014;28:544–50.
[18] Hamzah S, Yusof A. The ergogenic effects of Tongkat Ali (*Eurycoma longifolia*). Br J Sports Med 2003;37:465–6.

[19] Tambi MI. Glycoprotein water-soluble extract of *Eurycoma Longifolia* Jack as a health supplement in management of Health aging in aged men. In: Lunenfeld B, editor. Abstracts of the 3rd World Congress on the Aging Male, February 7–10. Germany: Berlin; 2002. *Aging Male* 2002;6 (Elsevier).

[20] Tambi MI. *Eurycoma Longifolia* jack: a potent adaptogen in the form of water-soluble extract with the effect of maintaining men's health. Asian J Androl 2006;8(1):49–50.

[21] Tambi MI. Standardized water soluble extract of *Eurycoma Longifolia* (LJ100) on men's health. Int J Androl 2005;28(1):27.

[22] Tambi MI. Standardized water soluble extract of *Eurycoma Longifolia* LJ100 maintains healthy aging in man. In: Lunenfeld B, editor. Abstracts of the 5th World Congress on the Aging Male, February 9–12. Salzburg: Austria; 2006. Aging Male 2006;9 (Elsevier).

[23] Low BS, Das PK, Chan KL. Standardized quassinoid-rich *Eurycoma longifolia* extract improved spermatogenesis and fertility in male rats via the hypothalamic-pituitary-gonadal axis. J Ethnopharmacol 2013;145:706–14.

[24] Low BS, Choi SB, Wahab HA, Das PK, Chan KL. Eurycomanone, the major quassinoid in *Eurycoma longifolia* root extract increases spermatogenesis by inhibiting the activity of phosphodiesterase and aromatase in steroidogenesis. J Ethnopharmacol 2013;149:201–7.

[25] Teh CH, Abdulghani M, Morita H, Shiro M, Hussin AH, Chan KL. Comparative X-ray and conformational analysis of a new crystal of 13α,21-dihydroeurycomanone with eurycomanone from *Eurycoma longifolia* and their anti-estrogenic activity using the uterotrophic assay. Planta Med 2011;77:128–32.

[26] Ismail SB, Wan Mohammad WMZ, George A, Nik Hussain NH, Musthapa Kamal ZM, Liske E. Randomized clinical trial on the use of PHYSTA freeze-dried water extract of *Eurycoma longifolia* for the improvement of quality of life and sexual well-being in men. Evid Based Complement Altern Med 2012;429268:10.

[27] Tambi MIBM, Imran MK. *Eurycoma longifolia* Jack in managing idiopathic male infertility. Asian J Androl 2010;12:376–80.

[28] Erasmus N, Solomon M, Fortuin K, Henkel R. Effect of *Eurycoma longifolia* Jack (Tongkat ali) extract on human spermatozoa in vitro. Andrologia 2012;44:308–14.

[29] Kotirum S, Ismail SB, Chaiyakunapruk N. Efficacy of Tongkat Ali (*Eurycoma longifolia*) on erectile function improvement: systematic review and meta-analysis of randomized controlled trials. Complement Ther Med 2014;23:693–8.

[30] Udani JK, George AA, Musthapa M, Pakdaman MN, Abas A. Effects of proprietary freeze-dried water extract of *Eurycoma longifolia* (Physta) and *Polygonum minus* on sexual performance and well-being in men: a randomized, double-blind, placebo-controlled study. Evid Based Complement Alternat Med 2014;2014.

[31] Tambi MIBM. Evaluation of Xgene TM, a *Eurycoma longifolia* extract enriched penis care cream, as a novel vehicle in creating penis consciousness and confidence in keeping and maintaining erection for penetrative sex. Andrology (Los Angel) 2017;6(2):189.

[32] Ezzat SM, Okba MM, Ezzat MI, Aborehab NM, Mohamed SO. Rho-kinase II inhibitory potential of *Eurycoma longifolia* new isolate for the management of erectile dysfunction. Evid Based Complement Alternat Med 2019;6:1–8.

[33] George A, Henkel R. Phytoandrogenic properties of *Eurycoma longifolia* as natural alternative to testosterone replacement therapy. Andrologia 2014;46:708–21.

[34] Tambi M, Imran M, Henkel R. Standardised water-soluble extract of *Eurycoma longifolia*, Tongkat Ali as testosterone booster for managing men with late-onset hypogonadism? Andrologia 2012;44:226–30.

[35] Talbott SM, Talbott JA, George A, Pugh M. Effect of Tongkat Ali on stress hormones and psychological mood state in moderately stressed subjects. J Int Soc Sports Nutr 2013;10:28.

[36] Kamel HK. Male osteoporosis. Drugs Aging 2005;22:741–8.

[37] Melton LJ, Atkinson EJ, O'Connor MK, O'Fallon WM, Riggs BL. Bone density and fracture risk in men. J Bone Miner Res 1998;13:1915–23.

[38] Melton LJ, Chrischilles EA, Cooper C, Lane AW, Riggs BL. How many women have osteoporosis? J Bone Miner Res 2005;20:886–92.

[39] Mohd EN, Mohamed N, Muhammad N, Naina MI, Shuid AN. *Eurycoma longifolia*: medicinal plant in the prevention and treatment of male osteoporosis due to androgen deficiency. Evid Based Complement Altern Med 2012;, 125761. 9 pages.

[40] Shuid AN, Abu Bakar MF, Abdul Shukor TA, Muhammad N, Mohamed N, Soelaiman IN. The anti-osteoporotic effect of *Eurycoma longifolia* in aged orchidectomised rat model. Aging Male 2011;14:150–4.

[41] Ali J, Saad J. Biochemical effect of *Eurycoma longifolia* Jack on the sexual behavior, fertility, sex hormone, and glycolysis [Ph.D. thesis]. Kuala Lumpur: University of Malaysia; 1993.

[42] Hooi HA, Cheang HS, Yusof APM. Effects of *Eurycoma longifolia* Jack (Tongkat Ali) on the initiation of sexual performance of inexperienced castrated male rats. Exp Anim 2000;49:35–8.

[43] Halliwell B, Gutteridge JM. Free radicals in biology and medicine. vol. 3. Oxford, Croydon: Oxford University Press; 1999.

[44] Wauquier F, Leotoing L, Coxam V, Guicheux J, Wittrant Y. Oxidative stress in bone remodelling and disease. Trends Mol Med 2009;15:468–77.

[45] Nicholson TM, Ricke WA. Androgens and estrogens in benign prostatic hyperplasia: past, present and future. Differentiation 2011;82:184–99.

[46] Imamoto T, Suzuki H, Utsumi T, Endo T, Takano M, Yano M, et al. Association between serum sex hormone levels and prostate cancer: effect of prostate cancer on serum testosterone levels. Future Oncol 2009;5:1005–13.

[47] Tong KL, Chan KL, AbuBakar S, Low BS, Ma HQ, Wong PF. The in vitro and in vivo anti-cancer activities of a standardized quassinoids composition from *Eurycoma longifolia* on LNCaP human prostate cancer cells. PLoS ONE 2015;10:e121752.

[48] Husen R, Pihie AHL, Nallappan M. Screening for antihyperglycaemic activity in several local herbs of Malaysia. J Ethnopharmacol 2004;95:205–8.

[49] Lahrita L, Kato E, Kawabata J. Uncovering potential of Indonesian medicinal plants on glucose uptake enhancement and lipid suppression in 3T3-L1 adipocytes. J Ethnopharmacol 2015;168:229–36.

Chapter 5.4.3

Herbal medicines (*Eleutherococcus senticosus, Astragalus membranaceus*) used to treat andrological problems: Asia and Indian Subcontinent

Chinyerum S. Opuwari

Department of Pre-Clinical Sciences, University of Limpopo, Polokwane, South Africa

1 Introduction

Infertility is defined as the inability to conceive after 1 year, following a regular, unprotected sexual intercourse, without the use of a contraceptive [1]. The male factor contributes to 35%–40% of the incidence of infertility in the world [2]. The number of couples as well as males reported to be infertile in Asia is unknown, however, couples in which the male factor is one of the involved multiple factors accounts for 37% of the cases [1]. However, the most common causes of male infertility are idiopathic male infertility and sperm dysfunction [3].

Eleutherococcus senticosus (also called "Ciwujia" in Chinese, "Shigoka" or "Ezo-ukogi" in Japanese, and "Siberian ginseng" in the Siberian Taiga region [4–6]) and *Astragalus membranaceus* (commonly referred to as Huangqi, bei qi, or huang hua huang qi in China or Radix astragali in Latin [7, 8]) have been used for thousands of years as a traditional remedy in TCM. Both plants are primarily described to be adaptogens, which generally have the following properties: (1) they are harmless to the host, (2) they have a general or nonspecific effect, (3) they increase resistance to stressors such as physical, biological, or chemical stressors to the individual, and (4) they maintain homeostasis [9–12].

Traditional Chinese medicine is a medical philosophy that has been in practice in China for over 5000 years [13]. Its practice is based on the "Yin-Yang" theory that describes a balance between anabolic and catabolic processes for the diagnosis and treatment of diseases [13–15]. The active principle of the normal physiology and metabolism in the human body depends on the "Qi," which is the vital energy that flows all over the body [13, 14]. Each organ has its specific pattern of Qi that is responsible for performing its specific function. For instance, the kidney and liver are essential in the normal functioning of the reproductive functions [14]. The kidney stores Qi, corresponding to male and female gametes in the modern concept. The liver on the other hand stores blood, which is considered the reproductive essence [13, 14]. Both, Qi and blood are Yin in nature, indicating that the liver and kidney are of the same source. Consequently, a weakness in one organ is linked to an imbalance in the other [13]. Thus, an imbalance in the pathway of Qi or in the components of Qi-Yang and blood-Yin may result in the occurrence of a disease [14]. As a result, infertility problems are thought to be brought about by kidney-Qi deficiency, weakness of Qi and blood or spleen, stagnation of liver-Qi, and obstruction of damp phlegm, besides congenital defects [14].

The diagnosis and treatment of diseases in TCM is focused on identifying patterns of disharmony in one or a number of organs as well as the balance of relationships between the organs in the disease, habitus of the patient, pulse, diet, appearance of the tongue, external environment, and lifestyle [13, 14]. Furthermore, herbs used for treatment are seldom used singly, but usually in combination to maintain reproductive health, as well as for the treatment of infertility and endocrine deficiencies [14].

1.1 *Eleutherococcus senticosus*

The rhizome and root of *E. senticosus* (Rupr. et Maxim.) Maxim, also known as *Acanthopanax senticosus* (Rupr. Et Maxim.) Harms are used as a tonic and anti-fatigue agent in Northeastern Asia and Eastern Russia [16]. *E. senticosus* is popularly

Herbal Medicine in Andrology. https://doi.org/10.1016/B978-0-12-815565-3.00017-5

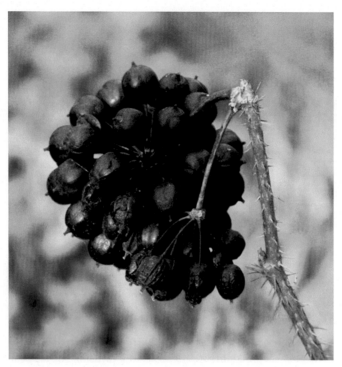

FIG. 1 *Eleutherococcus senticosus. Creator: Doronenko; License: CC BY 2.5; Source: Wikimedia Commons.*

known as Siberian ginseng due of its ginseng-like adaptogenic effect that is similar to the Chinese *Panax ginseng* [6, 17]. *E. senticosus*, belonging to the family Araliaceae, consists of about 84 genera and is innate to Asia, the Malay peninsula, Polynesia, Europe, North Africa, and the Americas [18]. *E. senticocsus* is a hardy shrub of height about 2 m (Fig. 1) and grows in the far eastern parts of Russia taiga and the northern regions of Korea, Japan, and China [4, 5]. "Shigoka" was first listed in Japanese Pharmacopeia from the 15th edition (2006) and was medicinally prescribed for the health benefits of the rhizomes and root of *E. senticosus*. In the Chinese Pharmacopeia (2005), the rhizomes, roots as well as the stem were medicinally used part. [19, 20]

The active compounds in *E. senticocsus* are mostly found in the roots and include eleutherosides A-M, saponins, eleutherans, beta sitosterol, isofraxidin, syringin, chlorogenic acid, sesamins, and friedelin [5, 21, 22]. Eleutherosides I, K, L, and M were also identified and isolated from the leaves of *E. senticosus* [21].

E. senticosus is efficient in revitalizing the liver and kidney, replenishing vital essence, and strengthening bones [5]. Its liquor is also widely used as a health supplement for weakness, rheumatism, impotence, and hemorrhoids in Northeast China by soaking it in alcohol liquor. It is now commonly used as dietary supplement beyond Asia such as in the United States and European countries in the form of capsules, powder, or tea bags [6]. The whole or sliced dried root of *E. senticosus* has been used in TCM, while the dried and ground roots are used in Western herbal medicine for tinctures or teas and in capsules [6].

E. senticosus is described as an adaptogen due to its ability to increase nonspecific body resistance to stress and fatigue [23, 24]. A study demonstrated that *E. senticosus* has vascular relaxation properties that is endothelium dependent and mediated by nitric oxide [25]. These properties point toward a potential use in conditions such as peripheral vascular disease, hypertension, coronary ischemia, and erectile dysfunction, which are characterized by endothelial dysfunction [26].

1.2 *Astragalus membranaceus*

A. membranaceus (Fisch.) Bunge (AM), Maxim of the Leguminosae family (Fig. 2), grows mostly in Northeast, North, and Northwest China, Mongolia, and Korea. [7] The dried root of *A. membranaceus* comprises 2′4′-dihydroxy-5,6-dimethoxyisoflavone, triterpenes, kumatakenin, choline, betaine, polysaccharides (astragalans), saponins, glucuronic acid, sucrose, amino acids, traces of folic acid, and astraisoflavanin [27–32].

A. membranaceus has been revealed to successfully treat a variety of diseases, and has consequently been vastly used as a tonic to improve the body's defense system [33]. *A. membranaceus* possesses hepatoprotective, diuretic, and expectorant properties as well as exhibits immunomodulatory, antihyperglymic, antinflammatory, antioxidant, antiapoptotic, antifibrotic, and antiviral activities [8, 34].

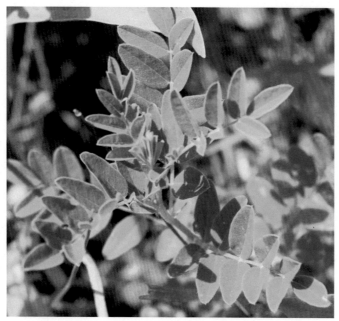

FIG. 2 *Astragalus membranaceus. Creator: Doronenko; License: CC BY 2.5; Source: Wikimedia Commons.*

2 Medicinal plants and infertility treatment

Several plants are traditionally used to treat different aspects of male infertility such as sexual asthenia, libido, erectile dysfunction, ejaculatory disorders, and sperm abnormalities such as azoospermia and oligozoospermia [35]. Despite the many health benefits of *E. senticosus* and *A. membranaceus*, there is limited study on the effect of both plants in treating these andrological problems.

2.1   *E. senticosus* and *A. membranaceus* on erectile dysfunction

Erectile dysfunction (ED) is a persistent or recurrent failure to achieve penile erection, leading to an unsatisfactory sexual performance [36]. It is the most common disorders of male sexual function and an underlying cause for infertility [36]. Administration of medicinal plants may bring about erection by inhibiting phosphodiesterase or stimulating the production and release of nitric oxide synthase [36]. Aphrodisiac agents cause the hypothalamus to release nitric oxide, which activates guanylate cyclase to convert nucleotide guanosine triphosphate (GTP) to cGMP, and in turn causes the relaxation of the smooth muscle cells in the penis leading to dilation of penile blood vessels with an increased blood influx into the corpora cavernosa and eventually to an erection. cGMP is then hydrolyzed by phosphodiesterase type-5 enzyme (PDE-5) to inactive GMP and thus terminate penile erection. Aphrodisiacs inhibit the hydrolysis of PDE-5, resulting in the accumulation of cGMP and maintaining erection thereof [37–39].

Mowrey suggested that *E. senticosus* might increase sexual performance as it increases stamina in athletes [40]. *E. senticosus* was demonstrated to have aphrodisiac effects in animals and might have such invigorative and tonic effect in humans [41]. Another study demonstrated that phenols from *E. senticosus* have effects similar to a "Viagra effect," by momentarily inhibiting nitric oxide by preventing transduction of cyclic GMP signal [42].

Testosterone plays a role in sustaining the growth of cavernosal smooth muscle as well as functional integrity through the upregulation of phosphodiesterase type 5 inhibitor (PDE-5 inhibitor) [43, 44]. Studies have demonstrated that *E. senticosus* and *A. membranaceus* may be used to increase testosterone production [34, 45].

2.2   *E. senticosus* and *A. membranaceus* on sperm parameters in vitro

Table 1 summarizes the effects of *E. senticosus* and *A. membranaceus* extracts on various sperm parameters. Administration of 5–10 mg/mL aqueous extracts of *E. senticosus* to asthenozoospermic infertile male from 15 to 180 min increased sperm viability and motility [33, 46]. The optimal concentration of this herbal extract to increase sperm motility in asthenozoospermic patients was suggested to be 10 g/L in vitro [46].

TABLE 1 Effects of *Eleutherococcus senticosus* and *Astragalus membranaceus* on various sperm parameters and TM3 cells.

Plant	Animal model	Dose	Duration of treatment	Effect obtained	References
Eleutherococcus senticosus	Asthenozoospermic infertile male	10 mg/mL	15, 60, and 180 min	Increased sperm viability and motility	[33]
	Asthenozoospermic infertile male	5, 10 mg/mL	30, 60, 120, and 180 min	Increased sperm motility, percentage of progressive motile sperm, VCL, VSL, and VAP	[46]
Astragalus membranaceus	Asthenozoospermic males	10 mg/mL	15, 60, and 180 min	Increased sperm viability and motility	[33]
	Human sperm			Increased viability, percentage of grade A sperm, VCL, VSL, and swaying frequency of spermatozoa head in semen	[47]
	Asthenozoospermic males	10 g/L	0, 1 and 3 h	Increased sperm motility, percentage of progressive motile sperm, VSL and VCL	[48]
	Human sperm from healthy donors	5, 10, and 20 mg/mL	2 h	Increased sperm motility by 2.5-folds	[49]
	TM3 cells	20, 50, 100, and 500 μg/mL A.M injection	48 h	Increased cell viability, testosterone production, SOD, and GPx	[34]
	Boar sperm	0.25, 0.5, 0.75, and 1 mg/mL		Preserve sperm quality, acrosome integrity, mitochondrial membrane potential	[50]
	Boar sperm	0.5, 1, 5, and 10 mg/mL (APS)	1 h	Increased mitochondrial activity, penetration rate, total IVF rate efficiency, cleavage rate, and blastocyst rate. No effect on sperm viability, and motility	[51]

Administration of *A. membranaceus* extract (10 mg/mL) to asthenozoospermic infertile men was shown to increase sperm motility and viability in vitro [47, 48]. Likewise, *A. membranaceus* was shown to stimulate sperm motility in healthy donors [49]. Sperm velocity parameters are usually correlated with sperm viability and fertilizing capacity as well as with progressive motility. These parameters were also shown to be increased by both plant extracts. For instance, *A. membranaceus* increased number of progressive motile spermatozoa, curvilinear velocity (VCL), average path velocity (VAP), amplitude of lateral head displacement (ALH) and straight-line velocity (VSL) significantly, while *E. senticosus* improved sperm viability, VAP, and ALH [33, 48]. In addition, another study also demonstrated that *A. membranaceus* significantly enhanced the percentage of grade A sperm, VCL, VSL, and the swaying frequency of spermatozoa head sperm motility in vitro [47].

The significant stimulatory effect of *A. membranaceus* and *E. senticosus* on human sperm motility may be related to the metal elements (such as extracellular calcium) contained in both plant extracts [33, 47]. Both plants stimulated adenylate cyclase and increased intracellular levels of cAMP in different cell systems such as plasma, immune cells, and ischemic myocardium [33, 52, 53]. *A. membranaceus* and *E. senticosus* may enhance sperm motility through alterations of the intracellular levels of cAMP, as sperm motility has also been shown to increase with elevated intracellular cAMP [33, 54].

Lipid peroxidation can damage sperm membranes, which in turn can result in the loss of motility and viability [33]. Studies have indicated that *A. membranaceus* and *E. senticosus* have effect on anti-lipoperoxidative defense by the reduction in myocardial malondialdehyde (MDA) levels, with an increased level of superoxide dismutase (SOD) [55, 56]. There is a strong correlation between SOD activity and the time interval for complete loss of sperm motility [57]. Furthermore, an addition of exogenous SOD to the spermatozoa suspension greatly reduced motility loss and prevented the increase in MDA concentration as a result of lipid peroxidation [58]. No direct study has demonstrated the effect of *A. membranaceus* and *E. senticosus* on spermatozoa superoxide dismutase or lipid peroxidation level, however, it is assumed that both plants may be beneficial for antilipoperoxidative therapy in infertile men [33].

2.3 Effect of *E. senticosus* and *A. membranaceus* as a tonic on sperm parameters

2.3.1 Kan Jan

In vivo administration of 1.578 g of Kan Jan (a mixture of *Andrographis paniculata* and *E. senticosus*) increased the number of spermatozoa in the ejaculate, percentage of total motile spermatozoa, and fertility indexes following a 10-day treatment in healthy men (Table 2) [59].

2.3.2 Hochu-ekii-to

Hochu-ekki-to (also known as Bu-Zhong-Yigi-Tang or TJ-41) is widely used to treat idiopathic male infertility and sperm dysfunction [65–68]. *A. membranaceus* has been mentioned as a component of Hochu-ekki-to [3, 60]. It is composed of Astragalus root (4 g), *Atractylodes lancea* rhizome (4 g), Ginseng root (4 g), Japanese angelica root (3 g), Bupleurum root (2 g), Jujube fruit (2 g), *Citrus unshiu* peel (2 g), Glycyrrhiza root (1.5 g), Cimicifuga rhizome (1 g), and Ginger rhizome (0.5 g) [3, 60].

As demonstrated in Table 2, Hochu-ekki-to is known to improve semen quality [69]. Administration of Hochu-ekki-to to 45 patients with primary male infertility due to oligozoospermia for over 12 weeks showed a substantial increase in sperm concentrations, motility, and total counts of normal spermatozoa [61]. Following 3 months of administration of

TABLE 2 Effect of tonics containing either *Eleutherococcus senticosus* or *Astragalus membranaceus* on sperm motility.

Mixture	Animal model	Dose	Length of treatment	Effects obtained	References
Kan Jan	Healthy men	1.578 g	9 days	Increased number of spermatozoa, percentage of active forms of spermatozoa and fertility index; decreased dyskinetics	[59]
Hochu-ekii-to	14 healthy donors	1, 10, and 100 μg/mL	1, 2, 4, and 6 h	Increased sperm motility	[60]
	Patients with primary male infertility due to oligozoospermia		12 weeks	Increased sperm concentration, rate of motility and total count of normal spermatozoa	[61]
	22 males with idiopathic infertility		3 months	Increased sperm count and motility	[62]
	Patients with oligozoospermia and/or asthenozoospermia			Increased total sperm density and motility	[63]
	20 patients with oligozoospermia and/or asthenozoospermia	7.5 g	3 months	Increased sperm motility and maintained semen volume, sperm count, and normal morphology	[64]

Hochu-ekki-to to 22 male patients with idiopathic infertility, a significant increase in sperm count and motility was observed [62]. Administration of Hochu-ekki-to to patients with oligozoospermia and/or asthenozoospermia improved total sperm density and motility [63, 66]. Furthermore, daily administration of 7.5 g of Hochu-ekki-to to 20 patients with oligozoospermic and/or asthenozoospermic patients for 3 months increased sperm motility and maintained semen volume, sperm count, and normal morphology [64]. Incubation of sperm from 14 healthy volunteers with 1, 10, and 100 µg/mL of Hochu-ekki-to for 1, 2, 4, and 6 h, respectively, showed a significant dose-dependent (as from 10 to 100 µg/mL) increase in sperm motility throughout the incubation period. The lowest concentration (1 µg/mL) increased sperm motility from 4 h of incubation [60]. Hochu-ekki-to is hypothesized to increase sperm motility by promoting protein synthesis associated with the functional maturation of spermatozoa in the epididymis or by affecting certain cytokines in the seminal fluid [3, 64].

2.4 Ameliorative effects of *A. membranaceus*

As shown in Table 3, administration of *A. membranaceus* extract possesses ameliorative effects against reproductive toxicants. Following the administration of cyclophosphamide (CP; 100 mg/kg) and *A. membranaceus* extract (100, 500, and 1000 mg/kg) to mice for 5 weeks, the plant extract ameliorated relative testes weight, sperm parameters, and cAMP-responsive element modulator (CREM) expression against CP-induced reproductive toxicity [70]. Cyclophosphamide is an anticancer drug that reduces sperm counts as well as cause an absence of spermatogenic cycles in the testicular tissue, injures progeny, decreases the weight of the reproductive organs, and impairs fertility [72, 73]. In another study, intraperitoneal administration of 5 g/kg per day or 10 g/kg per day of *A. membranaceus* extract injections given to male rats for 7 days, followed by a simultaneous administration of cadmium chloride (0.2 mg Cd/kg body weight) for a further 15 days showed that *A. membranaceus* extract provided a protection against cadmium-induced genetic damage by significantly increasing testis coefficient, testicular sperm count, and daily sperm production compared to the cadmium group [71].

2.5 Role of *A. membranaceus* in cryopreservation for assisted reproductive therapy

Astragalus polysaccharide (APS), a main component of *A. membranaceus*, is often used in TCM as a semen extender supplementation owing to its antioxidant properties [50, 51]. Supplementation of thawing boar semen extender with APS (0.5, 1, 5, and 10 mg/mL) for 1 h enhanced mitochondrial activity, penetration rate, total IVF rate efficiency, cleavage rate, and blastocyst rate [51]. It, however, had no effect on sperm viability and motility but decreased ROS with increased activity of SOD and CAT [51]. The ability of APS to scavenge ROS, leading to their reduction could therefore inhibit mitochondrial injury by scavenging ROS [74].

Furthermore, supplementation with APS (0.25, 0.5, 0.75, and 1 mg/mL) was revealed to effectively preserve boar sperm quality, acrosome integrity, and mitochondrial membrane potential (MMP) at 4°C. This may be as a result of the removal of excessive mitochondrial ROS, with increased antioxidant capacities and enhanced ATP levels [50].

3 Conclusion

In traditional Chinese medicine, *E. senticosus* and *A. membranaceus* usage is claimed to be beneficial in the treatment of male infertility. The individual use of each plant as well as in combination with other ingredients as a tonic have been scientifically proven to increase sperm parameters such as motility, viability, concentration, and mitochondrial membrane potential. *E. senticosus* and *A. membranaceus* are thought to increase sperm motility through alterations in the intracellular

TABLE 3 Ameliorative effects of *Astragalus membranaceus* on male reproductive organs in animals.

Animal model	Dose	Duration of treatment	Effect obtained	References
Mice	1000 mg/kg CP followed by 100, 500, and 1000 mg/kg A.M.	5 weeks	Amelioration of reproductive toxicity induced by cyclophosphamide such as improving testes weight, sperm parameters, and CREM expression	[70]
Rats	5 g/kg.d and 10 g/kg.d followed by 0.2 mg Cd/kg BW	22 days	Increased testes coefficient, testicular sperm count, daily sperm production	[71]

levels of cAMP. Hence, these plants maybe be beneficial in the management of male infertility in men affected by asthenozoospermia. Both plants may also act as an aphrodisiac through the relaxation of the smooth cavernosal muscles. This is achieved by the upregulation of PDE-5 inhibitors that prevents the hydrolysis of cGMP-specific PDE-5 on cyclic GMP in the smooth muscles. Furthermore, human sperm cell preservation is an important part of assisted reproductive technology (ART) and studies revealed that the use of APS in TCM can be an important ingredient in semen extender supplementation.

To better understand the benefits and mechanism of action of *E. senticosus* and *A. membranaceus* in male infertility treatment, large size clinical studies and antioxidant studies on spermatozoa are recommended. In addition, further research using human semen is needed to better understand the role of both plants as well as their components in ART. Lastly, it will also be insightful to correlate the effects of these plants on the sperm parameters with functions of the liver and kidney to better understand the principles underlying the Traditional Chinese Medicine.

References

[1] Agarwal A, Mulgund A, Hamada A, Chyatte MR. A unique view on male infertility around the globe. Reprod Biol Endocrinol 2015;13. https://doi.org/10.1186/s12958-015-0032-1.

[2] Scarneciu I, Lupu S, Scarneciu C. Smoking as a risk factor for the development of erectile dysfunction and infertility in men; evaluation depending on the anxiety levels of these patients. Soc Behav Sci 2014;127(1):437–42. https://doi.org/10.1016/j.sbspro.2014.03.286.

[3] Nakayama T, Noda Y, Goto Y, Mori T, Tashiro S. Effects of Hochu-ekki-to, a Japanese Kampo medicine, on cultured hamster Epididymal cells. American Journal of Chinese Medicine 1994;22:301–7.

[4] Boon H, Smith M. Tlw botanical pharmacy. Kingston, ON: Quarry Press; 1994. p. 194.

[5] Huang L, Zhao H, Huang B, Zheng C, Peng W, Qin L. *Acanthopanax senticosus*: review of botany, chemistry and pharmacology. Pharmazie 2011;66:83–97.

[6] Zhu S, Bai Y, Oya M, Tanaka K, Komatsu K, Maruyama T, Goda Y, Kawasaki T, Fujita M, Shibata T. Genetic and chemical diversity of *Eleutherococcus senticosus* and molecular identification of *Siberian ginseng* by PCR-RFLP analysis based on chloroplast trnK intron sequence. Food Chem 2011;129:1844–50.

[7] Peng X, Chen S, Ning F, Li M. Evaluation of *in vitro* antioxidant and antitumour activities of *Astragalus membranaceus* aqueous extract. J Med Plants Res 2011;5:6564–70.

[8] Fu J, Wang Z, Huang L, Zheng S, Wang D, Chen S, Zhang H, Yang S. Review of the botanical characteristics, phytochemistry, and pharmacology of *Astragalus membranaceus* (Huangqi). Phytother Res 2014;28:1275–83.

[9] Brekhman II. Eleutherokokk (Eleutherococcus). In: Leningrad. USSR in Russia: Nauka Publishing House; 1968.

[10] Davydov M, Krikorian AD. *Eleutherococcus senticosus* (Rupr. & Maxim.) Maxim. (Arallaceae) as an adaptogen: a closer look. J Ethnopharmacol 2000;72:345–93.

[11] Yance DR. Adaptogens in medical herbalism: elite herbs and natural compounds for mastering stress, aging, and chronic disease. New York: Simon and Schuster; 2013. p. 103–17.

[12] Liao L, He Y, Li L, Meng H, Dong Y, Yi F, Xiao P. A preliminary review of studies on adaptogens: comparison of their bioactivity in TCM with that of ginseng-like herbs used worldwide. Chin Med 2018;13:57.

[13] Crimmel AS, Conner CS, Monga M. Withered Yang: a review of traditional Chinese medical treatment of male infertility and erectile dysfunction. J Androl 2001;22:173–82.

[14] Xu X, Yin H, Tang D, Zhang Z, Gosden RG. Application of traditional Chinese medicine in the treatment of infertility. Hum Fertil 2003;6:161–8.

[15] Unschuld PU. Huang Di Nei Jing Su wen nature, knowledge, imagery in an ancient Chinese medical text: With an appendix: The doctrine of the five periods and six qi in the Huang Di Nei Jing Su wen. California: University of California Press; 2003.

[16] Xiao PG. Xin Bian Zhong Yao Zhi. Beijing, China: Chemical Industry Publishing House; 2002. p. 567–73.

[17] Antoshechkin AG. Selective plant extracts and their combination as the nutritional therapeutic remedies. Journal of Nutritional Therapeutics 2016;5:1–11.

[18] Wielgorskaya T, Takhtajan A, editors. Dictionary of generic names of seed plants. New York: Columbia University Press; 1995.

[19] Chinese Pharmacopoeia Committee, Ministry of Public Health, The People's Republic of China. The Chinese pharmacopoeia, part I. Beijing, China: Chemical Industry Publishing House; 2005. p. 143–4.

[20] The Society of Japanese Pharmacopoeia. Japanese pharmacopoeia. 15th ed. Tokyo: Ministry of Health, Labour and Welfare of Japan; 2006. p. 1222.

[21] Tang W, Eisenbrand G. Chinese drugs of plant origin. Heidelberg. Germany: Springer Verlag; 1992. p. 9.

[22] Dcyama T, Nishibe S, Nakazawa Y. Constituents and pharmacological effects of Hucomniia and Siberian ginseng. Acta Pharmacol Sin 2001;22:1057–70.

[23] Steinmann GG, Esperester A, Joller P. Immunopharmacological *in vitro* effects of *Eleutherococcus senticosus* extracts. Arzneimittelforschung 2001;51:76–83.

[24] Szolomicki J, Samochowiec L, Wojcicki J, Drozdzik M, Szolomicki S. The influence of active components of *Eleutherococcus senticosus* on cellular defence and physical fitness in man. Phytother Res 2000;14:30–5.

[25] Kwan CY, Zhang WB, Sim SM, Deyama T, Nishibe S. Vascular effects of Siberian ginseng I (*Eleutherococcus senticosus*): endothelium-dependent NO- and EDHF-mediated relaxation depending on vessel size. Naunyn Schmiedebergs Arch Pharmacol 2004;36:473–80.

[26] Eleutherococcus senticosus. Alternative medicine review. vol. 11 (2); 2006. p. 151–5.

[27] Subarnas A, Oshima Y, Hikino H. Isoflavans and a pterocarpan from Astragalus mongholicus. Phytochemistry 1991;30(1):2777–80.

[28] Bensky D, Gamble A. Chinese herbal medicine. Materica Medica: Eastland Press Inc., Seattle; 1993.

[29] Lin ZL, He GX, Lindenmaier M, Nolan G, Yang J. Liquid chromatography–electrospray ionization mass spectrometry study of the flavonoids of the roots of Astragalus mongholicus and A. membranaceus. J Chromatogr A 2000;876(1–2):87–95.

[30] Ma Q, Shi Q, Duan A, Dong TT, Tsim KW. Chemical analysis of radix Astragali (Huangqi) in China: a comparison with its adulterants and seasonal variations. J Agric Food Chem 2002;50(17):4861–6.

[31] Wu FB, Chen XY. Pharmacological effects of Astragalus. J Chin Med Mater 2004;27:232–4.

[32] Aldarmaa J, Liu Z, Long J, Mo X, Ma J, Liu J. Anti-convulsant effect and mechanism of Astragalus mongholicus extract in vitro and in vivo: protection against oxidative damage and mitochondrial dysfunction. Neurochem Res 2010;35(1):33–41.

[33] Liu J, Liang P, Yin C, Wang T, Li H, Li Y, Ye Z. Effects of several Chinese herbal aqueous extracts on human sperm motility in vitro. Andrology 2004;36:78–83.

[34] Jiang X, Cao X, Huang Y, Chen J, Yao X, Zhao M, Liu Y, Meng J, Li P, Li Z, Yao J, Smith GW, Lv L. Effects of treatment with Astragalus membranaceus on function of rat Leydig cells. BMC Complement Altern Med 2015;15:261.

[35] Nantia EA, Moundipa PF, Monsees TK, Carreau S. Medicinal plants as potential male anti-infertility agents: a review. Andrologia 2009;19:148–58.

[36] Singh S, Ali A, Singh R, Kaur R. Sexual abnormalities in males and their herbal therapeutic aspects. Pharmacologia 2013;4:265–73.

[37] Palmer E. Making the love drug. Chem Br 1999;35:24–6.

[38] Chew KK, Stuckey BGA, Thompson PL. Erectile dysfunction, sildenafil and cardiovascular risk. Med J Aust 2000;172:279–83.

[39] Sharma M, Arya D, Bhagour K, Gupta RS. Natural aphrodisiac and fertility enhancement measures in males: a review. Curr Med Res Pract 2017;7:51–8.

[40] Mowrey DB. Herbal tonic therapies. New Canaan, CT: Keats Publishing; 1993.

[41] Rätsch C. Plants of love. The history of aphrodisiacs and a guide to their identification and use. Berkeley, CA: Ten Speed Press; 1997.

[42] Goldstein I, Lue TF, Padma-Nathan H, Rosen RC, Steers WD, Wicker PA. Oral sildenafil in the treatment of erectile dysfunction. N Engl J Med 1998;338:1397–404.

[43] Shabsigh R. The effects of testosterone on the carvenous tissue and erectile function. World J Urol 1997;15:21–6.

[44] Traish AM, Park K, Dhir V, Kim NN, Moreland RB, Goldstein I. The effects of castration and androgen replacement on erectile function in a rabbit model. Endocrinology 1999;140:1861–8.

[45] Merekar AN, Pattan SR, Kuchekar BS, Dighe NS, Laware RB, Nirmal SA, Parjane SK, Gaware VM. Male infertility and its treatment by alternative medicine: a review. Pharmacol Online 2009;3:956–72.

[46] Chen Z, Yin C-P, Liu J-H, Fang J-G, Wang W-Q, Shi C-Y. Extract of Acanthopanacis senticosus improves sperm motility of asthenospermia patients in vitro. Zhonghua Nan Ke Xue = Natl J Androl 2007;13(1):21–3.

[47] Jiang F, Wang YX, Sheng XF, Xia LC, Qian XM, Wu YL. Effect of Astragalus membranaceus additive on sperm quality in vitro. Chin J Androl 1998;2:74–7.

[48] Wu W, Liu JH, Yin CP, Zhang CH. A comparative study of the effects of Acanthopanacis senticosi injection, theophylline and caffeine on human sperm mobility in vitro. Natl J Androl 2009;15(3):278–81.

[49] Hong CY, Ku J, Wu P. Astragalus membranaceus stimulates human sperm motility in vitro. Am J Chin Med 1992;20:289–94.

[50] Fu J, Yang Q, Li Y, Li P, Wang L, Li X. A mechanism by which Astragalus polysaccharide protects against ROS toxicity through inhibiting the protein dephosphorylation of boar sperm preserved at 4 °C. J Cell Physiol 2018;233:5267–80.

[51] Weng X, Cai M, Zhang Y, Liu Y, Gao Z, Song J, Liu Z. Effect of Astragalus polysaccharide addition to thawed boar sperm on in vitro fertilization and embryo development. Theriogenology 2018;121:21–6.

[52] Liang HP, Wang ZG, Tian FQ, Geng B, Chen RD. Effects of Astragalus polysaccharides, Ginsenosides on cAMP, cGMP contents in plasma and immune cells of traumatized mice. Chin J Pathophysiol 1995;6:595–9.

[53] Zhou JY, Fan Y, Kong JL, Wu DZ, Hu ZB. Effects of components isolated from Astragalus membranaceus bunge on cardiac function injured by myocardial ischemia reperfusion in rats. China J Chin Mater Med 2000;25:300–2.

[54] Bhatnagar SK, Anand SR. Cyclic nucleotide phosphodiesterase activity in midpiece and tail of buffalo spermatozoa and its role in sperm motility. Biochim Biophys Acta 1982;716:133.

[55] Zhong L, Ye QR. Protective effects of Acanthopanecis senticasi on experimental ischemic myocardium. Chin J Pathophysiol 1995;4:366–9.

[56] Zhou SN, Shao W, Zhang WG, Gao FJ. Experiment studies of Astragalus membranaceus injection combined with Ligustrazine injection on protective and therapeutic effect on myocardial ischemia-reperfusion injury. Chin J Integr Tradit Western Med Intens Crit Care 2001;4:233–5.

[57] Alvarez JG, Storey BT. Evidence for increased lipid peroxidative damage and loss of superoxide dismutase activity as a mode of sublethal cryodamage to human sperm during cryopreservation. J Androl 1992;13:232–41.

[58] Kobayashi T, Miyazaki T, Natori M, Nozawa S. Protective role of superoxide dismutase in human sperm motility: superoxide dismutase activity and lipid peroxide in human seminal plasma and spermatozoa. Hum Reprod 1991;6:987–91.

[59] Mkrtchyan A, Panosyan V, Panossian A, Wikman G, Wagner H. A phase I clinical study of Andrographis paniculata fixed combination Kan Jang™ versus ginseng and valerian on the semen quality of healthy male subjects. Phytomedicine 2005;12:403–9.

[60] Amano T, Hirata A, Namiki M. Effects of Chinese herbal medicine on sperm motility and fluorescence spectra parameters. Arch Androl 1996;37(3):219–24.

[61] Yoshida H, Tanifuji T, Sakurai H, Tashiro H, Ogawa H, Imamura K. Clinical effects of Chinese herb medicine (hochu-ekki-to) on infertile men. Hinyokika Kiyo. Acta Urol Japonica 1986;32(2):297–302.

[62] Furuya Y, Akashi T, Fuse H. Treatment of traditional Chinese medicine for idiopathic male infertility. Hinyokika Kiyo. Acta Urol Japonica 2004;50(8):545–8.

[63] Manabe F, Yoshii S, Ishikawa H, Koiso K. Effect of Tsumura hochu-ekki-to on male infertility. Jpn J Fertil Steril 1991;36:683–9.

[64] Akashi T, Watanabe A, Morri A, Mizuno I, Fuse H. Effects of the herbal medicine hochuekkito on semen parameters and seminal plasma cytokine levels (TNF-(α), IL-6. RANTES) in idiopathic male infertility. J Tradit Med 2008;25:6–9.

[65] Ishikawa H, Manabe F, Zhongtao H, Yoshii S, Koiso K. The hormonal response to HCG stimulation in patients with male infertility before and after treatment with hochu-ekki-to. Am J Chin Med 1992;20:157–65.

[66] Mitsukawa S, Kimura M, Ishikawa H, Orikasa S. Treatment of male sterility by hochu-ekki-to. Jpn J Fertil Steril 1984;29:458–65.

[67] Tamaya T, Ohno Y, Okada H. Treatment of hochu-ekki-to for oligospermic patients and implications of their clinical signs for therapeutic efficacy. Jpn J Fertil Steril 1987;32:385–90.

[68] Hu M, Zhang Y, Ma H, Ng EHY, Wu X. Eastern medicine approaches to male infertility. Semin Reprod Med 2013;31:301–10.

[69] Clément C, Witschi U, Kreuzer M. The potential influence of plant-based feed supplements on sperm quantity and quality in livestock: a review. Anim Reprod Sci 2012;132:1–10.

[70] Kim W, Kim SH, Park SK, Chang MS. *Astragalus membranaceus* ameliorates reproductive toxicity induced by cyclophosphamide in male mice. Phytother Res 2012;26:1418–21.

[71] Liang P, Li H, Peng X, Xiao J, Liu J, Ye Z. Effects of *Astragalus membranaceus* injection on sperm abnormality in Cd-induced rats. Natl J Androl 2004;10(1):42–5. 48.

[72] Howell S, Shalet S. Gonadal damage from chemotherapy and radiotherapy. Endocrinol Metab Clin North Am 1998;27:927–43.

[73] Trasler JM, Hales BF, Robaire B. Chronic low dose cyclophosphamide treatment of adult male rats: effect on fertility, pregnancy outcome and progeny. Biol Reprod 1986;34:275–83.

[74] Huang Y, Lu L, Zhu D, Wang M, Yin Y, Chen D, Wei L. Effects of *Astragalus* polysaccharides on dysfunction of mitochondrial dynamics induced by oxidative stress. Oxid Med Cell Longev 2016. https://doi.org/10.1155/2016/9573291. Article ID 9573291, 13 p.

Chapter 5.4.4

Herbal medicines (*Zingiber officinale* and *Epimedium grandiflorum*) used to treat andrological problems: Asia and Indian subcontinent

Lourens Johannes Christoffel Erasmus[a] and Kristian Leisegang[b]

[a]*Physiology and Environmental Health, University of Limpopo, Mankweng, Limpopo Province, South Africa*, [b]*School of Natural Medicine, University of the Western Cape, Cape Town, South Africa*

1 Zingiber officinale

1.1 Introduction

The English botanist, William Roscoe gave the name *Z. officinale* to what is commonly known as ginger. Traditionally, ginger is used in Ayurveda, Siddha, Chinese, Arabian, African, Caribbean and many other medicinal systems to treat a variety of diseases [1–4]. In the Sanskrit text, dating back 2000 BC, Ayurvedic medicine describes the medicinal use of ginger rhizomes [5]. In Europe, the Greek physician Dioscorides, in the first century, mentioned the use of ginger for its digestive properties [6]. As a therapeutic agent, *Z. officinale* is also being accepted by modern physicians [7]. This can probably be attributed to proven therapeutic uses such as antioxidants, antiemetics, anti-inflammatory agents [8], as well as its capacity to affect reproductive functions [9]. Furthermore, its hepato- [7, 10], cardio- [11, 12], reno- [13], neuro- [14], and gastroprotective [11, 15] activities emphasize its wide acceptance in the management of general health.

1.2 Taxonomic classification

The family Zingiberaceae is one of the 10 largest monocotyledonous families in India. It comprises approximately 52 genera and 1400 species, of which 22 genera and 178 species are endemic to the Indo-Malayan region of Asia [16]. The taxonomical, classification of *Z. officinale* is summarized in Table 1. Ginger is a narrow blade bearing, herbaceous perennial plant that grows approximately 1 m tall.

1.3 Distribution and botanical description

The genus *Zingiber* is widely distributed in tropical to warm-temperate Asia and Far East Asia [18]. It has been under cultivation in India and China for more than two millennia [19], from where it was introduced to other parts of the world. Currently, the world market for ginger is dominated by India (32.75%) and China (21.41%) [20]. Ginger is predominantly exported in the form of whole, dry ginger. Even though it is cultivated all over the world, Nigeria ranks first with regard to area under ginger covering (56.23%), followed by India (23.6%) and China (4.47%). The major importers of ginger are Japan and United States [2].

Z. officinale is an herbaceous rhizomatous perennial herb, reaching up to 90 cm in height under cultivation. The rhizome is stout, tuberous, thick lobed, horizontal, aromatic, and white or pale yellow to brown in color [21, 22]. The stem is leafy and thick with an approximate height of 60 cm. Leaves are approximately 20 cm long and 2–3 cm wide. They are pointed, narrow or linear-lanceolate with sheathing bases clasping the stem. Cultivated plants rarely produce flowers. When they do these are rather small subtending with bracts and bracteoles. These pale green bracts, closely pressed against each other, are ovate with an approximate length of 2.5 cm [23]. While the calyx is three-lobed and short, the corolla presents as two greenish-yellow pointed segments with a shorter, oblong-ovate, dark purple lip spotted with yellow. This plant requires a hot, moist climate with a rich, well-drained soil [22].

Herbal Medicine in Andrology. https://doi.org/10.1016/B978-0-12-815565-3.00018-7

TABLE 1 Taxonomical classification of *Zingibar officinale* Rosc.1 [17].

Kingdom	Plantae
Subkingdom	Tracheobionta
Division	Magnoliophyta
Class	Liopsida
Subclass	Zingiberidae
Order	Zingiberales
Family	Zingibraceae
Genus	*Zingiber*
Species	*officinale*

1.4 Ethnobotanical information

Current literature supports the diverse use of ginger in the management of various ailments [4]. It seems unlikely that there are any organ systems that would not be affected by ginger [4]. However, it is possible that the symptoms of some ailments are alleviated via a secondary mechanism, for example, the management of chronic diseases can contribute to improved sexual functions. From a traditional perspective, very little evidence exists to indicate that ginger is outright used for its androgenic effect. In Unani medicine it is used to treat sexual debility (Zoafe Bah) [3]; though this term seems to be a generalization emphasizing weakness, fatigue, or tiredness. Ample evidence exists to support the use of ginger in the management of cardiovascular diseases [11, 24], inflammation [1, 24], and diabetes [25, 26]. It is fair to argue that in doing so underlying sexual dysfunctions can be restored. With India, China, and Japan as some of the biggest stakeholders in the ginger market, it is implied that ginger plays an important role in their medicinal practices.

Ginger, either fresh or dried, is used as an ingredient in traditional Indian drinks and is one the key spices in many of their vegetarian and nonvegetarian foods. In the Ayurveda system it is a common household remedy for the treatment of a vast array of illnesses [27, 28]. Among others, ginger is used as an appetizer, analgesic, diuretic, and as aphrodisiac [29]. The Chinese and Japanese medicinal systems consider ginger rhizomes to be a key element in their management of ailments [27]. They use ginger for its antiemetic, antitussive, antidiarrheal, and expectorant capabilities [30]. Clearly, ginger is an important therapeutic agent and spice used throughout Asia and has gained considerable global popularity.

1.5 Phytochemistry

Phytochemical assessment of the ginger rhizome indicate that it contains a variety of biologically active compounds. The major phytochemical groups are essential oils, phenolic compounds, flavonoids, carbohydrates, proteins, alkaloids, glycosides, saponins, steroids, terpenoids, and tannin [2]. While the composition of the essential oils can vary based on geography, the principal constituent sesquiterpene hydrocarbons remain fairly constant. These hydrocarbons are responsible for the characteristic aroma of ginger [31]. A summary of some of the major chemical constituents is presented in Table 2.

1.6 Andrology

In male reproductive physiology, many parameters can be employed to assess the ability of a medicinal plant to manage sexual dysfunction (SD). For as far as recorded history can inform, the devastating nature of SD prompted the use of natural products such as plants to treat infertility, impotence, and decreased libido. *Z. officinale* has been the focus of andrology studies for many years, using various models to specifically assess its role in reproductive endocrinology as well as alterations in sperm production.

When exploring the impact of any medicinal plant or extract on male reproductive functions, the focus must be on much more than gonadotropins and testosterone only. In an effort to understand possible mechanisms, the endocrine axis can in all probability be traced back to the contribution of Kisspeptin. It is expressed by neurons in the arcuate and anteroventral/periventricular nuclei within the hypothalamus [34]. The arcuate nucleus is also considered the putative GnRH pulse generator in primates [35]. There is an established link between Kisspeptin and GnRH, with specific reference in the literature to the initiation of male puberty [35]. Therefore, Kisspeptin regulates GnRH, which in turn regulates the gonadotropins, where luteinising hormone stimulates the Leydig cells to produce testosterone [8]. However, information on the Kisspeptin/

TABLE 2 Summary of major phytochemical compounds in the rhizomes of *Z. officinale* [32, 33].

Chemical constituent	
Proteins (2%–9%)	
Carbohydrates (up to 50%)	
Lipids (1%–8%)	Free fatty acids, lecithins, phosphatidic acid, triglycerides
Minerals	Calcium, magnesium, phosphorus, potassium
Vitamins	A, B3 (niacin), B6 (riboflavin), C.
Oleo-resin	Gingerol, shogaol, zingiberole
Volatile oils (1%–2%)	Bisabolene, gingerol, citral, citronellal, geranial, linalool, Limonene, camphene, borneol, cineole, phelandrene, zingiberene.

GnRH/*Z. officinale* relationship is lacking. Currently, most studies focus on the impact of *Z. officinale* on luteinizing and follicle-stimulating hormone. In vivo studies focussing on broiler breeder males [36] and male mice [37] observed an increase in gonadotropin levels following *Z. officinale* administration. Interestingly, no increase in their levels were observed when using a rat model [9]. Irrespective of the animal model, there seems to be agreement that the administration of ginger resulted in an increased testosterone level and testicular weight [9, 37, 38].

Concomitant with the increased testicular weight, attention is also drawn to events within the testis, more specifically semen parameters. However, due consideration should be given to the contribution of follicle-stimulating hormone and its role in spermatogenesis. The use of *Z. officinale* almost without exception exhibited pro-fertility properties: semen volume [36], sperm concentration [36], sperm count [36, 37, 39, 40], and sperm motility [37, 40] were increased. In addition, sperm morphology was either normal [38, 40] or/presented with a reduced number of abnormalities [36]. Even though uncertainty exist regarding the mechanisms involved in the improved sexual function associated with the administration of ginger; consensus is reached regarding it pro-fertility capabilities as well as its modulatory impact on reproductive endocrinology.

2 Epimedium grandiflorum

2.1 Introduction

In the traditional Chinese medicinal system, and elsewhere, some species from the genus *Epimedium* have an age-old history in the management of ailments. Among these *E. grandiflorum*, *Epimedium sagittatum* and others have been used to treat illnesses such as erectile dysfunction, joint pain, and fatigue [41]. Furthermore, it has been credited with improved cardiovascular and cerebrovascular functions, antitumor and antiaging effects as well as immunomodulatory functions [42, 43]. Colloquially, plants from this genus, more specifically *E. grandiflorum*, have been referred to as "horny goat weed" or "yin yang huo." The colloquial names are attributed to the legendary discovery of its aphrodisiac properties by a Chinese goat herder who noted an increased sexual activity in his herd after they consumed the plant's leaves [44]. Clearly, most of the interest in this genus can be attributed to its aphrodisiac properties [41]; however, existing literature illustrates that this genus has much more to offer [41–44].

2.2 Taxonomical classification

Epimedium, the largest herbaceous genus in the Family Berberidaceae, is an attractive genus and has been recognized horticulturally and botanically (Table 3). It comprises approximately 60 species, which is distributed in temperate mountainous regions stretching from Asia to Northwestern Africa; however, large distributional gaps have been reported in these regions [45–47].

2.3 Distribution and botanical description

This herbaceous, deciduous perennial plant is endemic to Southern China, Europe, and Central, Southern, and Eastern Asia [47]. Typically, their habitats range from dense mounds to wide-spreading ground covers. They are low-growing plants (30 cm) with heart-shaped leaves, the majority of which present with a four-parted "spider-like" flower during spring [42].

TABLE 3 Taxonomical classification of *Epimedium grandiflorum*.

Kingdom	Plantae
Subkingdom	Tracheobionta
Division	Magnoliaphyta
Class	Magnoliopsida
Subclass	Magnoliidae
Order	Ranunculales
Family	Berberidaceae
Genus	*Epimedium*
Species	*grandiflorum*

E. grandiflorum, an herbaceous member of the predominantly woody Barberidaceae Family, exhibits flowers in a wide range of colors. These can vary from white to yellow to rose, violet or even crimson; even combination thereof. As such, it offers the gardener an array of colors to consider for dry, shaded landscapes [48]. On nodding blooms, outer sepals are attached to the arching flower stem. The inner sepals, located adjacent to the outer sepals, characteristically extend perpendicular to the peduncle or flower stem. Furthermore, the true petals in different species have developed a variety of shapes, which can either be contained within or extend beyond the colorful sepals [48].

2.4 Phytochemistry

Numerous studies have explored the chemical richness of this genus, and many chemical compounds have been isolated and identified in it. Currently, most attention is on the various flavonoids and polysaccharides it contains. While the best known and described flavonoid is icariin, others such as apigenin, chrysoeriol, kaempferol, quercetin, and luteolin, epimedin A, epimedin B, epimedin C, and baohuoside have also been isolated and investigated [49–52]. In *Epimedium*, total flavonoids (TFE) are considered the main active components. They have been described to possess activities such as anti-aging, immunomodulatory, osteoclast inhibition, antidepressant, cardiovascular protection and cerebrovascular protection, as well as shown to enhance sex hormone secretion [53, 54] and improve the lipid profile in hyperlipidemia. In contrast to this, very few studies have explored the role of its polysaccharides on male sexual functions.

2.5 Andrology

The andrological value of this genus is widely appreciated, even though not all physiological mechanisms have been elucidated. There are some indications that the increased production of testosterone associated with the use of icariin may, even if only partially, explain the increased libido levels observed [55]. Interesting enough, the acknowledgement of the role of testosterone did not prompt focussed investigations into the effect of icariin on the activity of the gonadotropins or GnRH per se. Evidence exist in support of icariin promoting the proliferation of Sertoli cells through the activation of the ERK1/2 signaling pathway, an important concept as the number of Sertoli cells are directly associated with sperm count [56]. However, it is known that GnRH stimulation activates ERK, which involves two distinct signaling pathways which converge on the level of Raf-1 [57]. Furthermore, if the release of GnRH is promoted through the use of icariin, then it is plausible that the increased release of LH and FSH could explain the improved spermatogenesis as well as the testosterone mimetic properties noted with its use.

The ability of icariin to improve the condition of the reproductive organs is of particular interest. This is predominantly associated with the ability of icariin to protect against oxidative stress and apoptosis. It enhances endothelial nitric oxide synthase (eNOS) expression and nitric oxide (NO) production [58] within human endothelial cells, where NO promotes vasodilation. Moreover, in response to hydrogen peroxide production it reduces caspase-3 expression and suppresses the extent of cellular apoptosis [59, 60]. Complementing this is the capacity of *Epimedium* polysacchharides (EPS) not only to enhance epididymis sperm count and significantly increase testosterone levels, but also to increase superoxide dismutase (SOD) and glutathione peroxidase (GPx) activities, and to reduce the levels of malondialdehyde (MDA) [61]. The potential of icariin to alter the functionality of endothelial cells within the penile tissue accentuates its key application in the management of erectile dysfunction.

The erectogenic effect of icariin can be attributed to increased intra-cavernous pressure (ICP) [62], which results from the vasodilation of penile blood vessels. Icariin has an inhibitory effect on all three PDE-5 isoforms [63]. The inhibition of PDE-5 prevents the degradation of cyclic GMP and prolongs the vasodilatory effect of NO [64]. When icariin is combined with two hydoxyethyl ester moieties, its PDE-5 inhibitory effect is increased almost 80-fold, which makes it nearly as effective as sildenafil [65]. Overall, the use of *Epimedium*-based products to improve male sexual functions is not only an acceptable practice, but also scientifically proven.

References

[1] Grzanna R, Lindmark L, Frondoza C. Ginger—a herbal medicinal product with broad anti-inflammatory actions. J Med Food 2005;8(2):125–32.

[2] Dhanik J, Arya N, Nand V. A review on *Zingiber officinale*. J Pharmacogn Phytochem 2017;6(3):174–84.

[3] Imtiyaz S, Rahman K, Sultana A, Tariq T, Chaudhary SS. *Zingiber officinale* Rosc.: a traditional herb with medicinal properties. Assoc Human Tradit Med 2013;3(4):e26. https://doi.org/10.5667/tang.2013.0009.

[4] Irfan S, Ranjha MMAN, Mahmood S, Mueen-ud-Din G, Rehman S, Saeed W, Alam MQ, Zahra SM, Quddoos MY, Ramzan I, Rafique A, bin Masood A. A critical review on pharmaceutical and medicinal importance of ginger. Acta Sci Nutr Health 2019;3(1):78–82.

[5] Sakr SA, Badawy GM. Effect of ginger (*Zingiber officinale* R.) on metiram-inhibited spermatogenesis and induced apoptosis in albino mice. J Appl Pharmaceut Sci 2011;1(04):131–6.

[6] Kapoor LD. Handbook of Ayurvedic Medicinal Plants. Boca Raton, FL: CRC Press; 1990.

[7] Langner E, Greifenberg S, Grunwald J. Ginger: history and use. Adv Ther 1988;15:25–44.

[8] Ibrahim AAE-M, Al-Shathly MR. Herbal blend of cinnamon, ginger, and clove modulates testicular histopathology, testosterone levels and sperm quality of diabetic rats. Int J Pharmaceut Sci Rev Res 2015;30(2):95–103.

[9] Afzali A, Ghalehkandi JG. Effect of ginger, *Zingiber officinale* on sex hormones and certain biochemical parameters of male Wistar rats. Biosci Biotechnol Res Commun 2018;11(1):181–6.

[10] Ajith TA, Hema U, Aswathy MS. *Zingiber officinale* Roscoe prevents acetaminophen-induced acute hepatotoxicity by enhancing hepatic antioxidant status. Food Chem Toxicol 2007;45(11):2267–72.

[11] Rehman R, Akram M, Akhtar N, Jabeen Q, Saeed T, Shah SMA, Ahmed K, Shaheen G, Asif HM. *Zingiber officinale* Roscoe (pharmacological activity). J Med Plants Res 2015;5(3):344–8.

[12] Ghosh AK, Banerjee S, Mullick HI, Banerjee J. *Zingiber officinale*: a natural gold. Int J Pharma BioSci 2011;2(1):283–94.

[13] Kuhad A, Tirkey N, Pilkhwal S, Chopra K. 6-Gingerol prevents cisplatin induced acute renal failure in rats. Biofactors 2006;26(3):189–200.

[14] Ha SK, Moon E, Ju MS, Kim DH, Ryu JH, Oh MS, Kim SY. 6-Shogaol, a ginger product, modulates neuroinflammation: a new approach to neuroprotection. Neuropharmacology 2012;63(2):211–23.

[15] Nanjundaiah SM, Annaiah HN, Dharmesh SM. Gastroprotective effect of ginger rhizome (*Zingiber officinale*) extract: role of gallic acid and cinnamic acid in H^+, K^+-ATPase/*H. pylori* inhibition and anti-oxidative mechanism. Evid-Based Complement Altern Med 2011. https://doi.org/10.1093/ecam/nep060.

[16] Jain SK, Prakash V. Zingiberaceae in India: phytogeography and endemism. Rheedea 1995;5:154–69.

[17] Tauheed HA, Ali A, Zaigham M. Zanjabeel (*Zingiber officinale* Rosc.): a household rhizome with immense therapeutic potential and its utilization in Unani medicine. Int J Pharmaceut Sci Res 2017;8(8):3218–30.

[18] Wu TL, Larsen K. In: Wu ZY, Raven PH, editors. Zingiberaceae, 24. Flora of China; 2000. p. 322–77.

[19] Ravinderan PN, Nirmal BK, Shiva KN. Botany and crop improvement of ginger. In: Ravinderan PN, Nirmal BK, editors. Ginger: the Genus *Zingiber*. New York: CRC Press; 2005. p. 15–85.

[20] Vasala PA. Ginger. In: Peter KV, editor. Handbook of Herbs and Spices. Cambridge, UK: Woodhead Publishing; 2004.

[21] Kritikar KR, Basu BD. Indian Medicinal Plants. 2nd ed. vol. 4. Dehradun, India: International Book Distributers; 2007.

[22] Ross IA. Medicinal plants of the world. Vol. 3. New Jersey, USA: Humana Press; 2005.

[23] Kawai T. Anti-emetic principles of *Magnolia obovate* bark and *Zingiber officinale* rhizome. Planta Med 1994;60(1):17–20.

[24] Yassin NAZ, ElRokh E-SM, El-Shenawy SMA, Ibrahim BMM. The study of the antispasmodic effect of ginger (*Zingiber officinale*) *in vitro*. Pharm Lett 2012;4:263–74.

[25] Afshari AT, Shirpoor A, Farshid A, Saadatian R, Rasmi Y, Saboory E, Khanizadeh B, Allameh A. The effect of ginger on diabetic nephropathy, plasma antioxidant capacity and lipid peroxidation in rats. Food Chem 2007;101:148–53.

[26] Ali BH, Blunden G, Tanira MO, Nemmar A. Some phytochemical, pharmacological and toxicological properties of ginger (*Zingiber officinale* Roscoe): a review of recent research. Food Chem Toxicol 2008;46(2):409–20.

[27] Remadevi R, Surendran E, Ravindran PN. Properties and medicinal uses of ginger. In: Nirmal BK, Ravinderan PN, editors. Ginger: The Genus Zingiber, 2004. Boca Raton, FL, USA: CRC Press; 2004. p. 489–508.

[28] Kumar KMP, Asish GR, Sabu M, Balachandran I. Significance of gingers (Zingiberaceae) in Indian system of medicine—Ayurveda: an overview. Ancient Sci Life 2013;32:253–61.

[29] Jayashree E, Kandiannan K, Prasath D, Rashid P, Sasikumar B, Senthil Kumar CM, Srinivasan V, Suseela Bhai R, Thankamani CK. Ginger. In: ICAR-Indian Institute of spices research Kozhikode-673 012, Kerala. ICAR-Indian Institute of Spices Research: Kerala, India; 2015.

[30] Benskey D, Gamble A. Chinese Herbal Medicine: Materia Medica. Seattle, DC, USA: Eastland Press; 1986.

[31] Braun L, Cohen M. Herbs and Natural Supplements. An evidence-based guide. 2nd ed. Australia: Elsevier; 2007.

[32] Sharma Y. Ginger (*Zingiber officinale*)—an elixir of life a review. Pharma Innov J 2017;6(10):22–7.

[33] Barnes J, Andersen LA, Phillipson JD. Herbal Medicines. 3rd ed. Royal Pharmaceutical Society (RPS), Publishing: Pharmaceutical Press; 2007. p. 721.

[34] Tng EL. Kisspeptin signalling and its roles in humans. Singapore Med J 2015;56(12):649–56.

[35] Ramaswamy S, Guerriero KA, Gibbs RB, Plant TM. Structural interactions between kisspeptin and GnRH neurons in the mediobasal hypothalamus of the male rhesus monkey (*Macaca mulatta*) as revealed by double immunofluorescence and confocal microscopy. Endocrinology 2008;149:4387–95.

[36] Saeid JM, Shanoon AK, Marbut MM. Effects of *Zingiber officinale* aqueous extract on semen characteristic and some blood plasma, semen plasma parameters in the broilers breeder male. Int J Poultry Sci 2011;10(8):629–33.

[37] Alessia MS, Shalaby AA, Alkarim HA, Ibrahim NA, Hossain ABM, Stam G. Influence of ginger (*Zingiber officinale*) on sperms parameters, spermatogenesis and sexual hormones of male mice. J Adv Biol 2016;8(2):1607–11.

[38] Memudu AE, Akinrinade ID, Ogundele OM, Duru F. Investigation of the androgenic activity of ginger (*Zingiber officinale*) on histology of the testis of the adult Sprague Dawley rats. J Med Med Sci 2012;3(11):697–702.

[39] Morakinyo AO, Adeniyi OS, Arikawe AP. Effects of *Zingiber officinale* on reproductive functions in the male rat. Afr J Biomed Res 2008;11:329–34.

[40] Donkor YO, Abaidoo CS, Tetteh J, Darko ND, Atuahene OO-D, Appiah AK, Diby T, Maalman RS. The effect of *Zingiber officinale* (ginger) root ethanolic extract on the semen characteristics of adult male Wistar rats. Int J Anat Res 2018;6(3.2):5481–7.

[41] Shindel AW, Xin ZC, Lin G, Fandel TM, Huang YC, Banie L, Brever BN, Garcia MM, Lin CS, Lue TF. Erectogenic and neurotrophic effects of icariin, a purified extract of horny goat weed (*Epimedium* spp.) *in vitro* and *in vivo*. J Sex Med 2010;7(1):1518–28.

[42] Ma H, He X, Yang Y, Li M, Hao D, Jia Z. The genus *Epimedium*: an ethnopharmacological and phytochemical review. J Ethnopharmacol 2011;134:519–41.

[43] Makarova MN, Pozharitskaya ON, Shikov AN, Tesakova SV, Makarov VG, Tikhonov VP. Effect of lipid-based suspension of *Epimedium koreanum* Nakai extract on sexual behaviour in rats. J Ethnopharmacol 2007;114(3):412–6.

[44] Horny Goats Weed [Internet]. Available from: http://www.herbwisdom.com/herb-horny-goats-weed.html; 2013.

[45] Stearn WT. The genus *Epimedium* and other herbaceous Berberidaceae. Portland: Timber Press; 2002. p. 10–128.

[46] Xu YQ, Xu Y, Liu Y, Ge F. Progress and open problems in classical taxonomic research on *Epimedium* L. Chin Tradit Herb Drug 2014;45:569–77.

[47] Zhang YJ, Dang HS, Li SY, Li JQ, Wang Y. Five new synonyms in *Epimedium* (Berberidaceae) from China. PhytoKeys 2015;49:1–12.

[48] Rudy MR. Plant evaluation notes an evaluation report on Barrenworts for the shade garden. Chicago Botanic Garden 2003;20. www.chicagobotanic.org/downloads/planteval_notes/no20_barrenworts.pdf.

[49] Du Q, Xia M, Ito Y. Purification of icariin from the extract of *Epimedium segittatum* using high-speed counter-current chromatography. J Chromatogr A 2002;962(1–2):239–41.

[50] Luk JM, Wang X, Liu P, Wong KF, Chan KL, Tong Y, Hui CK, Lau GK, Fan ST. Traditional Chinese herbal medicines for treatment of liver fibrosis and cancer: from laboratory discovery to clinical evaluation. Liver Int 2007;27(7):879–90.

[51] May BH, Yang AWH, Zhang AL. Chinese herbal medicine for mild cognitive impairment and age associated memory impairment: a review of randomized controlled trials. Biogerontology 2008;10(2):109–23.

[52] Chen CY, Bau DT, Tsai MH, Hsu YM, Ho TY, Huang HJ, Chang YH, Tsai FJ, Tsai CH, Chen CY. Could traditional Chinese medicine be used for curing erectile dysfunction effective. In: Proceeding of the 2nd International Conference, Biomedical Engineering and Informatics, 17–19 October 2009, Tianjin; 2009, ISBN:978-1-4244-4132-7. https://doi.org/10.1109/BMEI.2009.5304967.

[53] Huang XL, Zhou YW, Wang W. Pharmacological research advances on total flavonoids of *Epimedium*. Chin Trad Patent Med 2005;27:719–21.

[54] Meng N, Kong K, Li SW. Advances in studies on chemical constituents and pharmaceutical activities in species of *Epimedium*. Acta Bot Boreali-Occidentalia Sin 2010;30:1063–73.

[55] Malo AF, Roldan ER, Garde J, Soler AJ, Gomendio M. Antlers honestly advertise sperm production and quality. Proc R Soc B: Biol Sci 2005;272:149–57.

[56] Wang S-C, Wang S-C, Chia-Jung Li C-J, Lin C-H, Hsiao-Lin Huang H-S, Tsai L-M, Chang C-H. The therapeutic effects of traditional Chinese medicine for poor semen quality in infertile males. J Clin Med 2018;7:239. https://doi.org/10.3390/jcm7090239.

[57] Benard O, Naor Z, Seger R. Role of Dynamin, Src and Ras in the PKC-mediated activation of ERK by gonadotropin-releasing hormone. J Biol Chem 2000;276(7):4554–63.

[58] Xiao H-B, Sui G-G, Lu X-Y. Icariin improves eNOS/NO pathway to prohibit the atherogenesis of apolipoprotein E-null mice. Can J Physiol Pharmacol 2017;95(6):625–33.

[59] Wang YK, Huang ZQ. Protective effects of icariin on human umbilical vein endothelial cell injury induced by H_2O_2 *in vitro*. Pharmacol Res 2005;52:174–82.

[60] Xu HB, Huang ZQ. Icariin enhances endothelial nitric-oxide synthase expression on human endothelial cells *in vitro*. Vascul Pharmacol 2007;47:18–24.

[61] Ni G, Zhang Y, Afedo SY, Rui R. *Epimedium* polysaccharides impacts the reproductive function of pubertal male mice. Acad J Pharm Pharmacol 2018;6(2):18–23.

[62] Lim PHC. Asian herbals and aphrodisiacs used for managing ED. Transl Androl Urol 2017;6(2):167–75.

[63] Ning H, Xin ZC, Lin G, Banie L, Lue TF, Lin CS. Effects of icariin on phosphodiesterase-5 activity *in vitro* and cyclic guanosine monophosphate level in cavernous smooth muscle cells. Urology 2006;68(6):1350–4.

[64] Wendlová J. Scientific medicine in integrative treatment of erectile dysfunction. J Integr Nephrol Androl 2015;2(1):5–18.

[65] Dell'Agli M, Galli GV, Dal Cero E, Belluti F, Matera R, Zironi E, Pagliuca G, Bosisio E. Potent inhibition of human phosphodiesterase-5 by icariin derivatives. J Nat Prod 2008;71:1513–7.

Chapter 5.4.5

Herbal medicine use to treat andrological problems: Asian and Indian subcontinent: *Ginkgo biloba*, *Curcuma longa*, and *Camellia sinensis*

Shubhadeep Roychoudhury[a,b], Saptaparna Chakraborty[a], Anandan Das[a], Pokhraj Guha[c], Ashok Agarwal[d], and Ralf Henkel[d,e,f]

[a]*Department of Life Science and Bioinformatics, Assam University, Silchar, India*, [b]*Department of Morphology, Physiology and Animal Genetics, Mendel University, Brno, Czech Republic*, [c]*Department of Zoology, Garhbeta College, Paschim Medinipur, West Bengal, India*, [d]*American Center for Reproductive Medicine, Cleveland Clinic, Cleveland, OH, United States*, [e]*Department of Medical Bioscience, University of the Western Cape, Bellville, South Africa*, [f]*Department of Metabolism, Digestion and Reproduction, Imperial College London, London, United Kingdom*

1 Introduction

Andrology (from Greek: ἀνήρ, anēr, genitive; ἀνδρός, andros, "man;" and -λογία, -logia) is the specialty of medical science that deals with male reproductive functions under physiological and pathological conditions [1]. The term andrology was coined by Habard Siebke in 1951 and initially the discipline developed in Germany from dermatology. However, modern day andrology is influenced more by urology, gynecology, and endocrinology [2]. Andrological problems have become both a common and a serious issue faced by at least 15% of couples worldwide [3]. The major problems covered by andrology include male infertility, male contraception, hypogonadism, erectile dysfunction, and male senescence [1]. Other issues such as testicular cancer and prostate disorders, for example, benign prostatic hyperplasia and carcinoma, delayed puberty, family planning and contraception, cryopreservation of semen and testicular tissue, hormone replacement therapy, forensic paternity problems, and as aging in the men come under the ambit of andrology [2].

In Asia, the male factor has been estimated to contribute to 37% of infertility cases [4]. Available data suggest 3.9%–16.8% primary infertility rate in India [5] with the male factor considered responsible in 23% of couples seeking treatment [6]. A vast array of management strategies of male infertility have evolved in course of time, which include the repair and reconstruction of varicocele, vas deferens, and the epididymis through microsurgical techniques [7]; assisted reproductive techniques (ART) such as intrauterine insemination (IUI), in vitro fertilization (IVF), and intracytoplasmic sperm injection (ICSI); combined administration of antibiotic and anti-inflammatory drugs to enhance semen quality of habitual tobacco smokers, etc. [8–10].

Community-based, primary-care, and screening studies have shown hypogonadism as one of the leading andrological problems in many Asian countries including the Indian subcontinent with variable prevalence rates of 9.5% in Hong Kong [11], 19.1% in Malaysia [12], 24.1% in Taiwan [13], and 24.2% in India [14]. Testosterone replacement therapy forms the major therapeutic option available in the management of clinical hypogonadism that includes intramuscular, subcutaneous, oral, and nasal formulations [15–18].

The prevalence rate of erectile dysfunction ranges from 9% to 73% in many Asian countries [19] with 8%–50% reports from Hong Kong, 13%–81% from Japan, 22.4%–59% from Malaysia, and 33%–65% from the Philippines [20]. The first line of treatment includes oral application of phosphodiesterase-5 inhibitors and vacuum erection devices [21, 22], whereas intracavernosal therapies and other surgical methods (e.g., penile prosthesis and penile revascularization surgery) constitute the second and third lines of therapeutic strategies, respectively [23].

Testicular cancer represents approximately 1% of all the malignancies diagnosed in men [24] and affects relatively younger generation between 20 and 40 years of age [25]. The incidence rates are low in Asia including India (1.3 per 100,000 men) and China (2.2); the overall testicular cancer mortality rate has also shown a declining trend in Asian populations,

Herbal Medicine in Andrology. https://doi.org/10.1016/B978-0-12-815565-3.00019-9

particularly China (−4.9%) [26]. Management procedures include orchiectomy, which is done in affected neoplastic cells and has high treatment success rate although low-dose radiotherapy constitutes another alternative therapeutic option [27].

In Asia, both the incidence as well as mortality rates of prostate cancer have been on the rise, which has been associated with the increasing consumption of red meat, fat, dairy, and eggs [28]. Age-standardized incidence as well as mortality rates have been higher in Singapore (33.1 and 4.5), Japan (30.4 and 5.0), and South Korea (30.3 and 4.6) in comparison to China (5.3 and 2.5) and India (4.2 and 2.7) [29]. Another nonmalignant growth of prostate gland termed "benign prostatic hyperplasia" is also seen among aged men [30–32] with particularly high occurrence among urban Chinese population over 40 years [33]. Modern techniques of treatment of high-risk prostate carcinoma include surgery, radiation therapy, cryosurgery, and androgen deprivation therapy [34–37], whereas prostatic urethral lift [38], transurethral resection of the prostate [39], prosthetic artery embolization [40], and vaporizing techniques [41] form the novel clinical options in the management of benign prostatic hyperplasia.

2 Herbal medicine

Among Asian populations including that of the Indian subcontinent, herbal remedies have been practiced since ancient times for the management of many complex diseases. In addition to the abovementioned therapeutic approaches, herbal medicines can also prove to be effective in the management of abovementioned andrological problems. Such medicines have been documented as folklore in various traditional systems based on geographical habitats and exposure to diseases. In the Asian continent the major traditional systems of herbal medicine include Ayurveda, Siddha, and Unani practiced widely in the Indian subcontinent and other parts of Asia; Chinese traditional medicine; and Koryo system of medicine prevalent in Korea to name a few. For treating such diseases, herbal remedies are still prescribed by traditional healers in many developing regions of Asia [30, 31, 42–44]. For instance, herbal tonics and preparations have been in use for improving the aging male's ability to have sexual drive or perform penetrative sex by increasing sexual stimulation, erectile, ejaculatory, orgasmic, and other responses for sexual function and satisfaction [30, 31]. The medicinal use of three such herbs *Ginkgo biloba*, *Curcuma longa*, and *Camellia sinensis* in the treatment of important andrological issues in Asia including the Indian subcontinent is focused in this chapter as given below.

2.1 *Ginkgo biloba*

G. biloba is an ancient medicinal plant belonging to its own division called Ginkgophyta because of the lack of its distinct relationship with any other plant group. It is regarded as a 'living fossil' because of the unchanged biological existence for 270 million years. Unveiling its use in modern medicine is currently underway owing to its bioactive triterpene lactones and flavonoids [45], including ginkgolides and bilobalides [46]. Perceived pharmacological action of *G. biloba* is attributed more to the synergistic effect of its bioactive components rather than the individual constituents [47]. A commercially available product called EGb761 prepared from the leaf extracts of *G. biloba* (which contains 24% ginkgo flavone glycosides and 6% terpene lactones) has been shown to improve memory functions [48, 49]. The leaf extract of *G. biloba* also plays a major role in the management of neurodegenerative diseases [50], and acts as cognitive enhancer in dementia [51]. It has also beneficial effects on glaucoma by increasing ocular blood flow [52], and gives positive results in the treatment of macular degeneration and altitude sickness [53, 54]. It is a medicinal plant of great andrological importance. Some of its major uses in the management of the abovementioned disorders are presented in Table 1 and are discussed in detail below.

2.1.1 *Male infertility*

Oral supplementation of *G. biloba* extract in rats at doses of 50, 100, and 200 mg/kg for 5 days have been able to ameliorate reproductive toxicity induced by an hour of cisplatin exposure, which include protection against testicular atrophy, cellular disorganization and degeneration [55]. A dose of 200 mg/kg body weight of *G. biloba* extract administered to rats by gavage for 12 weeks has been found to induce the production of antioxidant enzymes, which can reduce cellular ROS levels and inhibit sperm membrane lipid peroxidation [56]. Oral application of *G. biloba* extract in rats for a period of 3 months has been associated with an increase in mean weight of the cauda epididymis and the prostate at daily doses of 50 and 100 mg/kg. However, long-term treatment caused chromosomal aberrations and failed to increase the protein content in testicular cells [57]. Continuous production of free radicals in sperm is combated by the first line of antioxidant defense system, which may be further activated by the *G. biloba* extract. It has a potent buffering action that keeps the levels of ROS within check [56]. *G. biloba* extract can also lower the expression of NF-κB, thus acting as a link between oxidative damage and inflammation stimulated by oxidative stress [55]. However, detrimental chromosomal aberrations and cytotoxicity induced by *G. biloba* may be attributed to the potential allergenic, mutagenic, and carcinogenic properties of ginkgolic acid and related

TABLE 1 Clinical significance of *Ginkgo biloba* as herbal medicine in the management of andrological problems.

Andrological problem	Herbal medicine	Experimental model	Dosage	Calculated human dose[a]	Action	Reference
Male infertility	*Ginkgo biloba* extract	Rat	50, 100, and 200 mg/kg for 5 days	568, 1135, and 2270 mg	Protection against testicular atrophy, cellular disorganization and degeneration induced by cisplatin	[55]
			200 mg/kg for 12 weeks	2270 mg	Reduction of oxidative stress by producing antioxidant enzymes	[56]
			50 and 100 mg/kg for 3 months	568 and 1135 mg	Increase in mean weight of cauda epididymis and prostate	[57]
Hypogonadism	*Ginkgo biloba* extract	Rat	3.5, 7, and 14 mg/kg for 56 days	40, 80, and 149 mg	Increase in serum testosterone level	[58]
			70 mg/kg for 7 days	795 mg		[59]
			Single dose of 50 mg/kg	568 mg		[60]
		Rat (Leydig cell culture)	0.05, 0.1, 0.25, 0.5, and 1 mg/mL	–		[61]
Erectile dysfunction	*Ginkgo biloba* extract	Human	40–60 mg twice daily for 4 weeks	–	Improvement of sexual functions including erection	[62]
			80 mg thrice daily for 6 months	–	Regaining of penile rigidity	[63]
			80 mg twice a week for 36 months	–	Improvement in erectile functions	[64]
Prostate cancer	Ginkgetin	Human (PC-3 cell line)	40, 50, and 60 µmol/L for 24 h	–	Reduction in cell viability by increasing the expression of caspase-3 and reduction of regulatory proteins	[65]
		Human (DU-145 cell line)	5 µmol/L for 24 h	–	Suppression of signal transducer and activator of STAT3-dependent cancer cells	[66]
	Kaempferol	Human (PC-3 and LNCaP cell line)	10–40 µmol/L for 24 h	–	Reduction of malignancy by induction of caspase-3 and inhibition of genes required for the survival of cancer cells	[67]
Benign Prostatic Hyperplasia	Cerenin (Commercial *Ginkgo biloba* extract)	Rat	3.5 mg/mL for 4 weeks	40 mg	Suppression of inflammation	[68]

[a] *Reagan-Shaw et al. [68a].*

alkylphenols [69]. Supplementation of *G. biloba* extract may be associated with the induction of free radicals that activate the γ-aminobutyric acid, glutamic acid, aspartic acid, and glycine, thus causing sperm membrane depolarization [69].

2.1.2 Hypogonadism

Intragastric administration of *G. biloba* extract to rats at daily doses of 3.5, 7, and 14 mg/kg for 56 days showed a marked increase in serum testosterone level [58]. A daily dose of 70 mg/kg *G. biloba* extract supplemented for 7 days also showed more than 5-fold increment in testosterone levels in rats [59]. Ischemic male rats undergoing orchiectomy followed by oral supplementation of a single dose of 50 mg/kg *G. biloba* extract increased the serum-free testosterone level along with reduction of ischemia [60]. An in vitro culture of rat Leydig cells when administered with *G. biloba* extract at doses 0.05, 0.1, 0.25, 0.5, and 1 mg/mL improved testosterone release although the effect could not be confirmed in vivo [61].

G. *biloba* plays a crucial role in protecting the Leydig cells from oxidative damage by scavenging free radicals [70]. Its antioxidant property and increased tissue resistance are believed to be the primary causes of resilience of seminiferous tubule hemorrhage which is brought about by reduction in testosterone levels and ischemia [71]. However, *G. biloba* supplementation may not always yield the desired improvement in serum testosterone level possibly due to the negative feedback mechanism of androgen. Excessive testosterone level attenuates GnRH stimulation of luteinizing hormone (LH) and inhibits testosterone synthesis in vivo. [72].

2.1.3 Erectile dysfunction

A capsule containing 40–60 mg *G. biloba* extract (together with antidepressants such as fluoxetine, nefazodone, bupropion, sertraline, paroxetine, venlafaxine, phenelzine, and vivactil) when taken orally twice daily for 4 weeks turned out to be 84% effective in improving sexual function including erection in patients suffering from erectile dysfunction [62]. Oral supplementation of another capsule of 80 mg *G. biloba* extract thrice daily for 6 months (along with other intracavernosal drugs such as papaverine and phentolamine) was capable of sufficiently regaining the rigidity of penis in patients of <70 years age [63]. Erectile dysfunction patients of <58 years mean age when supplemented with 80 mg *G. biloba* extract (together with tadalafil) twice a week for 36 months has recently showed improvement in attaining erection [64].

The active compounds of *G. biloba*—ginkgolides, terpenoids, and flavonoids—inhibit platelet aggregation, neutrophil degranulation, and ROS production. They may be able to cause erection by enhanced vascular flow to the genitals through the inhibition of platelet-activating factor and prostaglandins to attain adequate erection, or serotonin- and norepinephrine-receptor-induced effects on the brain [47, 62]. *G. biloba* increases nitric oxide synthase (NOS) expression which is associated with better noncontact erection [73]. Moreover, *G. biloba* extract exhibits neuroprotective effects on the dorsal penile nerve supplying the corpus cavernosum facilitating better erection signal [74]. Higher doses of *G. biloba* may be beneficial in reducing apoptosis of the cavernosal cells and improving the content of smooth muscle cells [75].

2.1.4 Testicular cancer

Clinical utility of *G. biloba* in the management of testicular cancer is yet to be investigated, although *G. biloba* extract showed protective effects on the testis against cisplatin-, doxorubicin- and diethylstilbestrol-induced reproductive toxicity in animal models [55, 76–78].

2.1.5 Prostate disorders

In human prostate cancer cells PC-3, ginkgetin administration at doses of 40, 50, and 60 μmol/L has been able to decrease their viability after 24 h. Furthermore, the doses of 15 and 30 μmol/L induced apoptosis including cell shrinkage. At these doses, ginkgetin also increased the cleavage of caspase-3 and poly (ADP-ribose) polymerase, and suppressed the expression of regulatory proteins involved in the apoptosis signaling pathway such as Bcl-2, Bcl-x_L, survivin, and cyclin D1 [65]. In human prostate cancer cells DU-145, ginkgetin application at 5 μmo/L dose has been found to suppress the proliferation of signal transducer and activator of transcription-3 (STAT3)-dependent cancer cells after 24 h, including inhibition of interleukin-6-induced STAT3 phosphorylation [66].

Kaempferol, another important bioactive component of *G. biloba*, decreased the viability and increased apoptosis of human prostate cancer cells PC-3 and LNCaP at a dose range of 10–40 μmol/L after 24 h [67]. The ability of *G. biloba* to suppress malignancy largely depends on the ability of its bioactive compound ginkgetin to form apoptotic bodies by caspase-3 activation and inhibition of the genes required for survival of PC-3 cells. It also increases the sub-G1 population in PC-3 cells, induces cleavage of PARP and caspase-3, and downregulates the expression of Bcl-2, Bcl-x_L, survivin, and cyclin D1 [65]. Ginkgetin can also inhibit STAT3 activation particularly by interfering with STAT3 phosphorylation and reducing nuclear localization of STAT3. Such blocking of STAT3 upregulates p53 expression leading to p53-mediated tumor cell

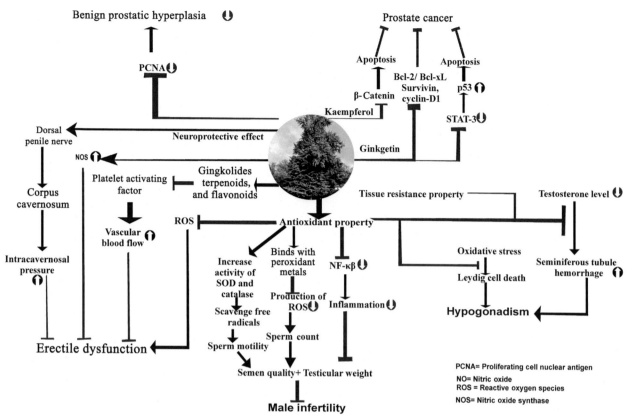

FIG. 1 Potential mechanism of action of *Ginkgo biloba* in the management of andrological problems. *Ginkgo biloba* extract with its potential to increase the activity of antioxidant enzymes superoxide dismutase and catalase along with the property of binding to peroxidant metals can reduce seminal oxidative stress and improve sperm motility. It also serves to enhance semen quality parameters by inhibiting the activity of NF-κB. Further, *Ginkgo biloba* extract inhibits oxidative stress in Leydig cells to regulate testosterone production. Various bioactive components of *Ginkgo biloba* extract, for example, ginkgolides show neuroprotective action against the dorsal penile nerve and increases NOS activity in the cavernous tissue to restore proper erectile function. Ginkgetin and kaempferol can also induce apoptosis by upregulation of apoptotic proteins and by downregulation of cell cycle proteins to reduce malignancy in prostate cancer cells. Also, *Ginkgo biloba* extract reduces the expression of proliferating cell nuclear antigen to relieve the effects of benign prostatic hyperplasia.

apoptosis [66]. Kaempferol is also capable of inducing apoptosis, inhibiting the β-catenin protein level and expression along with its downstream targets C-myc, cyclin D1, and survivin as well as inhibiting the β-catenin/TCF transcriptional activity in PC-3 and LNCaP cells [67].

In rats, a daily injection of a commercial *G. biloba* leaf extract Cerenin for 4 weeks at a dose of 3.5 mg/mL (240 mg/g flavonoids and 60 mg/g terpenoids) in a solution containing ethanol, sorbitol, and NaOH have been able to suppress inflammation [68]. The therapeutic potential of *G. biloba* in the management of benign prostatic hyperplasia is believed to be mediated mainly by the reduction of proliferating cell nuclear antigen thereby lowering the risk of the disease. It also ameliorates the upregulation of prostatic aromatase enzyme indicating its effectiveness in curing benign prostatic hyperplasia [68].

The potential mechanism of action of *G. biloba* in the management of andrological problems are presented in Fig. 1.

2.2 *Curcuma longa*

C. longa, commonly called turmeric, is a tuberous herbaceous perennial plant belonging to the family Zingiberaceae with yellow flowers and wide leaves [79]. *C. longa* has been traditionally known to possess beneficial properties for the prevention as well as treatment of several diseases in Asian populations for more than 2500 years [80]. The main components of the rhizome are turmerone, santalene, and curcumin [81]. Curcumin, an orange-yellow colored lipophilic polyphenolic substance, is the most studied for its beneficial medicinal properties [80]. Its ability to prevent skin diseases has been described in Ayurveda and Chinese pharmacopoeia, and the rhizomes of the herb act as a home remedy for curing burns, bites, and acne [82, 83]. It prevents neurodegenerative and cardiovascular diseases [84], and also possesses anticancer effects. The role of *C. longa* in the management of major andrological disorders are presented in Table 2 and discussed in detail below.

TABLE 2 Clinical significance of *Curcuma longa* as herbal medicine in the management of andrological problems.

Andrological problem	Herbal medicine	Experimental model	Dosage	Calculated human dose[a]	Action	Reference
Male infertility	Curcumin	Human	80 mg/kg for 10 weeks	–	Increase in sperm count, motility and concentration	[85]
	Curcuma longa extract	Rat	5 and 50 mg/kg for 15 days	57 and 568 mg	Increase in testicular weight, sperm count and motility	[86]
	Curcumin	Mouse	100 mg/kg for 3 months	568 mg	Increase in weight of cauda epididymis, sperm count and motility	[87]
Hypogonadism	Curcumin	Rat	100 mg/kg for 15 days	1135 mg	Increase in serum testosterone level	[88]
		Rat	100 mg/kg for 16 days	1135 mg		[89]
Erectile dysfunction	Curcumin	Rat	10 mg/kg for 7 days	114 mg	Increase in HO-1 and NOS gene expression as well as intracavernosal pressure	[90]
			2 mg/kg for 12 weeks	23 mg	Increase in cavernosal cGMP, HO-1 and NOS activity	[91]
			2 mg/kg for 2 weeks	23 mg	Increased intracavernosal pressure which facilitated better erection	[92]
Testicular cancer	Curcumin	Rat	200 mg/kg for 5 days	2270 mg	Increased expression of apoptotic proteins	[93]
		Mouse (F9 cell line)	1.15 mg/kg	–	Inhibited cell proliferation and induced apoptosis	[94]
		Human (NTera-2 cell line)	1.72 mg/kg for 32 h	–		
		Human NCCIT cell line	5 μmol/L for 72 h	–	Increase in expression of cellular apoptotic proteins	[95]
Prostate cancer	Turmeric powder	Human	100 mg for thrice daily for 6 months	–	Reduction in prostate specific antigen and inhibition of prostate cancer metastasis	[96]
	Curcumin	Human	6000 mg	–	Enhanced levels of prostate specific antigen	[97]
		Human (PC-3 cell line)	2500 μmol/L	–	Decline in metastatic cell colonies	[98]
		Human (RPWE-1, LNCaP, VCaP and PC-3 cell line)	5 μmol/L	–	Induction of apoptosis and reduction of malignant cell colonies	[99]
		Human (LNCaP cell line)	5–50 μmol/L for 3 days	–	Decrease in proliferative potential of cancer cells	[100]
		Human (LNCaP and C42B cell line)	50 μmol/L for 24–48 h	–	Inhibition of cell proliferation	[101]
Benign Prostatic Hyperplasia	Meriva (Commercial phytosome complex of curcumin)	Human	1000 mg daily for 24 weeks	–	Reduction in urogenital infection and urinary block	[102]
	Curcumin	Rat	50 mg/kg for 4 weeks	568 mg	Reduction in prostate weight and total serum protein	[103]

[a] Reagan-Shaw et al. [68a].

2.2.1 Male infertility

Supplementation of curcumin nanomicelle at an oral dose of 80 mg/day for 10 weeks have been found to improve semen quality parameters such as, sperm count, concentration, and motility in infertile oligoasthenoteratozoospermic men in the age range of 20–45 years. The findings of infertility alleviation has been supported by a marked increase in serum malondialdehyde level and serum total antioxidant capacity [85]. Curcumin at 5 and 50 mg/kg doses when administered orally for 15 days was able to increase testicular weight, sperm count, and motility in rats, whose reproductive performance was disrupted by a protein-deficient diet for 60 days [86]. In mice, ethanolic extract of *C. longa* at an oral dose of 100 mg/kg/day body weight administered for 3 months was able to increase the weight of cauda epididymis, sperm count, and motility [87]. In vitro doses of 0.1, 3.45, 5.75, and 11.5 mg/L prepared from a stock solution of 23 mg/L curcumin in ethyl alcohol has been able to recover di(2-ethylhexyl)phthalate-induced decline in sperm motility in mice [104]. The dose- and time-dependent beneficial effects of curcumin in improving fertility parameters in the men is mediated by its antioxidative action whereby curcumin is capable of scavenging free radicals directly facilitating enhanced activity of antioxidant enzymes [105]. Inhibition of ROS generation and/or improvement in the activity of superoxide dismutase and catalase is also mediated by binding of curcumin to peroxidant metals [106]. Neutralization of free radicals and/or chelation with metal ions further prevents lipid peroxidation of sperm membrane lipids and helps keep the integrity of sperm cell membrane intact [107]. Moreover, curcumin is able to downregulate the levels of inflammation-inducing mediators such as cyclooxygenase, TNF-α, INF-γ, and NF-κB [108].

2.2.2 Hypogonadism

Oral supplementation of curcumin after dissolving in olive oil at a dose of 100 mg/kg/day can improve the levels of serum testosterone, LH, and follicle-stimulating hormone (FSH) in rats exposed to chronic variable stress for 15 days [88]. The efficacy of the same dose of curcumin in enhancing serum testosterone level has earlier been reported, too, in rats exposed to metronidazole (an antiparasitic testosterone level lowering drug) for 16 days [89]. The recovery in the levels of male reproductive hormones by curcumin is mediated via the protection of Leydig cells through its antioxidative and antigenotoxic properties [109]. Various stressors act as endocrine disruptors potentially interfering with the pituitary-testicular axis [110] to undesirably alter the levels of testosterone, LH, and FSH [111]. Such stressors may act as strong mediators of Leydig cell death via intrinsic pathway of apoptosis which is associated with mitochondrial dysfunction leading to the release of cytochrome C into cytosol and caspase activation [112]. Curcumin, in turn, facilitates the translocation of cytochrome C from cytosol to the mitochondria thereby preventing mitochondrial disruption [113]. It also suppresses adrenocorticotropic hormone, inhibits cortisol secretion, and mediates transcription for the steroid-controlling protein [114].

2.2.3 Erectile dysfunction

Natural curcumin when supplemented at a dose of 10 mg/kg/day for 7 days showed an increase in hemeoxygenase-1 (HO-1) and NOS gene expression as well as intracavernosal pressure required for penile erection in rats exposed to a single intraperitoneal injection of streptozotocin [90]. Earlier, a much lower oral dose of 2 mg/kg/day curcumin for 12 weeks was able to bring improvement in intracavernosal pressure, cavernosal cGMP level, and activity of HO-1 and NOS in diabetic rats induced by a single intraperitoneal injection of streptozotocin [91]. A daily gentle massage of curcumin nanoparticles (in a coconut oil paste) on the rat skin containing 2 mg/kg curcumin until absorption for 2 weeks also increased intracavernosal pressure, HO, and NOS activity facilitating better penile erection [92]. The potential therapeutic property of curcumin in erectile dysfunction is regulated by increasing the activity of HO and NOS. Hyperglycemia is one of the causal factors of erectile dysfunction which activates protein kinase C thereby inducing phosphorylation of a guanine exchange factor [115], which, in turn, leads to a decrease in the bioavailability of NO [116]. Protein kinase C increases the concentration of ROS, too, affecting the activity of endothelial NOS [117]. Curcumin supplementation may improve diabetes-induced endothelial dysfunction by lowering superoxide production and inhibiting protein kinase C [118]. Furthermore, curcumin and its water-soluble protein conjugate act via upliftment of cavernosal cGMP level resulting in the induction of HO-1 enzyme activity and intracavernosal pressure [91].

2.2.4 Testicular cancer

Application of curcumin at 1.72 mg/kg doses to a human malignant testicular germ cell line NTera-2 when cultured in MEM alpha medium for 32 h inhibited cell proliferation and induced apoptosis [94]. Cultured human anterior mediastinal mixed germ cell tumor NCCIT when supplemented with 5 µmol/L curcumin in culture for 72 h resulted in two- to three-fold increase in the activity of cellular apoptotic caspases [95]. In mouse tetra-carcinoma cell line F9 cultured in DMEM medium, a 64.1% reduction in the colonies of cancer cells were seen after addition of curcumin at a dose of 1.15 mg/kg [94]. In a recent study, intraperitoneal administration of 200 mg/kg/day curcumin for 5 days has increased the expression of apoptotic proteins caspase 3, Bax, and Bcl-2 in rats exposed to antineoplastic drug cisplatin [93]. Curative potential of curcumin in testicular neoplasms is regulated via the upregulation of cellular apoptotic proteins caspase 9 and 8 through respective extrinsic and intrinsic pathways. Curcumin lowers the expression of AP-2γ, a protein, which is considered critical in the regulation of tumorigenesis and in the management of testicular cancer [94]. Moreover, curcumin targets multiple cell signaling pathways such as NF-κB, Wnt, MAP kinase, and Notch and thus play a crucial role in reducing malignancy [119].

2.2.5 Prostate disorders

Oral intake of a tablet consisting of 100 mg turmeric powder (along with broccoli powder, pomegranate whole fruit powder, green tea extract) three times a day for a period of 6 months reduced the level of prostate-specific antigen indicating inhibition of prostate cancer metastasis in men having an average age of 74 years [96]. Application of curcumin at a dose of 6000 mg/day has shown a similarly enhanced response in prostate-specific antigen levels [97]. At a dose of 2500 μmol/L, curcumin has been able to bring about significant decline in metastatic cell colonies of human prostate cancer cell line PC-3 cultured in an RPMI medium [98]. Similarly, human prostate cancer cell lines RPWE-1, LNCaP, VCaP, and PC-3 when supplemented with curcumin at a dose of 5 μmol/L also showed reduction in malignant cell colonies and induction of apoptosis [99]. When applied to androgen-sensitive human prostatic carcinoma cell line LNCaP for 3 days (that underwent batch change each day), curcumin supplementation exhibited a decrease in cell proliferative potential at a dose range of 5–50 μmol/L [100]. Supplementation of human prostate cancer cells LNCaP and C42B with 50 μmol/L dose of curcumin for 24–48 h resulted in 70%–80% inhibition of cell proliferation without affecting their viability. Interestingly, only 5–10 μmol/L dose of liposomal curcumin also showed a similar inhibition of cell proliferation without affecting their viability [101]. Further experimentation in this direction may open up the door for the development of liposomal formulation of curcumin for clinical management of such andrological problems.

The potential of C. longa and its major polyphenolic constituent curcumin in the management of prostate cancer may be mediated via downregulation of the apoptotic suppressor protein MDM2 and upregulation of proapoptotic proteins of Bcl-2 family as well as through activation of caspases [100]. Curcumin has also been associated with downregulation of NF-κB signaling pathway, thus lowering the expression of prostate cancer specific cell marker CXCL 1 and 2 [98]. Furthermore, it inhibits angiogenesis in vitro and in vivo thereby arresting cell cycle in the G1/S phase in prostate cancer cells [120]. Inhibition of NF-κB expression is also regulated by curcumin, which is linked with the decline in the growth of prostate cancer cells [121]. Curcumin has been associated with the decrease in the expression of the MAPK family of protein ERK 1/2, which may also reduce the chances of neoplastic growth [122].

Meriva, a commercially available lecithinized curcumin delivery system (containing 500 mg curcumin per tablet) when supplemented to benign prostatic hyperplasia patients at a dose of two tablets/day for 24 weeks showed a reduction in the number of episodes of urogenital infections and urinary block apart from an increase in prostate-specific antigen levels [102]. In benign prostatic hyperplasic rats (induced by subcutaneous testosterone injection for a month), oral administration of curcumin at a dose of 50 mg/kg for 4 weeks followed by orchiectomy resulted in a decline in prostate weight and total serum protein [103]. Potential therapeutic use of curcumin in benign prostatic hyperplasia may be associated with the inhibition of mitogenic effects of insulin-like growth factor-1 (IGF-1) and IGF-1-receptor signaling in hypertrophic cells [123], reduction in the expression of TGF-β [124], and T-cell-dependent inflammatory stress [125].

The potential mechanisms of action of C. longa in the management of andrological problems are presented in Fig. 2.

2.3 Camellia sinensis

C. sinensis, commonly known as tea, is a shrub belonging to the family Theaceae that can grow to a height of about 16 m [126]. Tea contains about 4000 metabolites among which polyphenols take the one-third share [127]. Catechins, the flavonols present in tea infusion constitute 20%–30% of tea's dry matter, and are responsible for the taste [128]. The most common types of tea include the black tea and the green tea, which differ from each other depending on the process of fermentation. Green tea contains catechin polyphenols called epicatechin (EC), epicatechin-3-gallate (ECG), epigallocatechin (EGC), and epigallactocatechin-3-gallate (EGCG), which when fermented gets converted to more complex compounds called theaflavins, thearubigins, and theobromines—the major chemical components of black tea [129, 130]. Catechins, however, are one of the best studied compounds of plant origin [131]. Other compounds present in tea include purine alkaloids, amino acids, carbohydrates, lipids, volatile compounds, pigments, vitamins, chlorophylls, and various minerals [132, 133].

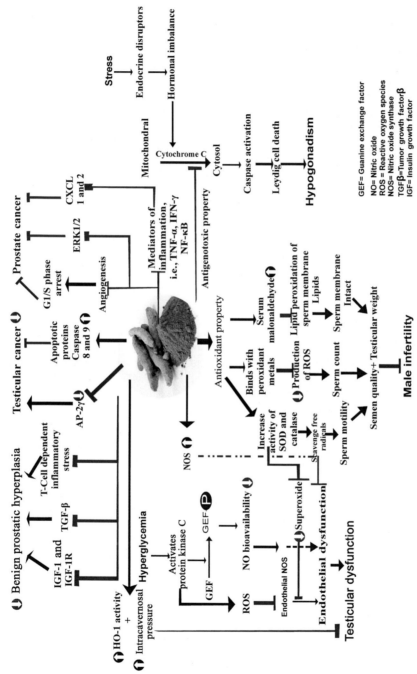

FIG. 2 Potential mechanism of action of *Curcuma longa* in the management of andrological problems. Curcumin has potent antioxidant properties which increases the enzymatic activity of superoxide dismutase and catalase to scavenge seminal free radicals. It also binds with peroxidant metals and serum malondialdehyde to reduce the production of ROS and to protect the sperm membrane from lipid peroxidation. Curcumin lowers the levels of hyperglycemia-induced protein kinase C which is responsible for ROS production. Furthermore, curcumin increases the HO-1 activity and intracavernosal pressure to restore normalcy in penile erection. Curcumin mediates the downregulation of inflammatory factors such as, TNF-α, INF-γ, and NF-κB and reduces angiogenesis to arrest metastatic cells in the G1/S phase. On the other hand, curcumin upregulates the expression of caspase 8, 9, and AP-2γ proteins and initiates cell death of neoplastic cells. It shows anti-genotoxic properties by reducing stress and hormonal imbalance-induced leakage of cytochrome C, which also results in Leydig cell death. Curcumin also reduces the expression of IGF-1, IGF-1R, and TGF-β, thus reducing the occurrence of benign prostatic hyperplasia.

Green tea possesses anticarcinogenic, anti-inflammatory, antimicrobial, and antioxidant properties [134]. The antioxidant and anti-inflammatory properties of green tea protect the neurons from degeneration and are also beneficial in cardiovascular diseases and diabetes [135, 136]. *C. sinensis* also plays a commendable role in the management of andrological disorders as shown in Table 3 and is discussed further in detail below.

2.3.1 Male infertility

In rats, an oral dose of 100 mg/kg green tea extract of *Camellia sinensis* when supplemented for 2 months showed improvement in epididymal weight, sperm motility, and viability [137]. Another oral dose of 15 mg/kg green tea extract of *C. sinensis* in boiling water when supplemented to rats have been able to increase the diameter of seminiferous tubules, number of spermatogonia, Sertoli cells, Leydig cells, and thickness of the germinal layer after 13, 25, and 49 days [138]. A dose of 150 mg/kg green tea extract of *C. sinensis* supplemented orally to male mice with γ-methrin-induced infertility for 28 days have shown improvement in sperm count and motility apart from reversing the negative effect of γ-methrin in testicular tissue degeneration [139]. In rats, an oral dose of 10 mg/mL white tea infusion administered to streptozotocin-induced diabetic rats for 2 months also increased epididymal sperm quality and testicular antioxidant potential while reducing testicular oxidative stress [140]. On the other hand, moderate and high oral doses of green tea extract of *C. sinensis* at 250 and 500 mg/kg resulted in lowering of testicular weight, sperm count, and motility in rats after 26 days of administration [150]. The abovementioned uses of *C. sinensis* in the management of male infertility may be attributed mainly to the antioxidant property exhibited by the green tea catechin polyphenols [151]. EGCG can scavenge free radicals by requisitioning metal ions by the catechin moieties in polyphenol molecules [152, 153]. EGCG is also found in rich quantity in white tea which serves as a protective agent against the deleterious effects of oxidative stress on sperm motility and testicular functioning [154]. ROS damages the phospholipid bilayer of Leydig cells and reduce their testosterone-producing efficiency, which is followed by the induction of infertility [155]. However, the inhibitory effect of higher doses of green tea extract on testosterone production by Leydig cells is probably regulated through the involvement in cell signaling pathway and decrease in the activity of steroidogenic enzymes [156].

2.3.2 Hypogonadism

In rats, black tea brew of *C. sinensis* at oral doses of 84, 167, and 501 mg/kg showed aphrodisiac activity (in terms of prolongation of latency of ejaculation, shortening of mount and intromission latencies) after 3 h and the ability to elevate serum testosterone level after 3 and 7 days [141]. However, Leydig cell culture of TM3 cells have been shown to reduce testosterone production 24 h after supplementation of 250–1000 μg/mL *C. sinensis* (green or black tea) without affecting cell viability, proliferation, and morphology (except for the cytotoxic dose of 5000 μg/mL) [157]. In spite of the beneficial effects, relatively high doses of *C. sinensis* extract (5.0% which is identical to 20 cups of tea/day) for 26 days impaired both the morphological and functional status of rat testis [158].

Black tea brew of *C. sinensis* contains theanine which possesses anxiolytic activity and thus enhances the ejaculatory time and level of serum testosterone. Black tea brew also increases the levels of serotonin and dopamine in the brain thereby elevating the serotoninergic and dopaminergic neurotransmitter signaling and uplifting the ejaculatory functions. Furthermore, the serotoninergic action of black tea brew of *C. sinensis* is known to mediate the synthesis of testosterone [141].

2.3.3 Erectile dysfunction

Daily intake of caffeine from tea and other beverages for 3–10 days at a dose range of 171–303 mg reduced the likelihood of reporting erectile dysfunction in men > 20 years age [142]. In rats, oral EGCG supplementation at doses of 10 and 100 mg/kg/day for 12 weeks have been able to recover erectile function and improve structural impairment in the corpus cavernosum [144]. Caffeine from *C. sinensis* administered to diabetic rats at 10 and 20 mg/kg doses for 8 weeks also increased the intracavernosal pressure and cavernosal cGMP levels [143].

The NO-cGMP pathway is crucial in the initiation of erection [159], and caffeine can increase the levels of cGMP and cAMP [160] apart from relaxing the smooth muscles of the corpus cavernosum [161]. Caffeine intake also increases the intracavernosal pressure and triggers vasodilation resulting in erection [162]. Moreover, catechins such as EGCG found in green tea can inhibit oxidative stress to regulate the PRMT1/DDAH/ADMA/NOS metabolic pathway. EGCG supplementation has been shown to restore superoxide dismutase activity and reduce malondialdehyde levels in the corpus cavernosum [144]. Green tea catechins have been also shown to function as potent hydrogen donors and free radical scavengers in a number of in vivo systems [163].

TABLE 3 Clinical significance of *Camellia sinensis* as herbal medicine in the management of andrological problems.

Andrological problem	Herbal medicine	Experimental model	Dosage	Calculated human dose[a]	Action	Reference
Male infertility	Green tea extract	Rat	100 mg/kg for 2 months	1135 mg	Improvement in epididymal weight, sperm motility, and viability	[137]
			15 mg/kg for 13, 25, and 49 days	170 mg	Increase in diameter of seminiferous tubules, number of spermatogonia, Sertoli cells, Leydig cells and thickness of germinal layer	[138]
		Mouse	150 mg/kg for 28 days	851 mg	Increment in sperm count and motility, recover the negative effect of deltamethrin in testicular tissue degeneration	[139]
	White tea infusion	Rat	10 mg/mL for 2 months	113.5 mg	Increase in epididymal sperm quality, testicular antioxidant potential, reduction in testicular oxidative stress	[140]
Hypogonadism	Black tea brew	Rat	84, 167, 501 mg/kg for 3 h, for 3 and 7 days	954, 1896, 5687 mg	Aphrodisiac activity, elevation of serum testosterone level	[141]
Erectile dysfunction	Caffeine from tea	Human	171–303 mg for 3–10 days	—	Likeliness of reduction in development of erectile dysfunction	[142]
		Rat	10 and 20 mg/kg for 8 weeks	114 and 227 mg	Increase in intracavernosal pressure and cavernosal cGMP levels	[143]
	EGCG	Rat	10 and 100 mg/kg for 12 weeks	114 and 1135 mg	Recovery in erectile function, improvement in structural impairment in corpus cavernosum	[144]
Testicular cancer	C. sinensis extract	Human (NT 2/DT cell line)	1000 mg for 24 h	—	Reduction in cancer invasion	[145]
Prostate cancer	Green tea extract	Human	2000 mg for 6 months	—	Reduction in oxidative stress markers, improvement in antioxidative status in erythrocytes	[146]
	Green tea polyphenol E	Human	1300 mg every day for 6 months	—	Decrease in serum level of prostate specific antigen, hepatocyte growth factor, vascular endothelial growth factor, IGF-1 and IGF binding protein-3	[147]
	Green tea	Human prostate cancer cell lines PC-3	5, 10, 25, 50 µg/mL for 24 h	—	Antiproliferative activity	[146]
	Green tea polysaccharide	Human prostate cancer cell lines PC-3	25, 50, 100 µg/mL for 48 h	—	Suppression of human prostate cancer cells	[148]
Benign Prostatic Hyperplasia	EGCG	Rat	50 and 100 mg/kg for 4 weeks	568 and 1135 mg	Reduction in level of glucose, total cholesterol, triglyceride, IGF-1, inflammatory cytokines	[149]

[a] *Reagan-Shaw et al. [68a].*

2.3.4 Testicular cancer

A nutrient mixture containing 1000 mg green tea extract of *C. sinensis* (along with vitamin C, L-lysine, L-proline, L-arginine, N-acetyl cysteine, selenium, copper, and manganese) showed reduction in cancer invasion in human testicular cancer cell line NT 2/DT after 24 h. Green tea extract consistently inhibited matrix invasion (matrix metalloproteins can degrade extracellular matrix components and induce tumor), proliferation, and migration of endothelial and vascular smooth muscle cells accompanied by a reduction of vascular endothelial growth factor, thus reducing the chances of angiogenesis [145].

2.3.5 Prostate disorders

Daily oral supplementation of 2000 mg green tea extract of *C. sinensis* for a period of 6 months has been found to reduce oxidative stress markers and improve antioxidative status in erythrocytes of prostate cancer patients with a median age of 71 years [146]. Another oral dose of 1300 mg *C. sinensis* polyphenol E per day for 6 months to prostate cancer patients during the interval between prostate biopsy and radical prostatectomy was able to decrease the serum level of prostate-specific antigen, hepatocyte growth factor, vascular endothelial growth factor, IGF-1 and IGF-binding protein-3 [147]. Human prostate cancer cells PC-3 when supplemented with 5, 10, 25, and 50 µg/mL green tea in culture media showed significant antiproliferative activity after 24 h [146]. At similar doses of 25, 50, and 100 µg/mL, green tea polysaccharide extracted from *C. sinensis* showed suppression of human prostate cancer cells PC-3 after 48 h [148]. In the rat model of benign prostatic hyperplasia, daily oral supplementation of 50 and 100 mg/kg EGCG for 4 weeks has been able to reduce the levels of glucose, total cholesterol, triglycerides, IGF-1, and inflammatory cytokines [149]. *C. sinensis* has the ability to regulate oxidative stress mainly through the antioxidant and antiproliferative properties [146] of catechin polyphenol EGCG as it can inhibit HGF/c-Met signaling pathways and possess downstream effects in prostate carcinoma cells. Polyphenol E also lowers serum prostate-specific antigen, IGF-1, and IGF-binding protein-3 levels [147]. Growth inhibitory effect of green tea polyphenols on human prostate cancer cells PC-3 is found to be mediated through induction of apoptosis (including enhanced expression of apoptosis-related proteins bax and caspase-3 but reduction in bcl-2 levels) ultimately leading to cell death [148]. In benign prostatic hyperplasia, the therapeutic potential of *C. sinensis* may be attributed to the potential of EGCG in restoring the altered levels of growth factors and inflammatory cytokines. EGCG may also reduce blood glucose, cholesterol, and triglyceride levels thereby relieving the prostate [149].

The potential mechanisms of action of *C. sinensis* in the management of andrological problems are presented in Fig. 3.

3 Perspective

In Asia, especially in the eastern and southern Asian countries including the Indian subcontinent, herbal medicine has been in use for thousands of years to treat many complex diseases. Despite the astounding success of modern medicine, a large number of Asian populations, predominantly the village dwellers still continue to prefer the traditional herbal remedies [164]. In the Indian subcontinent, use of herbal medicine has formed an ancient and important component of the healthcare system owing to the large repository of medicinal plants [165]. In traditional herbal medicine, usually a cocktail of a number of herbs are used as integrity therapy in several forms such as powders, capsules, tinctures, syrups, etc. [166]. Their efficacy is believed to depend largely on the synergistic interactions of the individual components because they are used mostly as whole extracts or sometimes as poly-herbal formulations [164]. In recent times, investigative studies have been taken up to validate the clinical efficacy and safety of individual herbal extracts, discrete chemical ingredients, and their active principles apart from elucidating their mechanism of action in the management of andrological problems. In this chapter, we have discussed various pharmacological effects of *G. biloba*, *C. longa* and *C. sinensis* that may be useful in the management of a wide range of andrological disorders such as male infertility, hypogonadism, erectile dysfunction, testicular cancer, prostate cancer, and benign prostatic hyperplasia. We have also attempted to provide their molecular mechanisms of action, to have a better understanding of how these herbal medicines exert their effects.

Thus far, a study conducted on infertile men indicated toward improvement of sperm quality parameters at 80 mg curcumin nanomicelle supplementation for a period of 2 months. In vivo studies conducted on rodent models also suggest dose-dependent beneficial properties of *G. biloba* and *C. sinensis* extracts in the treatment of male infertility; however, these studies have not looked at pregnancy rates, implantation rates, or live birth rates as end points of fertility treatments. Studies on erectile dysfunction patients indicate that supplementation of 40–80 mg *G. biloba* extract 2–3 times daily for 1 month to up to 3 years may benefit such men in the clinical management of the disease. Supplementation of a tablet containing 100 mg *C. longa* powder three times a day for 6 months may potentially benefit prostate cancer patients by decreasing the level of prostate-specific antigen and inhibiting metastasis of cancer cells, whereas supplementation of 1300–2000 mg green tea polyphenol of *C. sinensis* for 6 months holds potential in the treatment of prostate cancer as it can lower the levels of serum prostate-specific antigen, hepatocyte growth factor, vascular endothelial growth factor, IGF-1, and IGFBP-3.

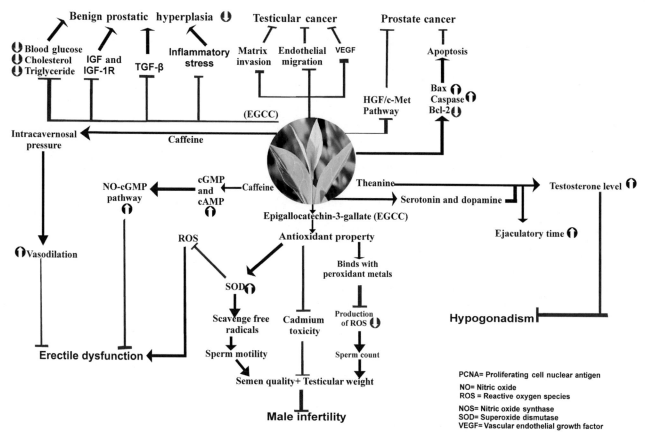

FIG. 3 Potential mechanism of action of *Camellia sinensis* in the management of andrological problems. EGCG from green tea possesses antioxidant properties which reduces cadmium toxicity, production of ROS, and increases activity of superoxide dismutase to scavenge free radicals ultimately leading to improvement in semen quality parameters. Theanine from black tea brew helps to increase the testosterone level and ejaculatory time by enhancing serotoninergic and dopaminergic activities. Moreover, caffeine content of black tea helps to increase cGMP and cAMP levels as well as intracavernosal pressure to improve erectile functions. Green tea extract also increases the expression of apoptotic proteins, thus reducing the chances of testicular and prostate cancer. Furthermore, EGCG reduces blood glucose, cholesterol, triglycerides, and several growth factors in order to hinder the occurrence of benign prostatic hyperplasia.

Supplementation of *G. biloba*, *C. longa*, and *C. sinensis* has the potential to reduce oxidative stress levels and poses a low-cost alternative that may uplift the health of reproductively compromised men. By combining these herbs with lifestyle modification and standard medical treatment, the clinician may be able to maximize the chances of restoring normal reproductive functioning of men with andrological problems. In this chapter, we have summarized the outcomes of already published reports on *G. biloba*, *C. longa*, and *C. sinensis;* however, we have not carried out any dose-response relationship or toxicological study. As such, more clinical intervention trials are needed to elucidate the exact mechanism of action of these herbs in humans. Carefully designed dose-response studies in humans are required to incorporate *G. biloba*, *C. longa*, and *C. sinensis* as potential alternatives in the clinical management of andrological problems.

References

[1] Nieschlag E. Scopes and goals of andrology. In: Nieschlag E, Behre HM, Nieschlag S, editors. Andrology: male reproductive health and dysfunction. 3rd ed. Springer; 2010. p. 1–3.

[2] Schill WB, Comhaire F, Hargreave TB. Andrology: definition, clinical issues and prevalence. In: Schill WB, Comhaire F, Hargreave TB, editors. Andrology for the clinician. Springer; 2006. p. 1–4.

[3] Bjorndahl L, Giwercman A, Tournaye H, Weidner W. Preface: clinical andrology EAU/ESAU course guidelines. European Association of Urology, CRC Press, Informa Healthcare; 2010. p. VI.

[4] Agarwal A, Mulgund A, Hamadaa A, Chyatte MR. A unique view on male infertility around globe. Reprod Biol Endocrinol 2015;13:37.

[5] NHP (National Health Portal, India). Infertility. Accessed online on 19th February, 2020 at https://www.nhp.gov.in/disease/reproductive-syatem/infertility; 2016, August 05.

[6] Zargar AH, Wani AI, Masoodi SR, Laway BA, Salahuddin M. Epidemiologic and etiologic aspects of primary infertility in the Kashmir region of India. Fertil Steril 1997;4:637–43.

[7] Esteves SC, Miyaoka R, Agarwal R. Sperm retrieval techniques for assisted reproduction. Int Braz J Urol 2011;37:570–80.

[8] Allahbadia GN. Intrauterine insemination: fundamentals revisited. J Obstet Gynaecol India 2017;67:358–92.

[9] Hommonai TZ, Sasson S, Paz G, Kraicer PF. Improvement of fertility and semen quality in men treated with a combination of anticongestive and antibiotic drugs. Int J Fertil 1975;20:45–9.

[10] Pajovic B, Pajovic L, Vukovic M. Effectiveness of antibiotic treatment in infertile patients with sterile leukocytospermia induced by tobacco use. Syst Biol Reprod Med 2017;67:391–6.

[11] Wong SYS, Chan DCC, Hong A, Woo J. Prevalence of risk factors for androgen deficiency in middle-aged men in Hong Kong. Metabolism 2006;55:1488–94.

[12] Khoo EM, Tan HM, Low WY. Erectile dysfunction and comorbidities in aging men: an urban cross-sectional study in Malaysia. J Sex Med 2008;5:2925–34.

[13] Liu CC, Wu WJ, Lee YC, Wang CJ, Ke HL, Li WM, Hsiao HL, Yeh HC, Li CC, Chou YH, Huang CH, Huang SP. The prevalence of and risk factors for androgen deficiency in aging Taiwanese men. J Sex Med 2009;6:936–46.

[14] Goel A, Sinha RJ, Dalela D, Sankhwar S, Singh V. Andropause in Indian men: a preliminary cross-sectional study. Urol J 2009;6:40–6.

[15] McCullough AR, Khera M, Goldstein I, Hellstorm WJ, Morgentalar A, Levine LA. A multi-institutional observational study of testosterone levels after testosterone pellet (Testopel) insertion. J Sex Med 2012;9:594–601.

[16] Miner MM, Sadovsky R. Evolving issues in male hypogonadism: evaluation, management, and related comorbidities. Cleve Clin J Med 2007;74:S38–46.

[17] Rogol AD, Tkachenko N, Bryson N. Natesto, a novel testosterone nasal gel, normalizes androgen levels in hypogonadal men. Andrology 2016;4:46–54.

[18] Thirumalai A, Berkseth KE, Amory JK. Treatment of hyogonadism: current and future therapies. F1000Res 2017;6:68.

[19] Ho CCK, Singam P, Hong GE, Zainuddin ZM. Male sexual dysfunction in Asia. Asian J Androl 2011;13:537–42.

[20] Park K, Hwang EC, Kim SO. Prevalence and medical management of erectile dysfunction in Asia. Asian J Androl 2011;13:534–49.

[21] Dunn ME, Althof SE, Perelman MA. Phosphodiesterase type 5 inhibitors' extended duration of response as a variable in the treatment of erectile dysfunction. Int J Impot Res 2007;19:119–23.

[22] Hatzirmouratidis K, Amar E, Eardley I, Giuliano F, Hatzirchristou G, Montorsi F, Vardi Y, Wespes E. Guidelines on male sexual dysfunction: erectile dysfunction and premature ejaculation. Eur Urol 2010;57:804–14.

[23] Pastuszak AW. Current diagnosis and management of erectile dysfunction. Curr Sex Health Rep 2014;6:164–76.

[24] Toni LD, Sabovic I, Garolla A. Testicular cancer: genes, environment, hormones. Front Endocrinol (Lausanne) 2019;10:408.

[25] Haresh KP, Benson R. Male reproductive cancers. In: Kumar A, Sharma M, editors. Basics of human andrology. Springer Nature; 2017. p. 477–90.

[26] Shanmugalingam T, Soultati A, Chowdhury S, Rudman S, Van Hemelrijck M. Global incidence and outcome of testicular cancer. Clin Epidemiol 2013;5:417–27.

[27] Rajpert-De Meyts E, Skakkebaek NE, Topari J. Testicular cancer pathogenesis, diagnosis and endocrine aspects. In: Feingold KR, Anawalt B, Boyce A, et al., editors. Endotext. South Dartmouth (MA): MDText.com, Inc.; 2018.

[28] Chung BH, Horie S, Chiong E. The incidence, mortality, and risk factors of prostate cancer in Asian men. Prostate Int 2019;7:1–8.

[29] Ferlay J, Soerjomataram I, Ervik M, Dikshit R, Eser S, Mathers C, Rebelo M, Parkin DM, Forman D, Bray F. Globocan 2012 cancer incidence and mortality worldwide: IARC cancerbase No. 11. International Agency for Research on Cancer: Lyon, France; 2013.

[30] Lim KB. Epidermology of clinical benign prostatic hyperplasia. Asian J Urol 2017;4:148–51.

[31] Lim PHC. Asian herbals and aphrodisiacs used for managing ED. Transl Androl Urol 2017;6:167–75.

[32] Roehrborn CG. Benign prostatic hyperplasia: an overview. Rev Urol 2005;7:3–14.

[33] Wang W, Guo Y, Zhang D, Tian Y, Zhang X. The prevalence of benign prostatic hyperplasia in mainland China: evidence from epidemiological surveys. Sci Rep 2015;5:13546.

[34] Chen F, Zhao X. Prostate cancer: current treatment and prevention strategies. Iran Red Crescent Med J 2013;15:279–84.

[35] Hayden A, Catton C, Pickles T. Radiation therapy in prostate cancer: a risk-adapted strategy. Curr Oncol 2010;17:S18–24.

[36] Lawrentschuk N, Trottier G, Kuk C, Zlotta AR. Role of surgery in high-risk localized prostate cancer. Curr Oncol 2010;17:25–32.

[37] Perlmutter MA, Lepor H. Androgen deprivation therapy in the treatment of advanced prostate cancer. Rev Urol 2007;9:S3–8.

[38] Garcia C, Chin P, Rashid P, Woo HH. Prostatic urethral lift: A minimally invasive treatment for benign prostatic hyperplasia. Prostate Int 2015;3:1–5.

[39] Sonksen J, Barbar NJ, Speakman MJ, Berges R, Wetterauer U, Greene D, Sievert KD, Chapple CR, Montorsi F, Patterson JM, Fahrenkrug L, Schoenthaler M, Gratzke C. Prospective, randomized, multinational study of prostatic urethral lift versus transurethral resection of the prostate: 12-month results from the BPH6 study. Eur Urol 2015;68:643–52.

[40] McVary KT, Roehrborn CG, Avins AL, Barry MJ, Bruskewitz RC, Donnell RF, Foster Jr HE, Gonzalez CM, Kaplan SA, Penson DF, Ulchaker JC, Wei JT. Update on AUA guideline on the management of benign prostatic hyperplasia. J Urol 2011;185:1793–803.

[41] Eken A, Soyupak B. Safety and efficacy of photoselective vaporization of the prostate using the 180-W green light XPS laser system in patients taking oral anticoagulants. J Int Med Res 2018;46:1230–7.

[42] Hopkins J. Asian aphrodisiacs: from bangkok to beijing – the search for the ultimate turn-on. North Clarendon: Tuttle Publishing; 2006.

[43] Thakur M, Thompson D, Connellan P, Deseo MA, Morris C, Dixit VK. Improvement of penile erection, sperm count and seminal fructose levels *in vivo* and nitric oxide release *in vitro* by ayurvedic herbs. Andrologia 2011;43:273–7.

[44] van Andel T, de Boer H, Towns A. Gynaecological, andrological and urological problems: an ethnopharmacological perspective. In: Heinrich M, Jager AK, editors. Ethnopharmacology. 1st ed. Wiley & Sons; 2015. p. 199–211.

[45] Isah T. Rethinking *Ginkgo biloba* L.: medicinal uses and conservation. Pharmacogn Rev 2015;9:140–8.

[46] Matsumoto T, Sei T. Antifeedant activities of *Ginkgo biloba* L components against the larvae of *Pierisrapaecrucivora*. Agric Biol Chem 1987;51:249–50.

[47] De Feudis FV. *Ginkgo biloba* extract (EGb 761): pharmacological activities and clinical applications. Paris: Elsevier. Eds Scientifiques; 1991. p. 1187.

[48] Chang JY, Chang MN. Medical uses of *Ginkgo biloba*. Todays Therapeut Trends 1997;15:63–74.

[49] De Feudis FV. *Ginkgo biloba* extract (EGb-761): from chemistry to the clinic. Wiesbaden: Ullstein Medical; 1998. p. 119–33.

[50] Zuo W, Yan F, Zhang B, Li J, Mei D. Advances in the studies of *Ginkgo biloba* leaves extract on aging-related diseases. Aging Dis 2017;8:812–26.

[51] Brondino N, DeSilvestri A, Re S, Lanati N, Thiemann P, Verna A, Emanuele A, Politi P. A systematic review and meta-analysis of *Ginkgo biloba* in neuropsychiatric disorders: from ancient tradition to modern-day medicine. Evid Based Complement Alternat Med 2013;2013:915691.

[52] Loskutova E, O'Brien C, Loskutov I, Loughman J. Nutritional supplementation in the treatment of glaucoma: a systematic review. Surv Ophthalmol 2019;64:195–216.

[53] Evans JR. *Ginkgo biloba* extract for age-related macular degeneration. Cochrane Database Syst Rev 2000;, CD001775.

[54] Sridharan K, Sivaramakrisnan G. Pharmacological interventions for preventing acute mountain sickness: a network meta-analysis and trial sequential analysis of randomized clinical trials. Ann Med 2018;50:147–55.

[55] Amin A, Abraham C, Hamza AA, Abdalla ZA, Al-Shamsi SB, Harethi SS, Daoud S. A standardized extract of *Ginkgo biloba* neutralizes cisplatin-mediated reproductive toxicity in rats. J Biomed Biotechnol 2012;362049.

[56] Zahran F, Tousson E, Shalapy MA. Oral supplementation of aqueous Moringa and Ginkgo leaf extracts abates oxidative stress and testicular injury associated with boldenone injection in rats. Pharmacologia 2016;7:381–9.

[57] Al-Yahya AA, Al-Majed A, Al-Bekairi AM, Al-Shabanah OA, Qureshi S. Studies on the reproductive, cytological and biochemical toxicity of *Ginkgo Biloba* in swiss albino mice. J Ethnopharmacol 2019;107:222–8.

[58] Oshio LT, Cristina TRC, Renato MM, Guerra MO, Luis PMS, Joao EPR, de Cassis dSSR, Campos LV, Vera MP. Effect of *Ginkgo biloba* extract on sperm quality, serum testosterone concentration and histometric analysis of testes from adult Wistar rats. J Med Plant Res 2015;9:122–31.

[59] Sugiyama T, Kutoba Y, Shinozuka K, Yamada S, Yamada K, Umegaki K. Induction and recovery of hepatic drug metabolizing enzymes in rats treated with *Ginkgo biloba* extract. Food Chem Toxicol 2004;42:953–7.

[60] Ahmed AI, Lasheen NN, El-Zawahry KM. Ginkgo Biloba ameliorates subfertility induced by testicular ischemia/reperfusion injury in adult Wistar rats: a possible new mitochondrial mechanism. Oxid Med Cell Longev 2016;2016:19.

[61] Yeh YK, Pu HF, Kaphle K, Lin SF, Wu SF, Lin JH, Tsai YF. Ginkgo biloba extract enhances male copulatory behavior and reduces serum prolactin levels in rats. Horm Behav 2008;53:225–31.

[62] Cohen AJ, Bartlik B. *Ginkgo Biloba* for antidepressant-induced sexual dysfunction. J Sex Marital Ther 1998;24:139–43.

[63] Sohn M, Sikora R. *Ginkgo biloba* extract in the therapy of erectile dysfunction. J Sex Edu Ther 2015;17:53–61.

[64] De La Hoz FJE. PM-04 impact of pregnancy on the sexuality of women in the ejecafetero. J Sex Med 2017;14:e381–2.

[65] You OH, Kim S, Kim B, Sohn EJ, Lee HJ, Shim B, Yun M, Kwon B, Kim S. Ginkgetin induces apoptosis via activation of caspase and inhibition of survival genes in PC-3 prostate cancer cells. Bioorg Med Chem Lett 2013;23:2693–5.

[66] Jeon YJ, Jung S, Yun J, Lee CW, Choi J, Lee Y, Han DC, Kwon B. Ginkgetin inhibits the growth of DU-145 prostate cancer cells through inhibition of signal transducer and activator of transcription 3 activity. Cancer Sci 2015;106:413–20.

[67] Zeng Y, Xiao D. *Ginkgo biloba*extract kaemferol induces apoptosis in human prostate cancer cells through downregulation of β-Catenin signaling. Cancer Res 2011;71.

[68] Peng C, Liu J, Chang C, Chung J, Chen K, Peng RY. Action mechanism of *Ginkgo biloba* leaf extract intervened by exercise therapy in treatment of benign prostate hyperplasia. Evid Based Complement Alternat Med 2013;2013:408734.

[68a] Reagan-Shaw S, Nihal M, Ahmad N. Dose translation from animal to human studies revisited. FASEB J 2008;22:659–61.

[69] Ahlemeyer B, Selke D, Schaper C, Klumpp S, Krieglstein J. Ginkgolicacids induce neuronal death and activate protein phosphatase type-2C. Eur J Pharmacol 2001;430:1–7.

[70] Turner TT, Bang HJ, Lysiak JL. The molecular pathology of experimental testicular torsion suggests adjunct therapy to surgical repair. J Urol 2004;172:2574–8.

[71] Unsal A, Eroglu M, Avci A, Cimentepe E, Guven C, Balbay MD, Durak I. Protective role of natural antioxidant supplementation on testicular tissue after testicular torsion and detorsion. Scand J Urol Nephrol 2006;40:17–22.

[72] Grumbach MM, Conte FA. Disorders of sex differentiation. In: Wilson J, Foster D, editors. Williams textbook of endocrinology. Philadelphia: WB Saunders; 1992. p. 853–951.

[73] Yeh KY, Wu CH, Tsai YF. Noncontact erection is enhanced by *Ginkgo biloba*treatment in rats: role of neuronal NOS in paraventricular nucleus and sacral spinal cord. Psychopharmacology (Berl) 2012;222:439–46.

[74] Laukeviciene A, Cecen S, Masteikova R. Reduction of small arteries contractility with improving the relaxation properties by *Ginkgo biloba*extract. J Med Plant Res 2012;6:4785–9.

[75] Ma K, Xu L, Zhan H, Pu M, Jonas JB. Dosage dependence of the effect of *Ginkgo biloba* on the rat retinal ganglion cell survival after optic nerve crush. Eye 2009;23:1598–604.

[76] Khafaga AF, Bayad AE. *Ginkgo biloba* attenuates hematological disorders, oxidative stress and nephrotoxicity induced by single or repeated injection cycles of cisplatin in rats: physiological and pathlogical studies. Asian J Anim Sci 2016;10:235–46.

[77] Wang W, Zhong X, Ma A, Shi W, Zhang X, Liu Y. Effects of *Ginkgo biloba*on testicular injury induced by diethylstilbesterol in mice. Am J Chin Med 2008;36:1135–44.

[78] Yeh YC, Liu TJ, Wang LC, Lee HW, Ting CT, Lee WL, Hung CJ, Wang KY, Lai HC, Lai HC. A standardized extract of doxorubicin-induced oxidative stress and 53-mediated mitochondrial apoptosis in rat testes. Br J Pharmacol 2009;156:48–61.

[79] Prasad S, Gupta SC, Tyagi AK, Aggarwal BB. Curcumin, a component of golden spice: from bedside to bench and back. Biotechnol Adv 2014;32:1053–64.

[80] Gupta SC, Patchva S, Aggarwal BB. Therapeutic roles of curcumin: lessons learned from clinical trials. AAPS J 2012;15:195–218.

[81] Singh G, Kapoor IP, Singh P, de Heluani CS, de Lampasona MP, Catalan CA. Comparative study of chemical composition and antioxidant activity of fresh and dry rhizomes of turmeric (*Curcuma longa* Linn.). Food Chem Toxicol 2010;48:1026–31.

[82] Deogade S, Ghate S. Curcumin: therapeutic applications in systemic and oral health. Int J Biol Pharm 2015;6:281–90.

[83] Hatcher H, Planalp R, Cho J, Torti FM, Torti SV. Curcumin: from ancient medicine to current clinical trials. Cell Mol Life Sci 2008;65:1631–52.

[84] Monroy A, Lithgow GJ, Alavez S. Curcumin and neurodegenerative diseases. Biofactors 2013;39:122–32.

[85] Alizadeh F, Javadi M, Karami AA, Gholaminezad F, Kavianpore M, Haghighian HK. Curcumin nanomicelle improves semen parameters, oxidative stress, inflammatory biomarkers, and reproductive hormones in infertile men: a randomized clinical trial. Phytother Res 2017;32:514–21.

[86] Ahmed Farid OAH, Nasr M, Ahmed RF, Bakeer RM. Beneficial effects of curcumin nano-emulsion on spermatogenesis and reproductive performance in male rats under protein deficient diet model: enhancement of sperm motility, conservancy of testicular tissue integrity, cell energy and seminal plasma amino acids content. J Biomed Sci 2017;24:66.

[87] Qureshi S, Shah A, Ageel A. Toxicity studies on *Alpiniagalanga* and *Curcuma longa*. Planta Med 1992;58:124–7.

[88] Mohamadpour M, Noorashan A, Karbalay-Doust S, Talaei-Khozani T, Aliabadi E. Protective effects of curcumin co-treatment in rats with establishing chronic variable stress on testis and reproductive hormones. Int J Reprod Biomed 2017;15:447–52.

[89] Karbalay-Doust S, Noorafshan A. Ameliorative effects of curcumin on the spermatozoon tail length, count, motility and testosterone serum level in metronidazole-treated mice. Prague Med Rep 2011;112:288–97.

[90] Zaahkouk AMS, Abdel Aziz MT, Rezq AM, Atta HM, Fouad HM, Ahmed HH, Sabry D, Yehia MH. Efficacy of anovel water-soluble curcumin derivative versus sildenafil citrate in mediating erectile function. Int J Impot Res 2015;27:9–15.

[91] Aziz MTA, Motawi T, Rezq A, Mostafa T, Fouad HH, Ahmed HH, Rashed L, Sabry D, Senbel A, Al-Malki A, El-Shafiey R. Effects of a water-soluble curcumin protein conjugate vs. pure curcumin in a diabetic model of erectile dysfunction. J Sex Med 2012;9:1815–33.

[92] Draganski A, Tar MT, Villegas G, Friedman JM, Davies KP. Topically applied curcumin-loaded nanoparticles treat erectile dysfunction in a rat model of type-2 diabetes. J Sex Med 2018;15:645–53.

[93] Gevrek F, Erdemir F. Investigation of the effects of curcumin, vitamin E and their combination in cisplatin-induced testicular apoptosis using immunohistochemical technique. Turk J Urol 2018;44:16–23.

[94] Zhou C, Zhao X, Li X, Wang C, Zhang X, Liu X, Ding X, Xiang S, Zhang J. Curcumin inhibits AP-2γ-induced apoptosis in the human malignant testicular germ cells in vitro. Acta Pharmacol Sin 2013;5:1192–200.

[95] Cort A, Timur M, Ozdemir E, Ozben T. Effects of curcumin on bleomycin-induced apoptosis in human malignant testicular germ cells. J Physiol Biochem 2013;69:289–96.

[96] Thomas R, Williams M, Sharma H, Chaudry A, Bellamy P. A double-blind, placebo-controlled randomised trial evaluating the effect of a polyphenol-rich whole food supplement on psa progression in men with prostate cancer—the U.K. NCRN Pomi-T study. Prostate Cancer Prostatic Dis 2014;17:180–6.

[97] Mahammedi H, Planchat E, Pouget M, Durando X, Curé H, Guy L, Van-Praagh I, Savareux L, Atger M, Bayet-Robert M, Gadea E, Abrial C, Thivat E, Chollet P, Eymard J. The new combination docetaxel, prednisone and curcumin in patients with castration-resistant prostate cancer: a pilot phase II study. Oncology 2016;90:69–78.

[98] Killian PH, Kronski E, Michalik KM, Barbieri O, Astigiano S, Sommerhoff CP, Pfeffer U, Nerlich AG, Bachmeier BE. Curcumin inhibits prostate cancer metastasis in vivo by targeting the inflammatory cytokines CXCL1 and −2. Carcinogenesis 2012;33:2507–19.

[99] Huang H, Chen X, Li D, He Y, Li Y, Du Z, Zhan K, DiPaola R, Goodin S, Zheng X. Combination of α-tomatine and curcumin inhibits growth and induces apoptosis in human prostate cancer cells. PLoS ONE 2015;10(12), e0144293.

[100] Dorai T, Gehani N, Katz A. Therapeutic potential of curcumin in human prostate cancer-I. Curcumin induces apoptosis in both androgen-dependent and androgen-independent prostate cancer cells. Prostate Cancer Prostatic Dis 2000;3:84–93.

[101] Thangapazham RL, Sharma A, Maheshwari RK. Multiple molecular targets in cancer chemoprevention by curcumin. AAPSJ 2006;8:443–9.

[102] Ledda A, Belcaro G, Dugall M, Luzzi R, Scoccianti M, Togni S, Appendino G, Ciammaichella G. Meriva(R), a lecithinized curcumin delivery system, in the control of benign prostatic hyperplasia: a pilot, product evaluation registry study. Panminerva Med 2012;54:17–22.

[103] Kim SK, Seok H, Park HJ, Jeon HS, Kang SW, Lee BC, Yi J, Song SY, Lee SH, Kim YO, Chung J. Inhibitory effect of curcumin on testosterone induced benign prostatic hyperplasia rat model. BMC Complement Altern Med 2015;15:380.

[104] Globmik K, Basta-Kaim A, Sikora-Polaczak M, Kubera M, Starowicz G, Styrna J. Curcumin influences semen quality parameters and reverses the di(2-ethylhexyl)phthalate (DEHP)-induced testicular damage in mice. Pharmacol Rep 2014;66:782–7.

[105] Panahi Y, Hosseini MS, Khalili N, Naimi E, Majeed M, Sahebkar A. Antioxidant and anti-inflammatory effects of curcuminoid-piperine combination in subjects with metabolic syndrome: a randomized controlled trial and an updated meta-analysis. Clin Nutr 2015;34:1101–8.

[106] Bengmark S. Curcumin, an atoxic antioxidant and natural NFκB, cyclooxygenase-2, lipooxygenase, and inducible nitric oxide synthase inhibitor: a shield against acute and chronic diseases. J Parenter Enteral Nutr 2006;30:45–51.

[107] Jha NS, Mishra S, Jha SK, Surolia A. Antioxidant activity and electrochemical elucidation of the enigmatic redox behavior of curcumin and its structurally modified analogues. Electrochem Acta 2015;151:574–83.

[108] Akram M, Shahab-Uddin AA, Usmanghani K, Hannan A, Mohiuddin E, Asif M. Curcuma longa and curcumin: a review article. Rom J Biol-Plant Biol 2010;55:65–70.

[109] Chen Y, Wang Q, Wang FF, Gao HB, Zhang P. Stress induces glucocorticoid-mediated apoptosis of rat Leydig cells in vivo. Stress 2012;15:74–84.

[110] Lipshultz LI, Witt MA. Mg Hamm. Infertility in male; 1993.

[111] Hari Priya P, Girish BP, Sreenivasula RP. Restraint stress exacerbates alcohol-induced reproductive toxicity in male rats. Alcohol 2014;48:781–6.

[112] Ilbey YO, Ozbek E, Cekmen M, Simsek A, Otunctemur A, Somay A. Protective effect of curcumin in cisplatin-induced oxidative injury in rat testis: mitogen-activated protein kinase and nuclear factor-kappa B signaling pathways. Hum Reprod 2009;24:1717–25.

[113] Woo J, Kim Y, Choi Y, Kim D, Lee K, Bae J, Min D, Chang J, Jeong Y, Lee Y, Park J, Kwon T. Molecular mechanisms of curcumin-induced cytotoxicity: induction of apoptosis through generation of reactive oxygen species, down-regulation of Bcl-XL and IAP, the release of cytochrome C and inhibition of Akt. Carcinogenesis 2003;24:1199–208.

[114] Smith JT, Young IR, Veldhuij D, Clark IJ. Gonadotropin-inhibitory hormone (GnIH) secretion into the ovine hypophsealortal system. Endocrinology 2012;153:3368–75.

[115] Xu J, Zou MH. Molecular insights and therapeutic targets fordiabetic endothelial dysfunction. Circulation 2009;120:1266–86.

[116] Romero MJ, Platt DH, Tawfik HE, Labazi M, El-Remessy AB, Bartoli M, Caldwell RB, Caldwell RW. Diabetes-inducedcoronary vascular dysfunction involves increased arginaseactivity. Circ Res 2008;102:95–102.

[117] Zhang C. The role of inflammatory cytokines in endothelialdysfunction. Basic Res Cardiol 2008;103:398–406.

[118] Rungseesantivanon S, Thenchaisri N, Ruangvejvorachai P, Patumraj S. Curcumin supplementation could improve diabetes-induced endothelial dysfunction associated with decreased vascular superoxide production and PKC inhibition. BMC Complement Altern Med 2010;10:57.

[119] Subramaniam D, Ponnurangam S, Ramamoorthy P, Standing D, Battafarano RJ, Anant S, Sharma P. Curcumin induces cell death in esophageal cancer cells through modulating notch signaling. PLoS ONE 2012;7, e30590.

[120] Deng G, Yu JH, Ye ZQ, Hu ZQ. Curcumin inhibits the expression of vascular endothelial growth factor and androgen-independent prostate cancer cell line PC-3 in vitro. Zhonghua Nan KeXue 2008;14:116–21.

[121] Mukhopadhyay A, Bueso-Ramos C, Chatterjee D, Pantazis P, Aggarwal BB. Curcumin downregulates cell survival mechanisms in human prostate cancer cell lines. Oncogene 2001;20:7597–609.

[122] Gioeli D, Mandell JW, Petroni GR, Frierson Jr HF, Weber MJ. Activation of mitogen-activated protein kinase associated with prostate cancer progression. Cancer Res 1999;59:279–84.

[123] Youreva V, Kapakos G, Srivastava A. Insulin-like growth-factor-1-induced PKB signaling and Egr-1 expression is inhibited by curcumin in A-10 vascular smooth muscle cells. Can J Physiol Pharmacol 2013;91:241–7.

[124] Kim M, Chun S, Choi J. Effects of turmeric (*Curcuma longa* L.) on antioxidative systems and oxidative damage in rats fed a high fat and cholesterol diet. J Korean Soc Food Sci Nutr 2013;42:570–6.

[125] Jacob A, Chaves L, Eadon MT, Chang A, Quigg RJ, Alexander JJ. Curcumin alleviates immune-complex-mediated glomerulonephritis in factor-H-deficient mice. Immunology 2013;139:328–37.

[126] Ferrera L, Montesano D, Senatore A. The distribution of minerals and flavonoids in the tea plant (*Camellia sinensis*). Farmacoterapia 2001;56:397–401.

[127] Sumpio BE, Cordova AC, Berke-Schlessel DW, Qin F, Chen QH. Green tea the "Asian Paradox", and the cardiovascular disease. J Am Coll Surg 2006;202:813–20.

[128] Wang H, Provan GJ, Helliwell K. Tea flavonoids: their functions, utilization and analysis. Trends Food Sci Technol 2000;11:152–60.

[129] Pauli ED, Scarmino IS, Tauler R. Analytical investigation of secondary metabolites extracted from *Camellia sinensis* L. leaves using a HPLC-DAD-ESI/MS data fusion strategy and chemometric methods. J Chemometr 2016;30:75–85.

[130] Zuo Y, Chen H, Deng Y. Simultaneous determination of catechins, caffeine and gallic acids in green, Oolong, black and puerh teas using HPLC with a photodiode array detector. Talanta 2002;57:307–16.

[131] Koch W, Zagórska J, Marzec Z, Kukula-Koch W. Applications of tea (*Camellia sinensis*) and its active constituents in cosmetics. Molecules 2019;24:4277.

[132] Juneja LR, Chu DC, Okubu T, Nagato Y, Yokogoshi H. L-Theanine-a unique amino acid of green tea and its relaxation effect in humans. Trends Food Sci Technol 1999;10:199–204.

[133] Zhu M, Xiao PG. Quantitative analysis of active constituents of green tea. Phytother Res 1991;5:239.

[134] Crew KD, Ho KA, Brown P, Greenlee H, Bevers TB, Arun B, Sneige N, Hudis C, McArthur HL, Chang J, Rimawi M, Cornelison TL, Cardelli J, Santella RM, Wang A, Lippman SM, Hershman DL. Effects of a green tea extract, Polyphenon E, on systemic biomarkers of growth factor signalling in women with hormone receptor-negative breast cancer. J Hum Nutr Diet 2015;28:272–82.

[135] Faria A, Pestana D, Teixeira D, Couraud P, Romero I, Weksler B, de Freitas V, Mateus N, Calhau C. Insights Into the Putative Catechin and Epicatechin Transport Across Blood-Brain Barrier. Food Funct 2011;2:39–44.

[136] Subramani C, Natesh RK. Molecular mechanisms and biological implications of green tea polyphenol, (−)-epigallocatechin-3-gallate. Int J Phar Biosci Technol 2013;1:54–63.

[137] Sha'hbani N, Sepideh M, Rafieian-kohpaye M, Namjoo AR. Survey of the detoxification effect of green tea extract on the reproductive system in the rats exposed to lead acetate. Adv Biomed Res 2015;4:155.

[138] Mahmoudi R, Arsalan A, Abedini S, Jahromi VH, Abidi H, Barmak MJ. Green tea improves rat sperm quality and reduced cadmium chloride damage effect in spermatogenesis cycle. J Med Life 2018;11:371–80.

[139] Bagherpour H, Malekshah AK, Amiri FT, Azadbakht M. Protective effect of green tea extract on the deltamethrin-induced toxicity in mice testis: an experimental study. Int J Reprod Biomed (Yazd) 2019;17:337–48.

[140] Oliveira PF, Tomás GD, Dias TR, Martins AD, Rato L, Alves MG, Silva BM. White tea consumption restores sperm quality in prediabetic rats preventing testicular oxidative damage. Reprod Biomed Online 2015;31:544–56.

[141] Ratnasooriya WD, Fernando TSP. Effect of black tea brew of *Camellia sinensis* on sexual competence of male rats. J Ethnopharmacol 2008;118:373–7.

[142] Lopez-Gutierrez N, Romero-Gonzalez R, Plaza-Bolanos P, Vidal JLM, Frenich A. Identification and quantification of phytochemicals in nutraceutical products from green tea by UHPLC-Orbitrap-MS. Food Chem 2015;173:607–18.

[143] Yang R, Wang J, Chen Y, Sun Z, Wang R, Dai Y. Effect of caffeine on erectile function via u-regulating cavernous cyclic guanosine monophosphate in diabetic rats. J Androl 2008;29:586–91.

[144] Chen D, Zhang KQ, Li B, Sun DQ, Zhang H, Fu Q. Epigallocatechin-3-gallate ameliorates erectile function in aged rats via regulation of PRMT1/DDAH/ADMA/NOS metabolism pathway. Asian J Androl 2017;19:291–7.

[145] Roomi MW, Ivanov V, Kalinovsky NA, Rath M. Inhibitory effects of a nutrient mixture on human testicular cancer cell line NT 2/DT matrigel invasion and MMP activity. Med Oncol 2007;24:183–8.

[146] Lassed S, Deus CM, Djebbari R, Zama D, Oliveira PJ, Rizvanov AA, Dahdouh A, Benayache F, Benayache S. Protective effects green tea (*Camellia sinensis* (L.) Kuntze) against prostate cancer: from in vitro data to Algerian patients. Evid Based Complement Alternat Med 2017;2017:1691568.

[147] McLarty J, Bigelow RLH, Smith M, Elmajian D, Ankem M, Cardelli JA. Tea polyphenols decrease serum levels of prostate-specific antigen, hepatocyte growth factor, and vascular endothelial growth factor in prostate cancer patients and inhibit production of hepatocyte growth factor and vascular endothelial growth factor in vitro. Cancer Prev Res 2009;2:673–82.

[148] Yang K, Gao ZY, Li TQ, Solng W, Xiao W, Zheng J, Chen H, Chen GH, Zou HY. Anti-tumor activity and the mechanism of a green tea (*Camellia sinensis*) polysaccharide on prostate cancer. Int J Biol Macromol 2019;122:95–103.

[149] Chen J, Song H. Protective potential of epigallocatechin-3-gallate against benign prostatic hyperplasia in metabolic syndrome rats. Environ Toxicol Pharmacol 2016;45:315–20.

[150] Das SK, Karmakar SN. Effect of green tea (*Camellia sinensis* L.) leaf extract on reproductive system of adult male albino rats. Int J Physio PathophysPharmacol 2015;7:178–84.

[151] Roychoudhury S, Agarwal A, Cho CL. Potential role of green tea catechins in the management of oxidative stress-associated infertility. Reprod Biomed Online 2017;34:487–98.

[152] Perron NR, Brumaghim JL. A review of the antioxidant mechanisms of polyphenol compounds related to iron binding. Cell Biochem Biophys 2009;53:75–100.

[153] Shi CY, Yang H, Wei CL, Yu O, Zhang ZZ, Jiang CJ, Sun J, Li YY, Chen Q, Xia T, Wan XC. Deep sequencing of the *Camellia sinensis* transcriptome revealed candidate genes for major metabolic pathways of tea-specific compounds. BMC Genomics 2000;12:131.

[154] Tipoe GL, Leung TM, Liong EC, Lau TYH, Fung ML, Nanji AA. Epigallocatechin-3-gallate (EGCG) reduces liver inflammation, oxidative stress and fibroisis in carbon tetrachloride (CCl_4) induced liver injury in mice. Toxicology 2010;273:45–52.

[155] Ko EY, Sabanegh Jr ES, Agarwal A. Male infertility testing: reactive oxygen species and antioxidant capacity. Fertil Steril 2014;102:1518–27.

[156] Figueiroa MS, César Vieira JS, Leite DS, Filho RC, Ferreira F, Gouveia PS, Udrisar DP, Wanderley MI. Green tea polyphenols inhibit testosterone production in rat Leydig cells. Asian J Androl 2009;11:362–70.

[157] Opwari CS, Monsees TK. Reduced testosterone production in TM3 Leydig cells treated with *Aspalathuslinearis* (Rooibos) or *Camellia sinensis* (tea). Andrologia 2015;47:52–8.

[158] Chandra AK, Ghose Roy Choudhury S, De N, Sarkar M. Effect of green tea (*Camellia sinensis* L.) extract on morphological and functional changes in adult male gonads of albino rats. Ind J Expt Biol 2011;49:689–97.

[159] Kandeel FR, Koussa VK, Swerdloff RS. Male sexual function and its disorders: physiology, pathophysiology, clinical investigation and treatment. Endocr Rev 2001;22:342–88.

[160] Moreland RB, Hsieh G, Nakane M, Brioni JD. The biochemical and neurologic basis for the treatment of male erectile dysfunction. J Pharmacol Exp Ther 2001;296:225–34.

[161] Lindaman BA, Hinkhouse MM, Conklin JL, Cullen JJ. The effect of phosphodiester inhibition on gallbladder motility in vitro. J Surg Res 2002;105:102–8.

[162] Moore CR, Wang R. Pathophysiology and treatment of diabetic erectile dysfunction. Asian J Androl 2006;8:888–93.

[163] Levites Y, Weinreb O, Maor G, Youdim MB, Mandel S. Green tea polypphenol (−)-epigallocatechin-3g-gallate prevents N-methyl-4-pphenyl-1,2,3,6-tetrahydropyridine-induced dopaminergic neurodegenration. J Neurochem 2001;78:1073–82.

[164] Kim SW. Phytotherapy: emerging therapeutic option in urologic disease. Transl Androl Urol 2012;1:181–91.

[165] Pandey MM, Rastogi S, Rawat AK. Indian traditional Ayurvedic system of medicine and nutritional supplementation. Evid-Based Compl Alt Med 2013; [Article ID 376327, 12 p.].

[166] Xin Z-C. Phytotherapy on sexual dysfunction in Asia: past, present and future. In: Proceedings of the 13th biennial meeting of the Asia-Pacific society for sexual medicine, Kaohsiung, Taiwan, November 16–20, 2011, vol. 9; 2012. p. 94–155. J Sex Med.

Chapter 5.5

Herbal medicine for the treatment of andrological diseases: Traditional Chinese Medicine

Xuesheng Ma[a] and Juliana Meredith[b]

[a]*School of Natural Medicine, Faculty of Community and Health Science, University of the Western Cape, Cape Town, South Africa,* [b]*Red Rose Dragon Chinese Medicine and Acupuncture Centre, Riebeeck Kasteel, South Africa*

1 Introduction of TCM theory in andrological diseases

1.1 TCM Yin-Yang theory

The concept of Yin and Yang is pivotal in understanding the theory of TCM in treating all diseases. It depicts the cycles of nature and life, and therefore movement. Yin represents cold, consolidation, and the quality of being at rest, while Yang represents heat, expansion, and activity.

In the human body, Yin is what is stable, maintains, endures, and nourishes, whereas Yang is active, generating, and expanding. An understanding of Yin and Yang from a conventional medicine perspective may reflect in anabolic and catabolic processes, respectively, and the balance thereof in the human body. Healthy male reproduction is a TCM state of homeostasis, which is a perfect balance between Yin and Yang.

The concept of Qi is widely applied in TCM, where Qi refers to the life force that drives various activities of the human body. Some conventional medicine researchers compare Qi to adenosine triphosphate, the energy molecule responsible for providing energy for physiological processes of the body, thus maintaining functions and activities of each organ.

1.2 TCM viscera theory

Viscera in TCM (Fig. 1) are based on traditional Chinese philosophy of Yin and Yang and the five elements (fire, earth, wood, water, and metal) and is more focused on the function of the viscera as illustrated in Fig. 1, instead of the anatomy and morphology, as is the case in conventional medicine. Each organ in TCM refers to the functional, physiological, and pathological unit in the human body. As such, the kidney in TCM includes the physiological and pathological section of water metabolism, the hypothalamic-pituitary-gonadal (HPG) axis. The function of the liver in TCM is related to bilirubin metabolism, neuropsychology, and the neuroendocrine system. The heart is related to the cardiovascular system, central nervous system, and the brain function, while the spleen relates to the digestive system, which is totally different from conventional medicine, which classifies the spleen as an immune organ.

1.3 Kidney and male physiology

The kidney in TCM refers to a functional genitourinary system and the HPG axis and rarely to the parenchymal organs as in conventional medicine. In TCM, the kidney consists of kidney Yang and kidney Yin.

All male reproductive and sexual physiological activities, including the growth of genital organs, development and maintenance of their functions, need the warmth that kidney Yang provides. When kidney Yang is deficient (low function and quantity), it will cause internal coldness, leading to impotence, infertility, and a loss of libido. In contrast, when kidney Yin is deficient, it will lead to excess heat and is responsible for low sperm, premature ejaculation, hypersexuality, prostate cancer, and benign prostatic hyperplasia (BPH). Kidney Yin nourishes the reproductive organs to maintain their functions.

Herbal Medicine in Andrology. https://doi.org/10.1016/B978-0-12-815565-3.00020-5

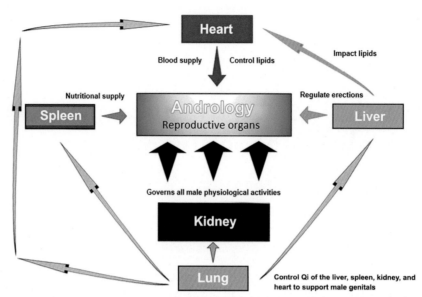

FIG. 1 Role of five major viscera (the heart, liver, spleen, kidney, and the lungs) on andrological diseases in TCM. The heart promotes the blood supply necessary for the health and function of the reproductive organs. The liver regulates erections. The spleen provides the necessary nutrition. The lungs control vital Qi of the heart, spleen, and liver to support male genitals and the kidney, the most important organ, is responsible to govern all reproductive activities.

1.4 Liver and male physiology

In TCM theory, optimal liver function is responsible for maintaining normal sexual activity. The liver has a soothing effect on mental and emotional activities as well as movement of the whole body. Specifically, for male physiology, liver Qi plays an important synergistic role in sexual activity. Disorders of the liver Qi caused by emotional depression will lead to low sexual desire, erectile dysfunction, and BPH.

1.5 Spleen and male physiology

The spleen is responsible for digestion and absorption of nutrition from the diet, which is the source of Qi and blood. Therefore, for the management of andrological diseases, the spleen plays an important nutritional role for the male reproductive organs to maintain and strengthen the reproductive function. Spleen deficiencies may cause testicular atrophy, BPH, low sexual desire, impotence, and infertility with low sperm count.

1.6 Heart and lung and male physiology

According to TCM theory, the heart manages spiritual activities, to which libido belongs and libido is dominated by the heart.

The lungs manage Qi movement of the whole body, which includes Qi to the reproductive organs. Disorders of the heart and lung can lead to low sexual desire, impotence, and infertility.

2 Common uses of Chinese herbs in andrological diseases

2.1 Herba Epimedii

Chinese medicine name: **Yin Yang Huo**

2.1.1 Introduction

The Herba Epimedii (Fig. 2) was first described in Shennong's Chinese Materia Medica (202 BC–220 AC) as dry leaves of *Epimedium brevicornu* Maxim., *Epimedium sagittatum* (Sieb. et Zucc.) Maxim., *Epimedium pubescens* Maxim., or *Epimedium koreanum* Nakai [1].

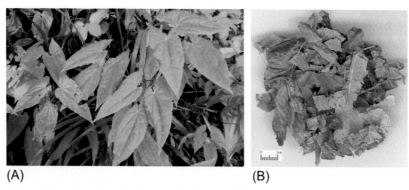

FIG. 2 (A) Fresh leaves of Herba Epimedii and (B) dried leaves of Herba Epimedii.

According to Chinese medicine, Herba Epimedii can tonify kidney Yang, strengthen the bones and sinews, and relieve joint pain. Usually dry leaves are used in herbal decoctions at a dose of 6–10 g daily, to treat kidney Yang deficiency, which is the cause of impotence, infertility, nocturnal emissions, bone and muscle atrophy, and rheumatism [1].

Scientific literature documented that the constituents of Herba Epimedii include flavonoids, phenol glycosides, and other types of compounds, the main active ingredients of Herba Epimedii include Icariin (ICA) and ICA derivatives, such as icaritin, icariside I, icariside II [2]. The pharmacological effects of Herba Epimedii include enhanced male reproductive function, osteoprotection, neuroprotection, cardioprotection, anticancer, and anti-inflammation [3–8].

2.1.2 Traditional use in the treatment of andrological diseases

In TCM practice, Herba Epimedii is best known as an aphrodisiac and tonic herb. Hongjing Tao (456–536 AC) first described Herba Epimedii as an aphrodisiac herb in the Chinese Materia Medica, Jizhu. Tao was informed by a shepherd that male goats on the farm could mate with the females more than 10 times a day, because it was observed that goats that eat the weed grown in that particular area. Therefore, this particular weed was popularly named Yin Yang Huo, which translates to Horny Goat Weed. Additionally, Shennong's and Rihuazi's Chinese Materia Medica also highlighted Herba Epimedii as an effective kidney Yang herbal tonic to treat impotence, male infertility, and pain in the male genital area.

2.1.3 Efficacies of Herba Epimedii

Protective effect on reproductive ability and spermatogenesis

Studies show that Herba Epimedii flavonoids, in particular ICA, can improve the morphology of the testes and increase sex hormone levels [3,9–11]. Chen found that ICA can increase the serum testosterone levels via regulating the mRNA expression of PBR StAR FSHR and Claudin-11 can increase the sperm count in healthy male rats. However, ICA is only beneficial to male reproductive functions at dosages of 50 and 100 mg/kg, while higher doses (200 mg/kg) may reduce testosterone levels and sperm count by increasing testicular oxidative stress [3]. Gao reported that ICA improved the testicular seminiferous tubule structure, reduced germ cell apoptosis, and promoted spermatogenesis and testosterone secretion of Leydig cells on cyclophosphamide-induced rats [9]. In an in vitro study by Nan et al. [10], ICA was shown to stimulate Sertoli cell proliferation in a dose-dependent manner. This effect was mediated by activating the ERK1/2 signal pathway, which might partially explain the protective role of ICA on male reproductive ability. In a recent study, it was found that the flavonoids of Herba Epimedii can reduce the inflammatory response of testes in aging rats and the underlying mechanism of this effect may be related to the regulation of AMPK/SIRT1/NF-κB signaling pathway [11].

Other studies demonstrate that Herba Epimedii can protect reproductive functions and be used to treat infertility, which may be caused by environmental pollution or alcohol abuse. Environmental pollutants such as microcystins (MCs) and di(2-ethylhexyl) phthalate (DEHP) impact spermatogenesis and contribute significantly to male infertility. Sun and coworkers indicate that ICA could protect mouse testes against DEHP-induced damage by inhibiting reactive oxygen species (ROS) accumulation and improving testosterone secretion as ICA was able to reverse the adverse effect of DEHP on Leydig cell proliferation and decreased ROS levels, elevated mitochondrial membrane potential ($\Delta\psi$m) levels, and upregulated the expression of transcription factor SF-1 and steroidogenic enzymes [12]. A study investigating the protective effect of ICA against MC-leucine-arginine (MC-LR) toxicity on gap junctions between Sertoli cells demonstrated that this compound significantly prevented the degradation of gap junction intercellular communication (GJIC) and the impairment of connexin43 (Cx43) induced by MC-LR by suppressing the PI3K (phosphatidylinositol 3-kinase) and Akt (protein kinase B) pathway, a transduction pathway that promotes survival and growth in response to extracellular signals [13]. Similarly, ICA could mitigate alcohol-induced mice spermatogenesis and seminiferous tubule structure disorders, and inhibit apoptosis of Leydig cells [14,15].

Effects on erectile dysfunction

Numerous studies have been conducted to investigate ICA on erectile dysfunction and related mechanisms. A study by Tian et al. revealed a dose-dependent improvement of the intracavernosal pressure (ICP) in normal rats after treatment with ICA without impacting the mean arterial pressure (MAP) [16]. Another study [17] revealed that after treatment with ICA, ICP and restoration of the eNOS expression were increased in the corpora cavernosa (CC) of arteriogenic erectile dysfunction (AED) in rats. The authors concluded that ICA can increase erectile function and that it can regulate the activity of nitric oxide/cyclic guanosine monophosphate (NO/cGMP) signaling pathway on CC to enhance erectile function.

Long et al. reported that ICA could improve the erectile function of spontaneous hypertensive rats (SHR). ICA treating SHR could increase ICPmax/MAP in SHR and the level of tetrahydrobiopterin (BH4), dihydrofolate reductase (DHFR) and guanosine triphosphate cyclohydrolase 1 (GTPCH1), decrease the ration of endothelial nitric oxide synthase (eNOS) monomers/dimmers, decrease the level of nitrotyrosine (NT), dihydrobiopterin (BH2), and nicotinamide adenine dinucleotide phosphate (NADPH) oxidase. Long concluded that inhibiting eNOS uncoupling may be an important mechanism of ICA to improve SHR erectile function [18].

Xu et al. investigated the effect of ICA combined with sildenafil on penile atrophy and erectile dysfunction in a rat model of bilateral cavernous nerve injury. The results of this study showed an increase in ICP/MAP ratio, increased circumference and mean width of the corpora cavernosa, as well as increased cavernous cGMP levels. It was concluded that the combined use of ICA and sildenafil is a potential therapy for neurogenic ED in the future [19].

Icariside II (ICA-II) is a bioactive compound of Herba Epimedii besides ICA. A study by Zhang et al. indicate that ICA-II is a promising compound for diabetic patients with erectile dysfunction as this compound can increase intracellular cGMP levels through the enhancement of nNOS expression and NOS activity in the corpora cavernosa of diabetic rats [20]. Further, treatment of erectile dysfunction in diabetes-induced rats with ICA-II resulted in an upregulation of smooth muscle cell proliferation and the NO-cGMP pathway as well as downregulation of advanced glycation end products (AGEs), autophagy, and the mTOR pathway [21]. ICA-II has also been shown to improve the function of human cavernous endothelial cells (HCECs) impaired by hyperglycemia [22]. ICA-II could also reverse the expression disorder of eNOS miR-155 and RAGE in HCECs induced by hyperglycemia [22]. Guan found that hyperglycemia could decrease the expression of miR-181c, while its targeting genes KLF6 and KLF9 expression were increased, which contribute to HCEC impairment; ICA-II can reverse these changes [23].

Effects on prostate cancer

Apart from its effects on the testes or the penis, the Herba Epimedii compounds ICA and icaritin affect the growth of PC-3 prostate cancer cells. Results of a study by Huang et al. [24] show that icaritin inhibits cell growth and causes a decline in mitochondrial transmembrane potential (Ψm), which was associated with a G1 and G2-M phase arrest in a dose-dependent manner. Icaritin also increases protein expressions of pRb, p27Kip1, and p16Ink4a, while decreased in phosphorylated pRb, cyclin D1, and CDK4. In addition, it appears that ICA has much lower effects on PC-3 cells and only cause a weak arrest of the G1-phase. The authors concluded that icaritin has antiprostate cancer activity through inducting cell cycle arrest, which is not associated with estrogen receptors in PC-3 cells.

Rao et al. [25] revealed an effective inhibitory effect of ICA on the proliferation of LNCaP prostate cancer cells with reduced cell invasion by inhibiting the activity of fatty acid synthase, arresting cells in the S-phase and inducing apoptosis and growth inhibition of cancer cells. ICA also inhibited LNCaP cell proliferation by inhibiting the phosphorylation of androgen receptor (AR) enhancing the expression of the PTEN gene (phosphatase and tensin homolog) [26].

2.2 Lycii Fructus

Chinese Medicine name: **Gou Qi Zi (Goji berries or Wolfberries)**

2.2.1 Introduction

The fruit of *Lycium barbarum* is known by many names but is most commonly known as either Goji berry or wolfberry (Fig. 3). It is one of the most famous Chinese medicinal plants used worldwide, both as a medicinal and a dietary

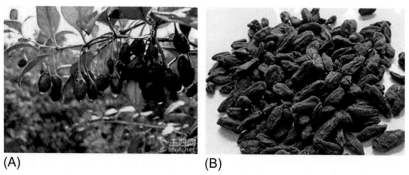

FIG. 3 (A) Plant and fruit of *Lycium barbarum* and (B) dried fruit of the *Lycium barbarum* commonly known as Goji berries or wolfberries.

supplement. As a Chinese indigenous herb, *L. barbarum* has a long history of use in China. Shennong's Chinese Materia Medica first recorded *L. barbarum* (202 BC–220 AC) as a top-grade medicinal material.

In the National Pharmacopoeia, some researchers also record the dry fruit of *L. barbarum* as the fruit of *Lycium chinense* Mill; according to botanical identification, *L. chinense* Mill and *L. barbarum* L. are the same plant [27]. Although the Lycium bark/root (called Di Gu Pi) is also used in Chinese medicine, it is considered as a completely different herb, with different actions and indications.

L. barbarum grows in the Ning Xia province in China and is regarded as the most indigenous and best quality in Chinese medicine. For identification purposes, the fruit are graded in five levels as indicated in Table 1.

The scientific literature has documented that *L. barbarum* fruit contains several chemical constituents, including polysaccharides, carotenoids, and related compounds (zeaxanthin) as well as various small molecules such as betaine, cerebroside, β-sitosterol, coumarins, and various vitamins (in particular, riboflavin, thiamine, and ascorbic acid). The most researched bioactive compounds are the polysaccharides, which have been established to comprise 5%–8% of the dry fruit (average 7.09%) [27].

2.2.2 Traditional use in the treatment of andrological diseases

In TCM theory and practice, *L. barbarum* fruit is neutral in temperature, sweet in flavor, can tonify the Liver and Kidney, and benefit the eyes. Therefore, it is used to treat liver and kidney deficiencies, with symptoms including dizziness, blurred vision, impotence, seminal emission, and lower back pain with a typical dose of 6–12 g/per day being prescribed (herbal mixture) for these conditions. Goji berries are also a popular food consumed by the Chinese in their daily life to promote general health. According to the Chinese Food and Drug Administration, it is one of the 87 TCM ingredients that can be used for both food and medicinal herbs, which is an indication of its effectiveness and safety.

In its long history, the Lycium fruit has an important reputation among the general Chinese population as an aphrodisiac and fertility-facilitating agent. There is an ancient saying, "the husband should not take Goji berries, when he is far away from his wife." This saying highlights the aphrodisiac effect of Goji berries on men. In the Variorum of Shennong's Chinese Materia Medica (480–496 AC), Hongjing Tao recorded that *L. barbarum* fruit can tonify Qi and strengthen reproductive

TABLE 1 Grade of *Lycium barbarum* fruit.

	Grade I	Grade II	Grade III	Grade IV	Grade V
Color	Bright red, purple red, or red	Bright red, purple red, or red	Brown red or pale red	Brown red or pale red	Various colors of red
Polysaccharides	High	High	Less	Less	Less
Quality	Soft and moist	Soft and moist	Soft and moist	Soft and moist	Soft and moist
Taste	Sweet	Sweet	Sweet	Sweet	Sweet
Quantity/50 g weight	<370 berries	<580 berries	<900 berries	<1100 berries	>1100 berries <30% broken berries

ability. Both, Yang Wang in the Essential of Materia Medica (1694 AC) and Gongxiu Hang in the Truth of Materia Medica (1769 AC), mentioned that Goji berries can tonify kidney and improve male reproductive function.

2.2.3 Efficacies of Lycium barbarum fruit

Protective effect on reproductive ability and spermatogenesis

Protective effect on spermatogenesis

Lycium polysaccharides have been reported to exert a protective effect on spermatogenesis, when the reproductive system of male mice was impaired after Cytoxan (chemotherapy medication) treatment. Studies show that Lycium polysaccharides can ameliorate Cytoxan-induced impairment on sperm density and motility, testis morphology, and serum testosterone levels [28]. Qian and coworkers tested serum cytokine levels of IL-2, IL-12, and TNF-α, superoxide dismutase (SOD) activity, and NO level of testes. She concluded that the spermatogenesis protective effect is related to its immune-modulating and antioxidant activity [29]. A study by Zhou et al. demonstrated that Lycium polysaccharides can promote spermatogenesis after the administration of busulfan (a cell cycle nonspecific alkylating antineoplastic drug) to mice, and increase the spermatogonia stem cells, quality of sperm in the epididymis and sperm count in the testes [30]. Luo and coworkers investigated Lycium polysaccharides on hemicastrated rats. The results indicated Lycium polysaccharides may adjust HPG axis to improve copulatory performance and reproductive function [31,32]. Zhang reported that Lycium polysaccharides can protect spermatogenic injuries induced by bisphenol A (BPA) in mice. Results showed that the weight of testes and epididymis and the levels of T, LH, and GnRH were increased; moreover, the activities of SOD and GSH-Px were increased, while malondialdehyde (MDA) was decreased [33].

Protective effect on reproductive ability and spermatogenesis against radiation, heat stress, psychological stress, and intensive physical exercise

Lycium polysaccharides can improve the weight and morphology of testes exposed to heat stress [31,34]. Lycium polysaccharides possess strong antioxidant activity and antiperoxidative effects [35]. The mechanism of heat stress protection may partly relate to this antioxidant activity. Lycium polysaccharides may also inhibit the Bax (apoptosis regulator) activation in germ cells, inhibit Cyc C released in the mitochondria, thereby protecting rat's germ cells against heat stress [34].

Administration of Lycium polysaccharides to rats can ameliorate chronic psychological stress induced by reproductive dysfunction, as evidenced by the improvement of testosterone levels, sperm count, and motility [36]. L. barbarum fruit juice has been confirmed to be effective in preventing low serum testosterone levels, induced by intensive physical exercise, as evidenced by a clinic trial including 28 healthy male university students [37].

Lycium polysaccharides has been reported to exert a protective effect against radiation-induced reproductive injury in male rats [38,39]. Lycium polysaccharides protected rats' testicles against radiation and improved mating function and organ coefficient of the testes, sperm count and mobility. It was also found that Lycium polysaccharides can reduce apoptosis of testicular cells induced by radiation and the mechanism was associated with regulation of P53 and HSP70 and the upregulation of Bcl-2, while downregulating the expression of Bax [38,39].

Protective effect on male sexual dysfunction and fertility caused by diabetes

Administration of Lycium polysaccharides to diabetic animals could assist in the recovery of impaired male fertility due to diabetes [40,41]. Shi et al. discovered when treating diabetic mice that Lycium polysaccharides can improve sexual behavior and histological changes of the testes and increase sexual hormone function of T, FSH, and LH. It was concluded that Lycium polysaccharides can regulate the endocrine activity of hypothalamic-pituitary-gonadal axis [40]. Study of Liu et al. also showed that Lycium polysaccharides can increase sperm count and motility in diabetic rats [41].

2.2.4 Effect on erectile dysfunction

Moon et al. [42] have found that L. barbarum fruit extraction treatments increased testosterone levels, increased GMP and expression of eNOS and nNOS in the penile tissue. Oxidative stress in the cavernosal tissue was decreased while SOD activity was increased, corporal fibrosis was decreased. Results indicated that L. barbarum fruit have a positive effect on erectile dysfunction and this may be related to the fruit's antioxidant effects [42]. An herbal formula (KH-204) including L. barbarum fruit was administered to spontaneous hypertensive male rats (SHR) and the results showed that the ICP/MAP ratio was increased; NOS activities of the penile tissue was increased. Expression levels of nNOS and eNOS in the penile tissue were increased. It showed that KH-204 enhanced intracavernous pressure and NO-cGMP activity in the penile tissue of rats [43].

2.2.5 Effect on prostate cancer

The influence of Lycium polysaccharides on human prostate cancer cells was investigated in vitro and in vivo by Luo et al. [44]. The in vivo studies showed that Lycium polysaccharides can inhibit the growth of both PC-3 and DU-145 human prostate cancer cells, on a dose- and time-dependent schedule. Lycium polysaccharides caused the breakage of cells of DNA strands and markedly induced PC-3 and DU-145 cell apoptosis by regulating the expression of Bcl-2 and Bax [44]. The in vivo experiment in nude mouse xenograft tumor model indicated that Lycium polysaccharides might inhibit PC-3 tumor growth. Both the tumor volume and weight were decreased [44].

2.3 Herba Cistanches

Chinese Medicine Name: **Rou Cong Rong (Broomrape)**

2.3.1 Introduction

The Herba Cistanches (Fig. 4) was first recorded in Shennong's Chinese Materia Medica (202 BC–220 AC, Han), as a top-grade medicinal material. It is the dried succulent stems of the *Cistanches deserticola* Y.C. Ma and *Cistanche tubulosa* (Schenk) R. Wight [45]. In Chinese Medicine practice, Herba Cistanches can tonify kidney Yang, nourish blood, lubricate intestines, and relieve constipation. It is used as a classic kidney Yang tonic herb and has even been named as "Ginseng of the deserts." In TCM, Herba Cistanches is used in herbal formulas as a mixture of decoctions at a dosage of 6–15 g daily to treat kidney Yang deficiency and deficiency of blood, which can cause impotence, seminal emission, and prostate disease.

Scientific literature documented that the main constituents of Herba Cistanches are polysaccharides and phenylethanoid glycosides (PhGs) such as cistanosides, echinacoside, and acteoside [46]. Its pharmacological effects include improvement of brain function, immune-boosting effects, antiaging, and aphrodisiac effects [47–50].

2.3.2 Traditional use in the treatment of andrological diseases

Herba Cistanches has been considered as a tonic agent on male reproductive function for thousands of years. Shennong's Chinese Materia Medica has recorded that Herba Cistanches can strengthen male reproductive function and improve fertility. Rihuazi's Chinese Materia Medica (618–907 AC) mentioned that Herba Cistanches can treat impotence and infertility of men, caused by Yang deficiency. In Medicinal Properties of Material Medica, Quan Zhen (541–643 AC) said Herba Cistanches is a remarkable tonic herb and has antiaging and aphrodisiac effects.

2.3.3 Efficacies of Herba Cistanches on reproductive ability and fertility improvement

Most of the studies on Herba Cistanches are focused on its effect on reproductive function and spermatogenesis. Wang investigated *C. tubulosa* extraction on healthy rats and the results showed that *C. tubulosa* could increase sperm count and motility, decrease abnormal sperm, increase serum progesterone and testosterone by improving testicular steroidogenic enzymes expression of cholesterol side-chain cleavage enzyme (CYP11A1), 17α-hydrolase (CYP17A1), and cytochrome P450 3A4 (CYP3A4) [51]. Shimoda have also found that the *C. tubulosa* extract induced the gene expression

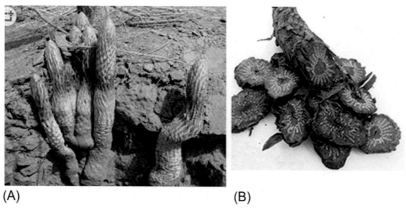

(A)   (B)

FIG. 4 (A) *Cistanche deserticola*, a parasitic desert plant and (B) dried fleshy stem of *Cistanche deserticola*.

of 3β-hydroxysteroid dehydrogenase and 5α-reductase-2 aldo-keto reductase to improve biosynthesis of steroidogenic enzymes. It also indicated that *C. tubulosa* extract had a positive effect on male hormone production [52].

Herba Cistanches has a protective effect on spermatogenesis, especially after impairment to sperm cells induced by different chemicals, such as hydrocortisone, Tripterygium glycosides, Bisphenol A (BPA is an estrogen-mimic environmental contaminant, which could induce oligoasthenozoospermia). *C. tubulosa* and Echinacoside could reverse BPA-induced abnormality in sperm characteristics and testicular structure and normalize serum testosterone, which is associated with increased expression of the key steroidogenic enzymes including steroidogenic acute regulatory protein (StAR), CYP11A1, 3β-hydroxysteroid dehydrogenase (3β-HSD), 17β-hydroxysteroid dehydrogenases (17β-HSD), and CYP17A1 [53]. A study by Wang et al. showed that total oligosaccharide, total phenyl ethanol glycosides, and total polysaccharide of *C. tubulosa* could ameliorate reproductive impairment induced by hydrocortisone, as evidenced by improving the sex behavior of rats, increasing T, FSH, and GnRH and by alleviating the pathological morphology of the testes [54]. Another study confirmed that it is in fact the main compounds in phenylethanoid glycosides, acteoside, and echinacoside that are responsible for improving sex behavior in rats [55]. Echinacoside could block the androgen receptor (AR) activity in the hypothalamus to increase the quantity of sperm and protect against BPA. The underlying mechanism of Echinacoside could inhibit negative feedback of sex hormone regulation and increase the secretion of luteinizing hormone (LH) and testosterone (T), subsequently enhancing the quantity of sperm [56].

C. deserticola is also very commonly used as Herba Cistanches in China. This herb could shorten erectile latency and prolong erectile duration, minimize the negative effects of castration on rats, and regulate serum LH to its normal level in castrated rats [57]. Other studies indicated that *C. deserticola* could alleviate spermatogenetic cell degeneration induced by hydroxyurea [49], reverse the reproductive toxicity in mice induced by Tripterygium glycoside [58], and reduce the impact of high-intensity exercise on serum testosterone [59].

2.3.4 Potential toxicity of Herba Cistanches

Wang et al. [51] reported that oral administration of 0.8 g/kg/day *C. tubulosa* extraction for 20 days caused mild hepatic edema; the liver index and ALT (alanine aminotransferase) were significantly increased compared with the normal control group. However, 0.2 g and 0.4 g/kg/day of *C. tubulosa* extract had no impact on the liver. Kim also reported that oral administration of 1 g/kg/day *C. tubulosa* extract for 35 days induced testes cytotoxicity and sperm count and the serum testosterone levels were decreased, while 0.25 mg/kg had no impact on the testes [60]. A dosage below 0.5 g/kg/day may be considered as a safe dosage for use.

2.4 Cuscutae Semen

Chinese Medicine name **Tu Si Zi** (Cuscuta Seed, Dodder Seed)

2.4.1 Introduction

Around 2000 years ago, Cuscutae Semen (Fig. 5) was first documented as a tonic herb in Shennong's Chinese Materia Medica. According to the National Pharmacopoeia 2015, dried seeds of the parasitic plant *Cuscuta chinensis* and *Cuscuta australis* are used as Cuscutae Semen (Tu Si Zi) in Chinese medicine practice [61]. The main chemical constituents of the *C. chinensis* and *C. australis* seeds are flavonoids, polysaccharides, alkaloids, steroids, volatile oils, and lignans [62,63].

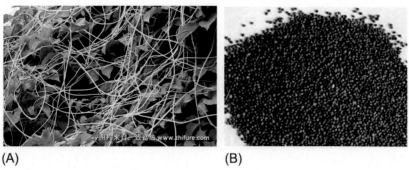

(A)   (B)

FIG. 5   (A) Growing plant of Cuscutae and (B) Cuscutae seed.

The pharmacology effects of Cuscutae seeds (CS) include antioxidant and antiaging activity, immune regulating, neuroprotection activity, anti-osteoporotic, and have a positive effect on the reproductive system [64–67].

2.4.2 Traditional use in the treatment of andrological diseases

In TCM, Cuscutae seeds can improve the function of the kidney and the liver, prevent abortion, improve vision, and stop diarrhea. It has been used to treat kidney deficiency, which can cause lumbago, impotence, spermatorrhea, frequent urination, infertility, abortion, and blurred vision. The recommended dosage is 6–12 g per day in the form of decoction [61]. In its 2000-year history, it was commonly documented as a tonic and an aphrodisiac herb in TCM, combined with other kidney herbs, to improve sexual function and treat impotence, male infertility, spermatorrhea, and premature ejaculation in clinics. In Ming Yi Bie Lu (220–450 AC), Hongjing Tao recorded that the seeds can strengthen the body, improve the male reproduction ability, treat pain in the penis and prostate, as well as difficult urination due to prostate problems. Ri Hua Zi's Materia Medica (618–907 AC) highlighted that it can treat spermatorrhea due to kidney deficiency. Zhumo Ni documented in the Collected Statement of Material Medica (1624 AC) that it can improve the function of the kidney and the liver and can treat male infertility, impotence, and spermatorrhea.

2.4.3 Efficacies of Cuscutae seed
Protective effect on reproductive ability and spermatogenesis

Studies demonstrated that CS improved sex hormone imbalances and male reproductive ability, which were impaired, after being induced by chemical drugs. Administration of total flavones from Cuscutae seeds (TFCS) to oligoasthenozoospermic rats induced by hydrocortisone, improved sperm quality, increased serum testosterone, and enhanced ACP, LDH, SDH activity in the testes; decreased the MDA; increased GSH and testosterone—SOD; and downregulated expressions of Fas (type I transmembrane protein) and FasL (Fas ligand) in the testes [68]. It also restored the reduction of testosterone level and AR mRNA and AR protein expression, induced by the hydrocortisone in the kidney and testicles [69]. It was concluded that TFSC can protect spermatogenesis against hydrocortisone. The effect may relate to released oxidative stress and inhibited Fas/FasL pathways in apoptosis, as well as regulate the AR gene expression [68,69].

Nan investigated the effect of CS extraction in infertile rats induced by adenine and results showed that CS extract increased the level of FSH, LH, T, E2 and increased sperm count in seminiferous tubules. Nan also found both CYP19 gene and aromatase (P450arom) expressed in Leydig cells in dolicho-nematoblasts in the testes [70]. Su and coworkers used CS aqueous extraction to treat rats, induced by estradiol and the results showed that CS extraction increased testis index, seminal vesicle index, seminal plasma fructose, GnRH, testosterone, and decreased the content of E2, FSH, and LH [71]. Ren et al. reported that TFSC can protect spermatogenic impairment induced by Tripterygium multiglycosides by inhibiting apoptosis and improving protein expression of stem cell factor/receptor (SCF/c-kit), master regulator of cell-cycle entry and proliferative metabolism transcription factor (C-myc) and (Creb)/cAMP response element modulator (CREM) [72].

Aqueous extraction of CS can protect reproduction and spermatogenesis against oxidative injury. Administration of CS extraction to human sperm in an ROS environment improved sperm acrosomal integrity and ultrastructure, improved SOD activity, and reduced the MDA of sperm. Yang et al. found that 0.25 mg/mL CS extract is more effective than vitamin C (0.25 mg/mL) in protecting sperm [73,74].

In another study, seminiferous tubules of rats treated with TFCS decreased ROS and MDA levels, increased antioxidant capacity, and inhibited cell apoptosis [75].

2.4.4 Effect on erectile dysfunction

Extract of CS enhanced sildenafil-induced penile corpus cavernosum (PCC) relaxation on rabbit PCC. Rabbit penises were precontracted with phenylephrine and treated with 1, 2, 3, 4, and 5 mg/mL of CS ethanol extraction. It was found that CS relaxed PCC phenylephrine-induced contraction in a dose-dependent manner and significantly increased sildenafil-induced PCC relaxation; pretreatment with a nitric oxide synthase (NOS) inhibitor, nitro-L-arginine-methyl ester (L-NAME), a guanylyl cyclase inhibitor 1H-[1,2,4]oxadiazolo[4,3-a]quinoxalin-1-one (ODQ), or a protein kinase A inhibitor (KT 5720) did not completely inhibit the relaxation. The treatment raised cGMP and cAMP levels in the PCC and it was concluded that CS has a relaxing effect on PCC, partly by activating the NO-cGMP pathway, which means CS can treat erectile dysfunction that do not completely respond to sildenafil [67].

2.5 *Morinda officinalis* Radix

Chinese medicine name: **Ba Ji Tian (Morinda root)**

2.5.1 Introduction

Morinda officinalis Radix (MOR) (Fig. 6) was first recorded in Shennong's Chinese Materia Medica (202 BC–220 AC). It is the dry root of *M. officinalis* [76]. In Chinese Medicine, MOR can tonify kidney Yang, strengthen the bones and sinews, and can relieve joint pain. Kidney Yang deficiency is responsible for impotence, spermatorrhea, infertility, irregular menstruation, pain in the lower abdomen, bone and muscle atrophy, and rheumatism [76].

The main active ingredients of the *M. officinalis* Radix include iridoid glucosides (namely monotropein), anthraquinones, polysaccharides, and oligosaccharides [77–79]. The pharmacological effects of *M. officinalis* Radix include anti-osteoporosis, improving reproductive capacity, neuroprotective, anti-rheumatoid, and antioxidant effects [80–83].

2.5.2 Traditional use in the treatment of andrological diseases

MOR is commonly used in TCM to treat many andrological diseases related with Kidney Yang deficiency. MOR dates back to 2000 years during the Han Dynasty. Shennong's Chinese Materia Medica (202 BC–220 AC) highlighted that it can treat impotence, strengthen health and tonify Qi. In Medicinal Properties of Materia Medica (Yao Xing Lun 541–643 AC), Quan Zhen mentioned that this plant can tonify and improve the reproductive capacity and treat spermatorrhea and nocturnal emissions. Both Hongjing Tao and Ming Yi Bie Lu (220–450 AC) and Yang Wang in Essentials of Materia Medica (Ben Cao Bei Yao 1694 AC) recorded that it can improve male reproductive activity.

2.5.3 Efficacies of Morinda officinalis *Radix*

Protective effect on spermatogenesis dysfunction

MOR can alleviate spermatogenesis impairment induced by Cytoxan in rats in a concentration-dependent manner. In several studies, Chen and coworkers showed that MOR extraction can improve testicular and epididymal indexes as well as the microstructure of testicular tissue, mean seminiferous tubule diameter (MSTD), testicular biopsy scores, improve follicle stimulating hormone receptor (FSHR) mRNA and androgen-binding protein (ABP) mRNA expression in the testes [84–86].

Zhang investigated the effects of *M. officinalis* polysaccharides (MOP) on spermatogenesis in a rat varicocele model. The authors found that MOP improved the mating behavior, alleviated damages seen in the seminiferous epithelium and in tight junctions (TJ), and increased the testosterone levels in the testicular tissue and serum. In addition, MOP reduced serum levels of GnRH, FSH, LH, and antisperm antibodies (AsAb) and decreased the levels of TGF-β3 and TNF-α, while it upregulated the expression of TJ proteins, vascular endothelial growth factor (VEGF), and matrix metalloproteinase 9(MMP9) [87,88].

Ding et al. reported that MOR could improve the expression of vimentin mRNA and vimentin protein in Sertoli cells of rats with varicocele [89]. The authors concluded that MOP promotes spermatogenesis and counteracts the varicocele-induced damage to the seminiferous epithelium and TJ, probably via decreasing cytokines and regulating the abnormal sex hormones in rats with varicocele. MOR extraction can improve reproductive capacity of Kidney Yang deficient mice induced by hydroxyurea, evidenced by MOR enhancing the mating behavior, increasing testosterone levels, improving sperm quality, and alleviating the histopathological impairment induced by hydroxyurea. It was found in this study that MOR protected the DNA of sperm against H_2O_2 injury [79].

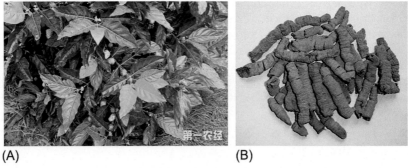

(A)   (B)

FIG. 6 (A) Fresh plant of *Morinda officinalis* Radix and (B) dried *Morinda officinalis* root.

Protective effect on radiation-induced reproductive impairment

The male reproductive system is highly susceptible to microwave radiations. Microwaves may lead to decreased sperm count, enzymatic and hormonal disorders, sperm DNA damage, and apoptosis [90].

Numerous studies have demonstrated that MOR exerted a protective effect on the male reproductive system against microwave radiation [91–94]. Intervention of MOR extraction on microwave-induced injuries in male rats could improve the mating behavior of rats, alleviate histopathological changes in the testis and the epididymis, increase sperm concentration, and decrease the malformation rate [92,95]. In addition, serum testosterone levels and the expression of StAR mRNA in the testis increased, while serum LH, serum GnRH, and the protein expression of GnRH in the hypothalamus and LHR expression in the testis decreased [91,93,94]. Thus, MOR can protect the reproductive system and spermatogenesis against microwave radiation-induced damage through regulating the hypothalamic-pituitary-testicular axis. Aqueous extraction exerted a better effect than ethanol extraction of MOR [91,95].

2.6 *Psoralea corylifolia* Fructus

Chinese Medicine name: **Bu Gu Zhi**

2.6.1 Introduction

Psoralea corylifolia Fructus (PCF) (Fig. 7) was first recorded by Lei Gong' Pao Zhi Lun (Lei Gong Treatise on the Herb Preparation, during the 5th century). It is the dry fruit of *P. corylifolia* L. [96]. In Chinese Medicine, Psoralea Fructus can tonify kidney Yang, replenish spleen Yang to stop diarrhea. It is also effective in treating impotence and spermatorrhea due to kidney Yang deficiency, as well lumbago, diarrhea, and dyspnoea caused by kidney Yang and spleen Yang deficiency [96].

Scientific literature documented well-researched active constituents of *P. corylifolia* Fructus including Bakuchiol, Bavachinin, Isobavachalcone, psoralen, and psoralidin [97–99]. Research shows that *P. corylifolia* Fructus has various pharmacological effects. In particular, antimicrobial activity, anticancer, antioxidant, and neuroprotective effects have been shown [98,100–102].

2.6.2 Traditional use in the treatment of andrological diseases

In TCM, *P. corylifolia* Fructus has a strong action in tonifying kidney Yang by consolidating sperm and is frequently used to treat andrological diseases, combined with other tonifying kidney Yang herbs in a Chinese herbal formula. Rihuazi's Chinese Materia Medica (618–907 AC) indicated that *P. corylifolia* Fructus has an aphrodisiac effect and can improve male reproductive activity. Kai Bao Ben Cao (Materia Medica of Kai Bao 973–974 AC) highlighted that *P. corylifolia* Fructus can treat spermatorrhea due to Kidney Yang deficiency. In Yu Qiu Yao Jie (AC 1754), Huang mentioned that *P. corylifolia* Fructus could treat spermatorrhea and nocturnal emissions.

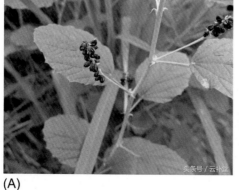
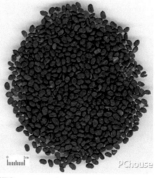

(A)   (B)

FIG. 7 (A) Fresh plant *Psoralea corylifolia* and (B) dry and mature fruit of *Psoralea corylifolia*.

2.6.3 Efficacy of Psoralea corylifolia Fructus

Antiprostate cancer effect

Lin investigated the anticancer effect of PCF in human PC-3 prostate cancer cells. Results indicated that the ethanol extraction of PCF induced morphological changes and cytotoxic effects, as well as chromatin condensation in PC-3 cells in a dose-dependent manner. PCF also induced apoptosis and autophagy in PC-3 cells and led to upregulations in 944 genes, while 872 genes were downregulated [101].

Other studies discovered the active constituents of PCF exerting the antiprostate cancer effect. One of the main active constituents, psoralen, could inhibit the proliferation of androgen-sensitive human prostate adenocarcinoma cells (LNCaP-AI cells) in a dose- and time-dependent manner. Results further showed that more cells were arrested at the G1 and G2 stage, but fewer at the S-stage. Psoralen also upregulated estrogen receptor-β (ERβ) mRNA, downregulated AR mRNA, as well as downregulated protein expression of the proliferating cell nuclear antigen (PCNA), AR, and nuclear protein Ki67 in LNCaP-AI cells [103,104]. Moreover, bakuchiol, as another active ingredient of PCF, could inhibit the androgen-induced proliferation of LNCaP cells through the suppression of androgen receptor (AR) transcription activity [105].

Miao et al. have shown that the half-maximal inhibitory concentration (IC50) of bakuchiol to AR is 8.87×10^4, which is similar with flutamide (10.00×10^4). The compound blocked testosterone-induced AR transcription activity of LNCaP cells, downregulated prostate-specific antigen (PSA) expression, and inhibited the cell proliferation induced by testosterone in LNCaP cells [105].

Psoralidin is one of the most researched active constituents of PCF in antiprostate effectiveness. Psoralidin was studied using cadmium-transformed prostate epithelial cells (CTPE) and results showed psoralidin treatment of cadmium-transformed prostate epithelial (CTPE) cells inhibited the growth of cells, decreased the expression of placenta-specific 8 (a lysosomal protein essential for autophagosome and autolysosome fusion), decreased the expression of pro-survival signaling proteins NF-kB and Bcl2 and increased the expression of apoptotic genes [106]. In vivo studies have shown that psoralidin effectively suppressed CTPE xenografts growth without any observable toxicity [106]. Psoralidin could also sensitize tumor necrosis factor-related apoptosis-inducing ligand (TRAIL)-resistant LNCaP cells, improve TRAIL-mediated apoptosis and cytotoxicity in LNCaP cells. Neobavaisoflavone extracted from PCF was also tested in this study and showed the same prostate cancer chemoprevention effect through enhancing TRAIL-mediated apoptosis [107].

Srinivasan indicated that psoralidin inhibited viability and induced apoptosis in androgen-independent prostate cancer (AIPC) cells. Further research showed psoralidin inhibited TNF-induced expression of TNF-α, inhibited its downstream pro-survival signaling molecules in AIPC such as NF-κB and Bcl-2 in AIPC cells, induced death receptor (DR)-mediated apoptotic signaling, and resultant induction of apoptosis of AIPC cell. Oral administration of psoralidin inhibits the expression of TNF-α and NF-κB/p65 in tumor sections, resulting in tumor regression in PC-3 xenografts [108].

Effect of Psoralea corylifolia Fructus on suppressing benign prostate hyperplasia

Jin et al. investigated herbal mixtures of Cornus officinalis and P. corylifolia, called HBX-6, and suppressed BPH. Results in mice showed that administration of the HBX-6 extract on testosterone propionate induced BPH, decreased prostate weight/body weight ratio and thickness of the prostatic epithelial tissue (TETP), decreased the expression of PCNA and PSA, and decreased the expression of cell cycle associated proteins E2F1, Rb, and cyclin D1 [109]. Further, studies by Yao and coworker indicated that psoralen could decrease prostatic weight, prostatic index and PCNA index, and decreased the expression of estrogen receptor (ER) and AR in prostatic cells in testosterone propionate-induced BPH in rats [110,111]. The authors concluded that psoralen can suppress benign prostatic hyperplasia through inhibiting expressions of ER and AR in prostatic cell.

2.6.4 Toxicity

Research has highlighted the possible toxic effects of PCF. Administration of PCF ethanol extract at a dose of 1.5, 1.0, and 0.5 g/kg for 28 days in rats could cause liver, prostate, seminal vesicle, and adrenal gland damage. Results have shown that enzymes related to adrenal steroid hormone synthesis, NET, VMAT2, and CYP11B1 were upregulated, while CYP17A1 was downregulated; cortisol and norepinephrine (NE) were increased, while serum adrenocorticotropic hormone (ACTH) and corticotropin-releasing hormone (CRH) were decreased. The authors concluded that the treatment caused abnormal enzyme and hormone production related to the HPA axis. The pathological sections showed liver and kidney toxicity and the metabolic trend was changed. The metabolic pathways involved were glycerol phospholipid metabolism, amino acid metabolism, and energy metabolism [112].

Psoralen and bakuchiol were reported to induce the toxicity of PCF. Administration of 60 mg/kg psoralen for 7 days in rats led to liver injury with the liver being the direct target of toxicity of psoralen. Psoralen also impaired amino acid metabolism in both serum and liver samples, such as valine, leucine, and isoleucine biosynthesis [113]. Li et al. indicated that intragastrically administered bakuchiol at 52.5 and 262.5 mg/kg for 6 weeks could cause hepatotoxicity in rats. Thereby, bakuchiol suppressed weight gain, increased weight of the liver, decreased mRNA expression of CYP7A1, 3-hydroxy-3-methyl-glutaryl-CoA (HMG-CoA) reductase, peroxisome proliferator-activated receptors (PPARα), and sterol regulatory element-binding protein 2 (SREBP-2). It was concluded that bakuchiol induced cholestatic hepatotoxicity [114].

In a clinical study involving 84 patients, Tian et al. reported in safety case reports of PCF that the adverse events were mainly liver damage (55.95%) and light toxic contact dermatitis (38.10%). This study indicated that PCF may lead to liver damage and phototoxicity. The authors proposed to strictly apply PCF in clinics and efforts should be made for safety monitoring of PCF and relevant preparations [115].

References

[1] Committee for the Pharmacopoeia. Herba Epimedii. In: Pharmacopeia of PR China, vol. 1. Beijing: Medical Science and Technology Press; 2015. p. 327–8.

[2] Ma H, He X, Yang Y, Li M, Hao D, Jia Z. The genus Epimedium: an ethnopharmacological and phytochemical review. J Ethnopharmacol 2011;134(3):519–41. https://doi.org/10.1016/j.jep.2011.01.001.

[3] Chen M, Hao J, Yang Q, Li G. Effects of icariin on reproductive functions in male rats. Molecules 2014;19(7):9502–14. https://doi.org/10.3390/molecules19079502.

[4] Nie J, Luo Y, Huang X, Gong Q, Wu Q, Shi J. Icariin inhibits beta-amyloid peptide segment 25-35 induced expression of beta-secretase in rat hippocampus. Eur J Pharmacol 2010;213–8. https://doi.org/10.106/j.jphar.2009.09.039.

[5] Qin L, Han T, Zhang Q, Cao D, Nian H, Rahman K. Antiosteoporotic chemical constituents from Er-Xian decoction, a traditional Chinese herbal formula. J Ethnopharmacol 2008;271–9. https://doi.org/1016/j.jep.2008.04.009.

[6] Ding L, Liang XG, Zhu DY, Lou YJ. Icariin promotes expression of PGC-1α, PPARα, and NRF-1 during cardiomyocyte differentiation of murine embryonic stem cells in vitro. Acta Pharmacol Sin 2007;28(10):1541–9. https://doi.org/10.1111/j.1745-7254.2007.00648.x.

[7] Xu C, Liu B, Wu J, Duan X, Cao Y. Icariin attenuates LPS-induced acute inflammatory responses: involvement of P13K/Akt and NF-kappaB signalling pathway. Eur J Pharmacol 2010;642(1–3):146–53.

[8] Lee K, Lee H, Ahn K, Kim S, Nam D. Cyclooxygenase-2/prostaglandin E2 pathway mediates icariside II induced apoptosis in human PC-3 prostate cancer cells. Cancer Lett 2009;93–100.

[9] Gao X, Lin S, Han M. Icariin regulates reproductive function of male rats. Chin J Anat 2013;36(4):740–3.

[10] Nan Y, Zhang X, Yang G, et al. Icariin stimulates the proliferation of rat Sertoli cells in an ERK1/2-dependent manner in vitro. Andrologia 2014;46(1):9–16. https://doi.org/10.1111/and.12035.

[11] Han S, Zhang C, Chen Q, Ma N, Yuan D, Zhao H. Total flavonoids of Epimedium reduce inflammatory reaction via AMPK/SIRT/NFkB signalling pathway in testes of natural aging rats. Nat Prod Res Dev 2018;30(9):1489–93. https://doi.org/10.16333/j.1001-6880.2018.9.003.

[12] Sun J, Wang D, Lin J, et al. Icariin protects mouse Leydig cell testosterone synthesis from the adverse effects of di(2-ethylhexyl) phthalate. Toxicol Appl Pharmacol 2019;378(June):114612. https://doi.org/10.1016/j.taap.2019.114612.

[13] Zhou Y, Chen Y, Hu X, et al. Icariin attenuate microcystin-LR-induced gap junction injury in Sertoli cells through suppression of Akt pathways. Environ Pollut 2019;251:328–37. https://doi.org/10.1016/j.envpol.2019.04.114.

[14] Liu Z, Tian H, Pan X. Effect of icariin on apoptosis of spermatogenic cells in alcohol treated testis of mice. Chin J Matern Child Health 2014;29:2438–40.

[15] Liu Z, Li Z, Tian H, Pan X. Effects of icariin on reproductive damage in alcohol-treated male mice. Chin J Androl 2014;28(12):3–6. https://doi.org/10.3969/j.issn.1008-0848.2014.12.001.

[16] Tian L, Xin Z, Yuan Y, Fu J, Liu W, Wang L. Effects of icariin on intracavernosal pressure and systematic arterial blood pressure of rat. Chin Med J (Engl) 2004;84(2):142–5.

[17] Tian L, Xin Z, Liu W, et al. Effects of icariin on the erectile function and expression of nitrogen oxide synthase isoforms in corpus cavernosum of arteriogenic erectile dysfunction rat model. Chin Med J (Engl) 2004;84(11):954–7.

[18] Long H, Jiang J, Xia J, Jiang R. Icariin improves SHR erectile function via inhibiting eNOS uncoupling. Andrologia 2018;50(9):1–7. https://doi.org/10.1111/and.13084.

[19] Xu Y, Xin H, Wu Y, et al. Effect of icariin in combination with daily sildenafil on penile atrophy and erectile dysfunction in a rat model of bilateral cavernous nerves injury. Andrology 2017;5(3):598–605. https://doi.org/10.1111/andr.12341.

[20] Zhang J, Wang YB, Ma CG, et al. Icarisid II, a PDE5 inhibitor from Epimedium wanshanense, increases cellular cGMP by enhancing NOS in diabetic ED rats corpus cavernosum tissue. Andrologia 2012;44(Suppl. 1):87–93. https://doi.org/10.1111/j.1439-0272.2010.01144.x.

[21] Zhang J, Li AM, Liu BX, et al. Effect of icarisid II on diabetic rats with erectile dysfunction and its potential mechanism via assessment of AGEs, autophagy, mTOR and the NO-cGMP pathway. Asian J Androl 2013;15(1):143–8. https://doi.org/10.1038/aja.2011.175.

[22] Guan R, Lei H, Yang B, Wang L, Guo Y, Xin Z. Effect of icariside II on miR-181c and its targeting genes, KLF6, KLF9, KLF10 and KLF15 in a diabetic-like human cavernous endothelial cell. Chin J Clin (Electron Ed) 2016;10(1):56–7.

[23] Guan R, Lei H, Yang B, et al. Icariside II improves human cavernous endothelial cell function by regulating miR155/eNOS signal pathway. Chin J Clin (Electron Ed) 2016;10(6):826–7.

[24] Huang X, Zhu D, Lou Y. A novel anticancer agent, icaritin, induced cell growth inhibition, G1 arrest and mitochondrial transmembrane potential drop in human prostate carcinoma PC-3 cells. Eur J Pharmacol 2007;564(1–3):26–36. https://doi.org/10.1016/j.ejphar.2007.02.039.

[25] Rao H, Wu F, Chen D. Effects of icariin signalling pathway of phosphatidylinositol 3-kinase (PI3K)/protein kinase B (Akt) and E-cadherin in prostate cancer tissues of BALB/c-nu nude mice. J Emerg Tradit Chin Med 2018;27(5):789–90.

[26] Chen S, Rao H, Chen D. Effects of icariin on signalling pathway of androgen receptor of androgen-dependent BALB/c-nu nude mice with prostate cancer. J Chang Univ Chin Med 2018;34(3):436–7.

[27] Committee for Chinese Materia Medica in State administration of Traditional Chinese Medicine. Lycii Fructus. In: Chinese Materia Medica. Shanghai: Shanghai Science and Technology Press; 1999. p. 267–73.

[28] Qian L, Yu S. Protective effect of polysaccharides from *Lycium barbarum* on spermatogenesis of mice with impaired reproduction system induced by cyclophosphamide. Am J Reprod Immunol 2016;76(5):383–5. https://doi.org/10.1111/aji.12558.

[29] Qian L. Modulation of cytokine level and sperm quality of mice by *Lycium barbarum* polysaccharides. Int J Biol Macromol 2019;126:475–7. https://doi.org/10.1016/j.ijbiomac.2018.12.250.

[30] Zhou B, Bao G, Wang S, Wang N, Zhang S, Gu Y. Function of spermatogenic promotion of *Lycium barbarum* polysaccharide on mice with spermatogenesis impairment. Chin J Reprod Contracept 2017;37(7):566–73. https://doi.org/10.3760/cma.j.issn.2096-2916.2017.07.009.

[31] Luo Q, Li Z, Huang X, Yan J, Zhang S, Cai YZ. *Lycium barbarum* polysaccharides: Protective effects against heat-induced damage of rat testes and H$_2$O$_2$-induced DNA damage in mouse testicular cells and beneficial effect on sexual behavior and reproductive function of hemicastrated rats. Life Sci 2006;79(7):613–21. https://doi.org/10.1016/j.lfs.2006.02.012.

[32] Luo C, Huang X, Li Z, ML Y, Yan J. Effect of *Lyciumbarbarum* polysaccharides on sexual function and reproductive function of male rats. Acta Nutr Sin 2006;(1):62–5.

[33] Zhang C, Wang A, Sun X, et al. Protective effects of *Lycium barbarum* polysaccharides on testis spermatogenic injury induced by bisphenol a in mice. Evid Based Complement Alternat Med 2013;2013. https://doi.org/10.1155/2013/690808.

[34] Tan Q, An C, Xiao Y. Effectiveness of *Lycium barbarum* polysaccharide on the expressions of Bax and cytochrome c of germ cells in rat exposed to heat stress. Chin J Androl 2013;27(1):6–11.

[35] Amagase H, Farnsworth NR. A review of botanical characteristics, phytochemistry, clinical relevance in efficacy and safety of *Lycium barbarum* fruit (Goji). Food Res Int 2011;44(7):1702–17. https://doi.org/10.1016/j.foodres.2011.03.027.

[36] Li LY. Effects of *Lycium barvarum* polysaccharides on reproductive system in rats with chronic psycologic stress. Carcina Genes Teratog Mutagen 2008;20(3):220–3.

[37] Weng X, Lin J, Xu G, Meng Y, Lin W. Preventing exercise-induced low blood testosterone by supplementation of Chinese wolfberry juice. Chin J Sport Med 2016;35(4):344–8.

[38] Luo Q, Li J, Cui X, Yan J, Zhao Q, Xiang C. The effect of *Lycium barbarum* polysaccharides on the male rats' reproductive system and spermatogenic cell apoptosis exposed to low-dose ionizing irradiation. J Ethnopharmacol 2014;154(1):249–58. https://doi.org/10.1016/j.jep.2014.04.013.

[39] Geng T, Luo Q, Wang A, Yan J, Caui X, Li J. Effects of *Lycium barbarum* polysaccharide on testicular cell apoptosis induced by low dose ionizing radiation in male rats. Acta Nutr Sin 2014;36(6):608–11.

[40] Shi GJ, Zheng J, Wu J, et al. Protective effects of *Lycium barbarum* polysaccharide on male sexual dysfunction and fertility impairments by activating hypothalamic pituitary gonadal axis in streptozotocin-induced type-1 diabetic male mice. Endocr J 2017;64(9):907–22. https://doi.org/10.1507/endocrj.EJ16-0430.

[41] Liu H, Li H, Zhang D, Kou H. Protective effect of *Lycium barbarum* polysaccharides on reproductive damage in male rats with diabetes. Lishizhen Med Mater Medica Res 2011;9:2166–8.

[42] Moon HW, Park JW, Lee KW, et al. Administration of Goji (*Lycium chinense* Mill.) extracts improves erectile function in old aged rat model. World J Mens Health 2017;35(1):43. https://doi.org/10.5534/wjmh.2017.35.1.43.

[43] Sohn DW, Kim HY, Kim SD, et al. Elevation of intracavernous pressure and NO-cGMP activity by a new herbal formula in penile tissues of spontaneous hypertensive male rats. J Ethnopharmacol 2008;120(2):176–80. https://doi.org/10.1016/j.jep.2008.08.005.

[44] Luo Q, Li Z, Yan J, Zhu F, Xu R, Cai Y. *Lycium barbarum* polysaccharides induce apoptosis in human prostate cancer cells and inhibits prostate cancer growth in a xenograft mouse model of human prostate cancer. J Med Food 2009;12(4):695–703. https://www.ncbi.nlm.nih.gov/pubmed/19735167. [Accessed 19 January 2020].

[45] Committee for the Pharmacopoeia. Herba Cistanches. In: Pharmacopeia of PR China, vol. 1. Beijing: Medical Science and Technology Press; 2015. p. 135–6.

[46] Jiang Y, Tu PF. Analysis of chemical constituents in Cistanche species. J Chromatogr A 2009;1216(11):1970–9. https://doi.org/10.1016/j.chroma.2008.07.031.

[47] Luo L, Aerziguli T, Wang X. Protective effects of glycosides of Cistanche on apoptosis of PC12 cells induced by aggregated β-amyloid protein. Chin J New Drugs Clin Rem 2010;29:115–8.

[48] Choi JG, Moon M, Jeong HU, Kim MC, Kim SY, Oh MS. Cistanches Herba enhances learning and memory by inducing nerve growth factor. Behav Brain Res 2011;216(2):652–8. https://doi.org/10.1016/j.bbr.2010.09.008.

[49] Gu L, Xiong W, Wang C, Sun H, Li G, Liu X. Cistanche deserticola decoction alleviates the testicular toxicity induced by hydroxyurea in male mice. Asian J Androl 2013;15:838–40. https://doi.org/10.1038/aja_2013.7.

[50] Xu H, Wei X, Ou Q, et al. Desertliving Cistanche anti-aging action: a comparative study. Heilongjiang Med Pharm 2011;34(1):1–2.

[51] Wang T, Chen C, Yang M, Deng B, Kirby GM, Zhang X. *Cistanche tubulosa* ethanol extract mediates rat sex hormone levels by induction of testicular steroidgenic enzymes. Pharm Biol 2015;54(3):481–7. https://doi.org/10.3109/13880209.2015.1050114.

[52] Shimoda H, Ranaka J, Takahara Y, Takemoto K, Shan S, Su M. The hypocholesterolemic effects of *Cistanche tubulosa* extract, a Chinese traditional crude medicine, in mice. Am J Chin Med 2009;1125–38. https://doi.org/10.1142/50192415.

[53] Jiang Z, Wang J, Li X, Zhang X. Echinacoside and *Cistanche tubulosa* (Schenk) R. wight ameliorate bisphenol A-induced testicular and sperm damage in rats through gonad axis regulated steroidogenic enzymes. J Ethnopharmacol 2016;193:321–8. https://doi.org/10.1016/j.jep.2016.07.033.

[54] Wang Q, Chen Z, Luo H, Lu W, Li C, Tu P. Effect of different fractions of Cistanches Herba extracting in improving sexual ability of Kidney-Yang deficiency rats. Chin J Exp Tradit Med Formulae 2018;24(22):95–101.

[55] Ma J, Zhao F, Sun Y. The effects of acteoside on nourishing kidney and strengthening Yang in Yang deficient mice. J Yangzhou Univ (Agric Life Sci Ed) 2009;30(1):22–5.

[56] Jiang Z, Zhou B, Li X, Kirby GM, Zhang X. Echinacoside increases sperm quantity in rats by targeting the hypothalamic androgen receptor. Sci Rep 2018;8(1):1–11. https://doi.org/10.1038/s41598-018-22211-1.

[57] Gu L, Xiong WT, Zhuang YL, Zhang JS, Liu X. Effects of *Cistanche deserticola* extract on penis erectile response in castrated rats. Pak J Pharm Sci 2016;29(2):557–62. http://www.ncbi.nlm.nih.gov/pubmed/27087079. [Accessed 19 January 2020].

[58] Li J, Huang D, He L. Effect of Roucongrong (*Herba Cistanches Deserticolae*) on reproductive toxicity in mice induced by glycoside of Leigongteng (*Radix et Rhizoma Tripterygii*). J Tradit Chin Med 2014;34(3):324–8. https://doi.org/10.1016/S0254-6272(14)60097-2.

[59] Zhou H, Cao J, Lin Q. Effects of Herba Cistanche on testosterone content, substance metabolism and exercise capacity in rats. Chin J Pharm 2012;47(13):1035–6.

[60] Kim SW, Yoo SH, Lee HJ, et al. Cistanches herba induces testis cytotoxicity in male mice. Bull Environ Contam Toxicol 2012;88(1):112–7. https://doi.org/10.1007/s00128-011-0428-3.

[61] Committee for the Pharmacopoeia. Cuscutae Semen. In: Pharmacopeia of PR China, vol. 1. Beijing: Medical Science and Technology Press; 2015. p. 309–10.

[62] Ye M, Yan Y, Ni X, Qiao L. Studies on the chemical constituents of the herba of *Cuscuta chinensis*. J Chin Med Mater 2001;24:339–41.

[63] Lin HB, Lin JQ, Lu N, Lin JQ. Study of quality control on *Cuscuta chinensis* and *C. australia*. J Chin Med Mater 2007;30:1446–9.

[64] Yang L, Chen Q, Wang F, Zhang G. Antiosteoporotic compounds from seeds of *Cuscuta chinensis*. J Ethnopharmacol 2011;135(2):553–60. https://doi.org/10.1016/j.jep.2011.03.056.

[65] Lin MK, Yu YL, Chen KC, et al. Kaempferol from Semen cuscutae attenuates the immune function of dendritic cells. Immunobiology 2011;216(10):1103–9. https://doi.org/10.1016/j.imbio.2011.05.002.

[66] Liu JH, Jiang B, Bao YM, An LJ. Effect of *Cuscuta chinensis* glycoside on the neuronal differentiation of rat pheochromocytoma PC12 cells. Int J Dev Neurosci 2003;21(5):277–81. https://doi.org/10.1016/S0736-5748(03)00040-6.

[67] Sun K, Zhao C, Chen XF, et al. Ex vivo relaxation effect of Cuscuta chinensis extract on rabbit corpus cavernosum. Asian J Androl 2013;15(1):134–7. https://doi.org/10.1038/aja.2012.124.

[68] Sun JJ, Wu XJ, Bao J, et al. Pharmaceutical effects and mechanisms of total flavones from Semen cuscutae on oligoasthenospermia induced by Hydrocortisone in rats. West China J Pharm Sci 2016;31(1):14–7.

[69] Yang JX, Wang YX, Bao Y, Guo J. The total flavones from Semen cuscutae reverse the reduction of testosterone level and the expression of androgen receptor gene in kidney-yang deficient mice. J Ethnopharmacol 2008;119(1):166–71. https://doi.org/10.1016/j.jep.2008.06.027.

[70] Nan YY, Wang RZ, Lu FZ, et al. Expression of P450arom CYP19 ganodal hormone levels and influence of the number of spermium in the testis of infertile rats with Kidney yang deficiency after treated by extract of Cuscutae. J Liaoning Univ TCM 2012;14(2):14–25.

[71] Su J, Chen SH, Lu GY. Effects on reproduction and sex hormone treated by Cortex Eucommiae and Semen Cuscutae in Kidney yang deficiency rats. J Zhejiang Chin Med Univ 2014;38(9):1087–90.

[72] Ren XQ, Zheng GZ, Su H, et al. Influence of flavonoids from Cuscutae Semen on cell cycle arrest, apoptosis and protein expression of spermatogenic cells induced by multi-glycoside from *Tripterygium wilfordii*. Drug Eval Res 2018;41(1):55–60. https://doi.org/10.7501/j.issn.1674-6376.2018.01.009.

[73] Yang X, Ding CF, Zhang YH, Yan ZZ, Du J. Protection of extract from Cuscutae Japonica on human sperm acrosome and ultrastructure. China J Chinese Materia Medica 2006;31(5):422–5.

[74] Yang X, Ding CF, Zhang YH, Yan ZZ, Du J. Extract from *Cuscuta chinensis* against the structure of human sperm membrane and the oxidative injury of function. Chin J Pharm 2006;41(7):515–8.

[75] Wang S, Qin DN. Semen Cuscutae flavonoids protect cells of rat seminiferous tubule from apoptosis induced by serum withdraw. Chin Pharmacol Bull 2006;22(8):984–7.

[76] Committee for the Pharmacopoeia. *Morindae officinalis* Radix. In: Pharmacopeia of PR China, vol. 1. Beijing: Medical Science and Technology Press; 2015. p. 81–2.

[77] Chen Y, Xue Z. Study on chemical constituents of *Morinda officinalis* how. Bull Chin Mater Med 1987;12:27–9.

[78] Xiang W, Song O, Zhang H, Guo S. Antimicrobial anthraquinones from *Morinda angustifolia*. Fitoterapia 2008;79:501–4.

[79] Wu ZQ, Chen DL, Lin FH, et al. Effect of bajijiasu isolated from *Morinda officinalis* F. C. how on sexual function in male mice and its antioxidant protection of human sperm. J Ethnopharmacol 2015;164:283–92. https://doi.org/10.1016/j.jep.2015.02.016.

[80] Zhang P, Chen D, Lin L. Effects of radix *Morindae officinalis* decoction on contents of monoamine neurotransmitters in brain tissues of natural aging mice. J Med Res 2014;43:79–81.

[81] Zhang H, Li J, Xia J, Lin S. Antioxidant activity and physiochemical properties of an acidic polysaccharide from *Morinda officinalis*. Int J Biol Macromol 2013;58(7):7–12.

[82] Ye W, Gong M, Zou Z. Metobonomic study of anti-inflammatory effect of *Morinda officinalis* on acute inflammation induced by carrageenan. Pharm Clin Chin Mater Med 2013;4:124–6.

[83] Wang X, Zhang X. Effects of radix *Morinda officinalis* ethanolic extracts on immune function in rats induced by D-galactose. China Med Herald 2013;17–9.

[84] Chen TJ, Wang W. *Morinda officinalis* extract repairs cytoxan-impaired spermatogenesis of male rats. Natl J Androl 2015;21(5):436–42.

[85] Chen TJ, Xiang JM, Wang W. The impact of *Morinda officinalis* extract on sertoli cells of adult male rats with cytoxan-induced impaired spermatogenesis. Guangdong Med J 2016;37(19):2855–9.

[86] Chen TJ, Xiang J, Wang W. Effect of *Morinda officinalis* extract on model rat with cytoxan induced testis injury. Chin J Anat 2016;39(4):422–7.

[87] Zhang LH, Zhao XZ, Wang F, Lin Q, Wei W. Effects of *Morinda officinalis* polysaccharide on experimental varicocele rats. Evid Based Complement Alternat Med 2016;2016. https://doi.org/10.1155/2016/5365291.

[88] Zhu Z, Zhao XZ, Huang F, Wang F, Wang W. *Morinda officinalis* polysaccharides attenuate varicocele-induced spermatogenic impairment through the modulation of angiogenesis and relative factors. Evid Based Complement Alternat Med 2019;2019. https://doi.org/10.1155/2019/8453635.

[89] Ding J, Tang Y, Tang Z, et al. Icariin improves the sexual function of male mice through the PI3K/AKT/eNOS/NO signalling pathway. Andrologia 2018;50(1):1–6. https://doi.org/10.1111/and.12802.

[90] Kesari K, Kumar S, Nirala J, Siddiqui M, Behari J. Biophysical evaluation of radiofrequency electromagnetic field effects on male reproductive pattern. Cell Biochem Biophys 2013;65(2):85–96.

[91] Song B, Wang F, Wang W. Effect of aqueous extract from *Morinda officinalis* F. C. How on microwave-induced hypothalamic-pituitary-testis axis impairment in male Sprague-Dawley rats. Evid Based Complement Alternat Med 2015;2015:10. https://doi.org/10.1155/2015/360730.

[92] Wang FJ, Wang W, Li R, Song B, Zhou YX. *Morinda officinalis* how extract improves microwave-induced reproductive impairment in male rats. Chin J Androl 2013;4:340–5.

[93] Liu XQ, Yan YY, Gao YB, Zeng T, Lin X, Wang W. Effect of *Morinda officinalis* on male rats spermatogenic dysfunction induced by microwave. Anat Res 2013;35(6):431–4.

[94] Li R, Yang WQ, Chen HQ, Zhang YH. *Morinda oflicinalis* how improves cellphone radiation induced abnormality of LH and LHR in male rat. Natl J Androl 2015;21(9):824–7.

[95] Li R, Liu LC, Wang FJ, Wang W. Effect of *Morinda officinalis* how on improving cellphone radiation-induced reproductive dysfunction of male rats. Guangdong Med J 2015;36(1):58–60.

[96] Committee for the Pharmacopoeia. *Psoraleae corylifolia* Fructus. In: Pharmacopeia of PR China, vol. 1. Beijing: Medical Science and Technology Press; 2015. p. 187–8.

[97] Chen J, Chen C, Lai R, Chen H, Kuo W, Liao T. New isoflavones and bioactive constituents from the fruits of *Psoralea corylifolia*. Planta Med 2011;77(12). https://doi.org/10.1055/s-0031-1282523.

[98] Ali S, Anwar H, Ali S, et al. Phytochemical studies and antimicrobial screening of non/less-polar fraction of *Psoralea corylifolia* by using GC-MS. J Basic Appl Sci 2015;11:159–62. https://doi.org/10.6000/1927-5129.2015.11.23.

[99] Yin S, Fan CQ, Dong L, Yue JM. Psoracorylifols A-E, Five novel compounds with activity against *Helicobacter pylori* from seeds of *Psoralea corylifolia*. Tetrahedron 2006;62(11):2569–75. https://doi.org/10.1016/j.tet.2005.12.041.

[100] Liu X, Nam JW, Song YS, et al. Psoralidin, a coumestan analogue, as a novel potent estrogen receptor signaling molecule isolated from *Psoralea corylifolia*. Bioorg Med Chem Lett 2014;24(5):1403–6. https://doi.org/10.1016/j.bmcl.2014.01.029.

[101] Lin CH, Funayama S, Peng SF, Kuo CL, Chung JG. The ethanol extraction of prepared Psoralea corylifolia induces apoptosis and autophagy and alteres genes expression assayed by cDNA microarray in human prostate cancer PC-3 cells. Environ Toxicol 2018;33(7):770–88. https://doi.org/10.1002/tox.22564.

[102] Lee KM, Kim JM, Baik EJ, Ryu JH, Lee SH. Isobavachalcone attenuates lipopolysaccharide-induced ICAM-1 expression in brain endothelial cells through blockade of toll-like receptor 4 signaling pathways. Eur J Pharmacol 2015;754:11–8. https://doi.org/10.1016/j.ejphar.2015.02.013.

[103] Li S, Cai J, Weng M, Yao H, Chen S, Wu W. Effect of Psoralen on the proliferation and cell cycle regulation of prostate cancer LNCaP-AI cell as well as its expression of estrogen-related receptor B. Chin J Cell Stem Cell (Electron Ed) 2018;8(1):1–2.

[104] Chen S, Weng M, Wang S, Lu J, Tan J. Investigation of effect of psolaren on proliferation of prostate cancer LNCaP-AD cells and its underlying molecular mechanism. Chin J Cell Stem Cell (Electron Ed) 2017;7(4):219–20.

[105] Miao L, Ma S, Fan G, Wang H, Chai L. Bakuchiol inhibits the androgen induced-proliferation of prostate cancer cell line LNCaP through suppression of AR transcription activity. Tianjin J Tradit Chin Med 2013;30(5):293.

[106] Pal D, Suman S, Kolluru V, et al. Inhibition of autophagy prevents cadmium-induced prostate carcinogenesis. Br J Cancer 2017;117(1):56–64. https://doi.org/10.1038/bjc.2017.143.

[107] Szliszka E, Czuba ZP, Sędek Ł, Paradysz A, Król W. Enhanced TRAIL-mediated apoptosis in prostate cancer cells by the bioactive compounds neobavaisoflavone and psoralidin isolated from *Psoralea corylifolia*. Pharmacol Rep 2011;63(1):139–48. https://doi.org/10.1016/S1734-1140(11)70408-X.

[108] Srinivasan S, Kumar R, Koduru S, Chandramouli A, Damodaran C. Inhibiting TNF-mediated signaling: a novel therapeutic paradigm for androgen independent prostate cancer. Apoptosis 2010;15(2):153–61. https://doi.org/10.1007/s10495-009-0416-9.

[109] Jin B, Kim H, Seo J, et al. HBX-6, Standardized *Cornus officinalis* and *Psoralea corylifolia* L. extracts, suppresses benign prostate hyperplasia by attenuating E2F1 activation. Molecules 2019;24(9):1–14.

[110] Yao L, Yang Z, Li S, Guo Y. Effect of Psolaren on cell proliferation of benign prostatic hyperplasia. Chin J Basic Med TCM 2005;11(8):601–2.

[111] Yao LQ, Li SM, Guo YH, Nie LA. Therapeutic effect of psoralen on prostatic hyperplasia and its influences on ER and AR of prostatic cells in SD rats. J Beijing Univ Tradit Chin Med 2005;12(4):8–10.

[112] Wang Y, Zhang H, Jiang JM, et al. Multiorgan toxicity induced by EtOH extract of Fructus Psoraleae in Wistar rats. Phytomedicine 2019;58. https://doi.org/10.1016/j.phymed.2019.152874.

[113] Zhang Y, Wang Q, Wang ZX, et al. A study of NMR-based hepatic and serum metabolomics in a liver injury Sprague-Dawley rat model induced by Psoralen. Chem Res Toxicol 2018;31(9):852–60. https://doi.org/10.1021/acs.chemrestox.8b00082.

[114] Li ZJ, Abulizi A, Zhao GL, et al. Bakuchiol contributes to the hepatotoxicity of *Psoralea corylifolia* in rats. Phyther Res 2017;31(8):1265–72. https://doi.org/10.1002/ptr.5851.

[115] Tian W, Lan S, Zhang L, et al. Safety evaluation and risk control measures of *Psoralea corylifolia*. China J Chinese Materia Medica 2017;42(21):4059–66.

Chapter 5.6

Herbal medicine used to treat andrological problems: Europe

Kristian Leisegang

School of Natural Medicine, University of the Western Cape, Bellville, Cape Town, South Africa

1 Introduction

Both *Pinus pinaster* (French maritime pine) and *Urtica dioica* (stinging nettle) have traditional association with andrological applications, with increasing laboratory and clinical interest. *P. pinaster*, produced and marketed as Pycnogenol, has some studies suggesting improvement in male infertility parameters on semen analysis, with more significant indications for erectile dysfunction. *U. dioica* has more significant focus and evidence relevant to prostate pathology, including benign prostatic hyperplasia and prostate cancer. These benefits are mediated through various mechanisms. Although poorly understood, these exactions may modulate oxidative stress and inflammatory pathways as common mechanisms of action. Numerous isolates have been identified which require further investigation and standardization for clinical application. This chapter reviews the current evidence for the clinical application of these herbal medicines and associated standardized and registered extractions.

2 *Pinus pinaster* and pycnogenol (maritime bark extract)

P. pinaster Ait. subsp. *Atlantica* (Maritime pine) is a tree that is found predominantly in Southwestern France (Fig. 1). The pine bark is harvested, powdered, and typically extracted via a patented methodology to produce Pycnogenol (Horphag Research, Geneva, Switzerland) [1]. Pycnogenol is manufactured by Horphag Research Ltd. (Route de Belis, France), and is therefore a patented preparation of *P. pinaster* standardized to $70 \pm 5\%$ procyanidins [2, 3]. Procyanidins are biopolymers of catechin and epicatechin subunits (Fig. 2), important components of human nutrition, with studies increasingly suggesting that this standardized extract has favorable pharmacological properties [3]. Importantly, procyanidins are considered powerful antioxidants found in significant quantities in foods including grapes, berries, and red wine, and are marketed widely through various different health promotional products for various chronic disorders [5]. Additional important constituents include taxifolin, the phenolic acids cinnamic, freulic, caffeic, and benzoic acid.

Pycnogenol has been shown to have beneficial effects in a variety of chronic diseases, including obesity, metabolic syndrome and type 2 diabetes mellitus, alongside associated dyslipidemia and hypertension [2]. Evidence further suggests beneficial effect in UV-induced radiation damage, asthma, and systemic lupus erythematosus, alongside improvements in osteoarthritis, cognitive function, specifically attention deficit disorder (ADD) [1, 3, 5]. Pycnogenol is considered safe with low toxicity in acute or chronic exposures [3]. The dosages recommended currently through clinical trials range from 100 to 360 mg per day [1].

2.1 Mechanisms of actions

Pycnogenol has significant antioxidant properties, protecting against oxidative stress (OS)-induced cellular and molecular damage. This is mediated via direct savaging of reactive oxygen species (ROS), increased synthesis of endogenous antioxidant enzymes (including superoxide dismutase, glutathione peroxidase and catalase), and increased regeneration of the exogenous antioxidants, vitamin C, and vitamin E [6–8]. These mechanisms confer protection of OS-induced damage to lipids and proteins, including cell membranes and mitochondria, as well the DNA [1]. Closely related to OS, antiinflammatory and immune-regulating activities have also been established. This is mediated, at least partly, through the activation of the nuclear-factor-kappa β (NF-kβ) pathway, which determines a reduction in IL-1 and TNFα synthesis, and reduced expression of cellular adhesion molecules in endothelial cells in vitro [9–11]. Further established mechanisms of action

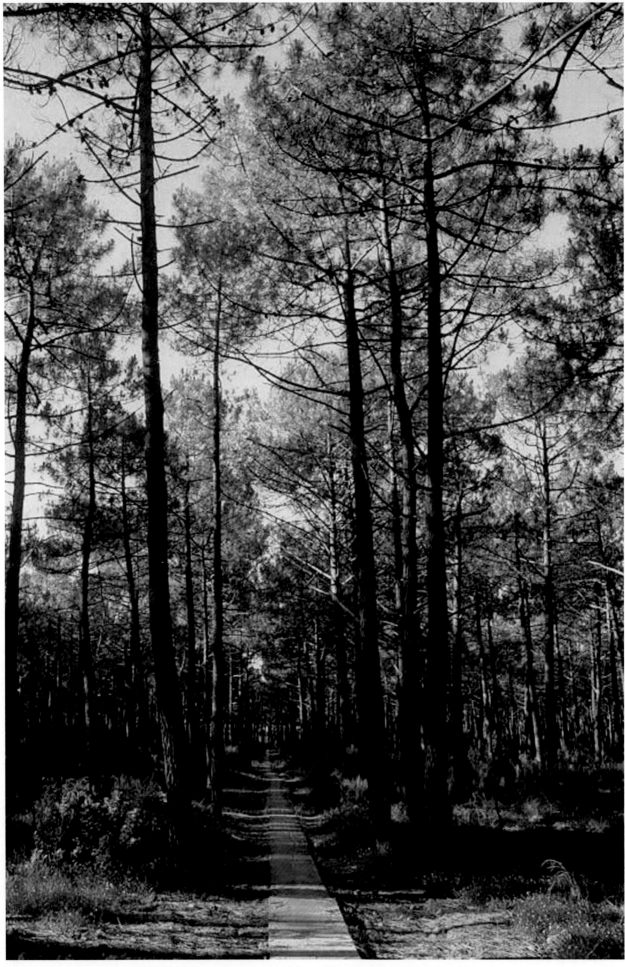

FIG. 1 *Pinus pinaster* trees within the natural habitat (http://www.folp.free.fr/Open.php?getTabSigIdeImg=1380).

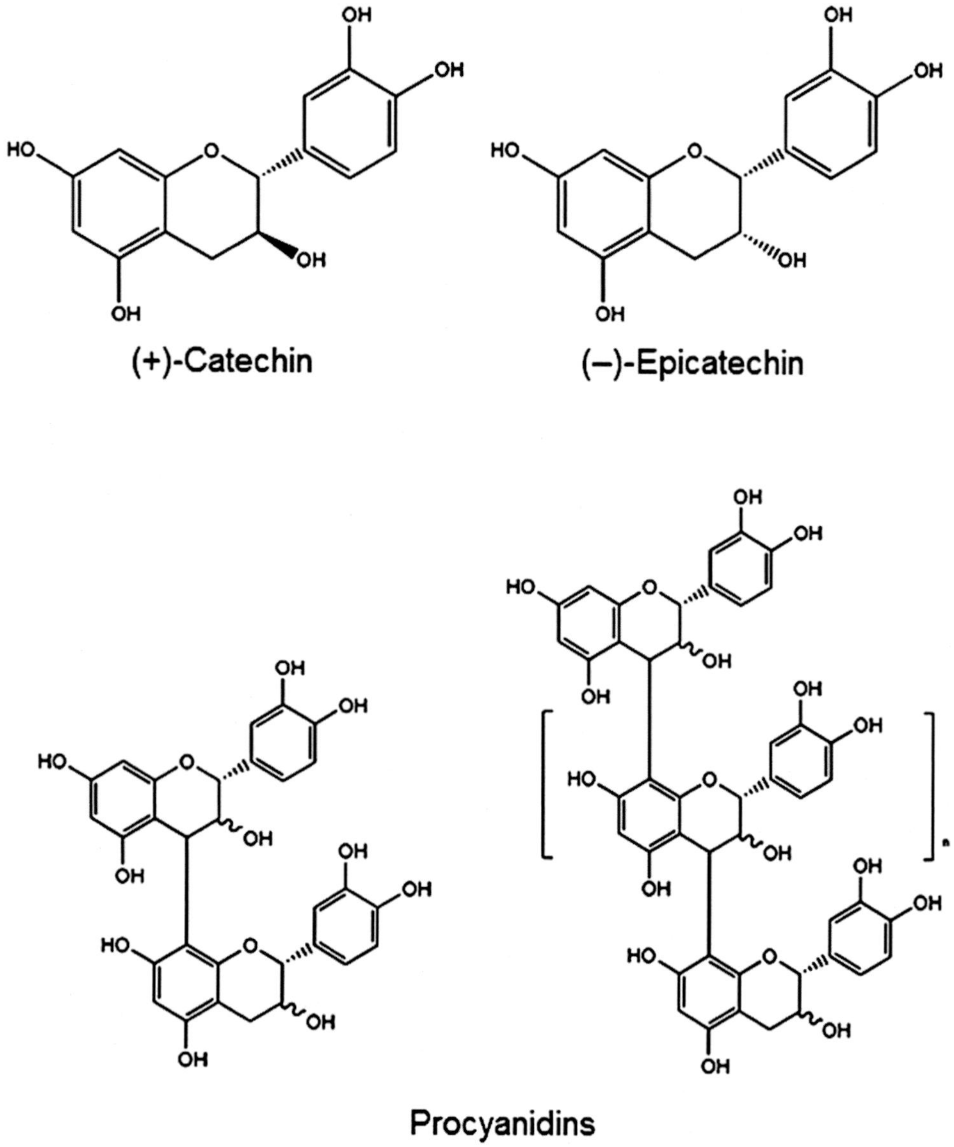

OH

OH

HO

O

OH

OH

(+)-Catechin

OH

OH

HO

O

OH

OH

(−)-Epicatechin

Procyanidins

FIG. 2 Proancyanidins as biopolymers of epicatechin and catechin subunits [4].

include antagonistic activity on catecholamines, vasodilation through increased nitric oxide synthase activity, reduction in platelet aggregation through reduced thromboxane synthesis and inhibition of angiotensin converting enzyme (ACE), antispasmodic activity on muscle and neurotransmitter alterations (particularly in ADD) [1, 3].

2.2 Male reproduction

There is generally a paucity of studies for Pycnogenol in male reproduction, particularly in preclinical studies. These suggest a positive impact on semen quality. However, there is more substantial evidence for the use of Pycnogenol in erectile dysfunction.

In a rat model, spermatotoxicity was induced through the administration of 30 mg/kg/day alpha-chlorohydrin (ACH) for 7 days, which resulted in reduced sperm motility, alongside histopathological changes, increased apoptosis with increased OS [increased malondialdehyde (MDA) with a reduction in glutathione] in the caput epididymis. Compared to a control, coadministration of Pycnogenol (20 mg/kg/day) showed a reduction in MDA, increased glutathione, catalase and peroxidase in the epididymis, improved histopathological changes, reduced apoptosis and resulted in an improvement in improved sperm motility [12].

A nonrandomized clinical trial investigated 19 subfertile men receiving 200 mg/day Pycnogenol for 3-months duration. Semen analysis showed improvement in capacitation (38%) and mannose receptor binding capacity (19%) compared to baseline (pretreatment), concluding that this treatment may improve natural or artificial reproductive outcomes in case of teratozoospermia. Prelox is a combination of Pycnogenol, alongside L-arginine, L-citrulline, and roburins. In a double-blind randomized control crossover trial, subfertile males ($n=50$) had monthly semen analysis through a pretreatment period (1-month duration), followed by treatment or placebo period (1-month duration), then a wash-out period (1-month duration), followed by the crossover period (1-month duration). Those receiving experimental treatment took two tablets per day for 4 weeks. The study found a significant improvement in sperm volume, concentration, motility, vitality, and morphology against placebo treatment, with an elevation in intracellular eNOS activity in spermatozoa [13].

Prelox showed an improvement in erectile function in a male cohort ($n=50$) over a 1-month treatment period in a randomized, placebo-controlled, double-blind, crossover study using the International Index of Erectile Function (IIEF) as a main outcome. Significant improvements in erectile function were reported compared to placebo [14]. This agreed with previous studies reporting the Prelox restored normal erectile dysfunction over 1-month treatment, alongside significant improvements in intercourse frequency (doubled) and increases in serum testosterone and spermatozoa eNOS [15, 16]. In an uncontrolled clinical trial, L-arginine alone resulted in a nonsignificant improvement in erectile function after 1 month in a cohort of 40 patients [17]. On the other hand, 80% of the patients in the same cohort achieved normal erectile function after the consumption of 40 mg Pycnogenol twice daily in combination with L-arginine for the following month. When Pycnogenol dose was doubled for the third month of the trail, 92% of the patients in the cohort reported normal erectile function [17]. This suggests that the Pycnogenol is critical in mediating the positive effects on IIEF observed in these studies of Prelox. A similar outcome was reported in an earlier RCT investigating the impact of Prelox on erectile function in 124 aging men using the IIEF [15]. This trial was conducted over 6 months, with baseline, 3 months, and endpoint reporting. In the Prelox group, a significant mean intra- and intergroup improvement in IIEF was observed compared to placebo. Furthermore, Prelox improved mean intra- and intergroup testosterone concentrations significantly after 6 months of treatment [15]. A double-blinded RCT on Japanese patients with mild-to-moderate erectile dysfunction investigated a treatment consisting of Pycnogenol (60 mg/day), L-arginine (690 mg/day), and aspartic acid (552 mg/day) over 8-week duration. This resulted in significant improvements in the IIEF, specifically with hardness of the erection and intercourse satisfaction. Moreover, a reduction in blood pressure, aspartate transaminase (AST), and gamma-glutamyl transpeptidase (GGT), as well as an increase in testosterone was been reported [18]. Taken together, these studies suggest some consistency for the impact of Pycnogenol on erectile dysfunction, however, they are combined with L-arginine, and therefore the impact of Pycnogenol alone is not clear.

3 *Urtica dioica* (stinging nettle)

U. dioica (UD) is a member of the Urticaceae family, commonly referred to as stinging nettle. Native to Europe, Asia, and Africa, UD is classified as a herbaceous perennial, with characteristic serrated leaves covered in hairs that produce a sting on contact with human skin (Fig. 3). As well as being a source of nutrition, recorded medicinal use of UD dates back to more than 4000 years ago, and has been traditionally used to treat cancers, cardiovascular disease, diabetes, urinary tract infections, kidney stones, hypertension, bronchitis, diarrhea, and rheumatoid arthritis [20–24]. Esposito et al. described the relevant use of UD on cancer, with evidence for potential therapeutic applications, especially in colon, lung, breast, cervical, and prostate cancers [25].

Over 123 plant compounds have been isolated in the genus, particularly the aerial parts of the plants (leaves), which are associated with health benefits from UD [23]. These include polyphenols, triterpenoids, sterols, flavonoids, and lectin [22, 23]. Further constituents identified include carotenoids (β-carotene, neoxanthin, violaxanthin, lutein, and lycopene), ascorbic acid, tocopherols, fatty acids (palmitic acid, *cis*-9,12-linoleic acid, and α-linoleic acid), essential amino acids, tannins, carbohydrates, polysaccharides, and minerals (selenium, zinc, and iron). The total phenolic content of the plant has been found to be 129 mg/g powdered leaves, higher than that of cranberry [24]. Chlorogenic acid and caffeic acid appear to make up 76% of total phenolic compounds, with rutin being the most dominant flavonol molecule [25]. Numerous additional plant metabolites have been isolated, including ferulic acid, ellagic acid, myriceti, and naringin as phenols, secoisolariciresinol, 9,90-bisacetyl-neoolivil and their glucosides as lignans, alongside β-sitosterol (sterol), *U. dioica* agglutinin (isolectin), and scopoletin (coumarin). The roots are particularly rich in oleanolic acid, sterols, and steryl glycosides [24]. However, all parts of the plants (roots, stems, and leaves) are rich in these beneficial constituents, which have been demonstrated to be higher in wild plants than in cultivated ones [25]. Hydroxycinnamic acid derivatives and flavonoids have been identified using high-performance liquid chromatography with photodiode-array detection (HPLC-DAD) analysis on an aqueous extract, and fatty acid esters and terpenes by gas chromatography–mass spectrometry (GC–MS) [26]. In a 45% hydroethanolic extract, Golalipour et al. reported high concentrations of phenolic and flavonoid molecules

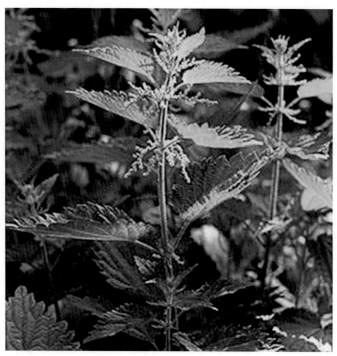

FIG. 3 *Urtica dioica* stems and leaves [19].

$(22.8 \pm 2.7$ and 41.2 ± 3.1 mg/g dry extract, respectively) [27]. These properties make UD an important source of molecules for functional foods, therapeutic supplementation, and pharmacological medicine development, converting a common weed into important therapeutic applications [24].

3.1 Mechanisms of action

Compounds in the plant can impact on diabetes and cardiovascular risk through reduced blood glucose and antihypertensive mechanisms, alongside antioxidant and anti-inflammatory properties. This is done via various molecular pathways, including increased nitric oxide synthesis (vasodilation), GLUT4 upregulation, inhibition of α-amylase and α-glycosidase, and pancreatic β-cell protection [22, 23, 26, 28]. These mechanisms have further been associated with numerous additional properties of UD, such as hepatoprotective, nephroprotective, diuretic, antiviral, and antinociceptive [23]. Antibacterial activity against Gram-positive and Gram-negative bacteria has also been established [24]. Furthermore, UD-isolated molecules with involvement in cancer regulation have been experimentally demonstrated, including oxyliptin (antiproliferative and inhibit cell cycle growth), *U. dioica* agglutinin (antiproliferative), β-sitosterol (antiproliferative and 5α-reductase inhibition), and scopelein (antiproliferative, antiinflammatory, proapoptosis, and 5α-reductase inhibition) [25]. Furthermore, Hartmann et al. demonstrated both 5α-reductase and aromatase inhibition of UD extractions [29]. Antioxidant activity is established through a direct scavenging of ROS as well as through increased expression of antioxidant defense mechanisms, including catalase, SOD, and glutathione [25]. An LC(50) dose established in rats is reportedly $> 1000\,\mu g/mL$ [26].

3.2 Male reproduction

3.2.1 Preclinical studies

Preclinical in vitro studies have focused on benign prostatic hyperplasia (BPH) and prostate cancer cell lines. A 20% methanolic extract of UD has been reported to have an antiproliferative concentration-dependent effect on an androgen-sensitive human prostate adenocarcinoma line cell (LNCaP), with no significant effect on hCPC stromal cells [30]. Similar results were observed when LNCaP cells were exposed to 20% methanolic extract of a polysaccharide fraction of the plant [31]. This was consistent with a previous study in which a 20% methanolic extract showed maximum antiproliferative effects on LNCaP cells [32]. Antiproliferative effects on pc3 prostate cancer cell line have also been reported [33]. More specifically, UD extractions protected against cell damage induced by a dichloromethane extract [34], which was reported to induce apoptosis in pc3 cells, determined by a reduced cell viability, increased DNA fragmentation (TUNEL), and caspase 3 and 9 activity alongside a reduction in bcl-2 mRNA expression and cell cycle arrest at G2. Prostate cancer samples collected from 10 men were incubated with an aqueous extract of UD, resulting in the inhibition of adenosine deaminase. This is proposed to be one the mechanisms to explain the observed benefit of UD in prostate cancer [35]. In tissue obtained from a patient with benign prostatic hyperplasia, the membrane Na^+,K^+-ATPase fraction was isolated and exposed to various extractions of UD, specifically hexane, ether, ethyl acetate, and butanol extractions. This resulted in up to 81% inhibition of enzyme activity, mediated by steroidal molecules stigmast-4en-3-one, stigmasterol, and campesterol. This suggests that lipophilic constituents such as steroids in the roots inhibit the Na^+,K^+-ATPase activity, reducing prostate cell growth and hyperplasia [36].

Hydroethanolic extracts of UD have been suggested to protect against nicotine impaired spermatogenesis in rats. Intraperitoneal injections of nicotine, coadministered with the extract (10, 20, and 50 mg/kg dosage over 28 days), significantly improved sperm count, motility, vitality, normal morphology of sperm cells, increased seminiferous tubule diameter and serum testosterone levels [28]. In a rat model of BPH induced through 28-day testosterone administration, petroleum ether and ethonolic extracts of UD, alongside β-sitosterol as an isolated compound, improved BPH. This was determined through prostate-to-body weight ratio, weekly urine output, serum testosterone, and prostatic specific antigen changes compared to control [37]. The proposed mechanism of action is based on the inhibition of 5α-reductase activity, which results in a reduction of dihydrotestosterone (DHT) and an increase in testosterone [38, 39].

A hydroethonolic extract of UD leaves (100 mg/kg/day), administered daily for 5 days prior to streptozotocin induction of diabetes, showed protective effects on testes [40]. Specifically, these included seminiferous tubule diameter and epithelial cell height, alongside protection against tubercular cell disintegration, Sertoli cell and spermatogonia cell vacuolization, and reduced sperm concentration associated with diabetes [40]. However, in a similar model in which UD extract was administered 1 week after the induction of diabetes for 28 days, there was no significant difference in these same outcomes compared to the control group [40].

UD has further demonstrated protection against ischemia-induced reperfusion injury in the testes in a rat model [41]. Specifically, UD extraction reduced structural damage induced by ischemic reperfusion, with a reduction in apoptosis, induced DNA fragmentation, and a rise in proliferating cell nuclear antigen in testicular tissues. This appears to be mediated through a reduction in OS, demonstrated through a significant reduction in MDH and an increase in endogenous antioxidants including catalase, SOD, and glutathione peroxidase in the experimental group [41].

WS1541 is a combination of UD and *S. serrulata* (saw palmetto) that is approved in numerous countries for the treatment of lower urinary tract symptoms (LUTS) and BPH. This has been investigated in Pb-PRL male mice as a well-established model for prostate epithelial hyperplasia with associated increase in stromal cellularity, inflammation, and LUTS. Compared to finasteride as a conventional 5α-reductase inhibitor serving as a negative control, WS1541 (300, 600, or 900 mg/kg/day) reduced prostate weight with reduced cell proliferation more than finasteride, and reduced inflammation, whereas finasteride increased inflammation [42].

3.2.2 Clinical studies

A recent review on phytotherapy and male reproduction has underlined the beneficial effects of UD for prostate health [43]. A separate review of herbal medicines in prostate cancer found UD to be of benefit in BPH, and in combination with *S. serrulata* showed equal equivalence to finasteride with few side effects [20]. A combined product of *S. serrulata* (320 mg), *UD* (120 mg), and *P. pinaster* (5 mg) showed a reduction in lower urinary tract symptoms (LUTS) in 85% of participants ($n = 80$) in an uncontrolled clinical trial. This was particularly reported for improvement in pain, urgency, hesitancy, and nocturia. No change in prostate volume was found [44]. This study however is limited due to inconsistent time lengths (1–12 months), lack of placebo control, and a relatively small sample group.

β-Sitosterol, a constituent derived from UD, has shown benefit in LUTS in the context of BPH in a multicenter randomized controlled trial involving 200 patients treated with 20 mg/day for 6 months. There was a decrease in the modified Boyarsky score and International Prostate Symptom Score (IPSS), with increased peak urinary flow and mean residual urinary volume. No effect on prostate volume was observed [45]. This was confirmed in systematic reviews of β-sitosterol clinical trials consisting of 519 patients with symptomatic BPH, in which there is symptomatic improvement with IPSS scores, and improvement in residual volume and urinary flow rates, with no effect on prostate size [46, 47].

Safarinejad et al. conducted a 6-month long randomized control trial, with a partial crossover design, involving 558 patients with LUTS secondary to BPH [48]. The experimental group showed significant improvements in LUTS symptoms, IPSS and maximum urinary flow rate, postvoid residual volume, and prostate size (evaluated by transrectal ultrasound). No significant differences were found for testosterone and PSA levels. Only patients who continued treatment maintained these improvements at 18 months follow-up.

PRO160/120 is a combination of *S. serrulata* (160 mg) and UD (120 mg). This product has been investigated in numerous clinical studies. Lopatkin et al. investigated this combination in elderly men ($n=219$ completed follow-ups) with moderate or severe LUTS caused by BPH. This was a randomized, double-blind trial of over 24 weeks, followed by 24 weeks wash-out period, and then extended to 48 weeks in which all participants received the herbal medicine. A significant reduction was reported for IPSS and residual volume, and an increase in peak and average urinary flow over 96 weeks [49]. In a similarly designed previous trail, PRO160/120 also improved BPH-induced LUTS compared to placebo as measured by the IPSS [50]. Both studies reported no significant adverse effects and good tolerability of PRO160/120. The same formulation showed benefit in 2050 patients in a prospective observation study involving over 200 urological centers, with efficacy and tolerability rated as very good by practitioners involved in patient in BPH management [45]. PRO160/120 has been further found to mediate benefit through 5α-reductase activity, equivalent to finasteride with better tolerability, and few adverse events [51]. A different combination of UD with soy and avocado oil (Pluvio) has been also shown to have similar benefits in symptomatic BPH, with improvements in IPSS scores, urinary flow rate, postvoid residual volume, and nocturia compared to blinded and randomized control patients [52].

4 Conclusions

Pycnogenol is a standardized commercial product, produced from *P. pinaster* extractions. Consisting of a significant proportion of procyanidins, the product has been found to be beneficial in numerous pathologies, including obesity and diabetes, cardiovascular risks, and various inflammatory and even neurological disorders. This is predominantly reported to be mediated through a reduction in OS and immune-modulating properties. However, relatively few preclinical or clinical studies have been conducted on *P. pinaster* extractions in andrology. The limited studies suggest a role in protection against induced spermatotoxicity through improved OS markers. It is also suggested to be useful in teratozoospermic patients. Combined with L-arginine, L-citrulline, and roburins (Prelox), pycnogenol may improve fertility outcomes of subfertile males. However, the most significant clinical indication of this combination has been demonstrated for erectile dysfunction. This is seemingly independent of the influence of the amino acid L-arginine and mediated through vasodilation. There remains a paucity of studies for the use of Pycnogenol for subfertility, with good evidence for the use of Prelox in erectile dysfunction. Based on the current evidence, further studies for use of Pycnogenol in andrology, particularly in OS-induced infertility and erectile dysfunction, is warranted.

UD is a perennial plant that grows wild as a weed and is cultivated for nutritional and therapeutic purposes. The use of the plant dates back thousands of years. Within this context, the plant has received significant attention, particularly in cardiovascular disease, diabetes, cancer, and specifically prostate health including BPH and cancer. Numerous molecules relevant to human health have been isolated, including various polyphenols, triterpenoids, sterols, flavonoids, lectins, and fatty acids. Mechanisms of action relevant to the clinical indications include antioxidant and antiinflammatory activity. Specific mechanisms include 5α-reductase and aromatase inhibition, as well as antiproliferative and cell cycle arrest in cancers. Preclinical studies have shown benefit in both BPH and prostate cancer cell lines, alongside animal models. Animal studies further report potential benefit in the prevention of diabetes-induced reproductive dysfunction and testicular histological changes, alongside ischemic reperfusion injury in the testes. Clinical studies predominantly combine UD with *Serenoa repens* in BPH-induced LUTS. This combination has shown benefit in numerous clinical trials particularly in IPSS scores, improved residual volume, peak, and maximal urinary flow rates. There remains little clinical evidence to suggest a change in prostate size and serum testosterone. UD and various isolates show specific promise for BPH and prostate cancer, in which further studies are warranted.

References

[1] Oliff BHS, Blumenthal M. Scientific and clinical monograph for PYCNOGENOL®; 2019.

[2] Gulati OP. Pycnogenol(R) in metabolic syndrome and related disorders. Phytother Res 2015;29(7):949–68. https://doi.org/10.1002/ptr.5341.

[3] Rohdewald P. A review of the French maritime pine bark extract (Pycnogenol), a herbal medication with a diverse clinical pharmacology. Int J Clin Pharmacol Ther 2002;40(4):158–68. https://doi.org/10.5414/cpp40158.

[4] D'Andrea G. Pycnogenol: a blend of procyanidins with multifaceted therapeutic applications? Fitoterapia 2010, October;81:724–36. https://doi.org/10.1016/j.fitote.2010.06.011.

[5] Schoonees A, Visser J, Musekiwa A, Volmink J. Pycnogenol® (extract of French maritime pine bark) for the treatment of chronic disorders (Review). Cochrane Datab System Rev 2012;4. https://doi.org/10.1002/14651858.CD008294.pub4.

[6] Bayeta E, Lau BHS. Pycnogenol inhibits generation of inflammatory mediators in macrophages. Nutr Res 2000;20(2):249–59. https://doi.org/10.1016/S0271-5317(99)00157-8.

[7] Cossins E, Lee R, Packer L. ESR studies of vitamin C regeneration, order of reactivity of natural source phytochemical preparations. Biochem Mol Biol Int 1998;45(3):583–97.

[8] Noda Y, Anzai K, Mori A, Kohno M, Shinmei M, Packer L. Hydroxyl and superoxide anion radical scavenging activities of natural source antioxidants using the computerized JES-FR30 ESR spectrometer system. Biochem Mol Biol Int 1997;42(1):35–44.

[9] Cho KJ, Yun CH, Yoon DY, Cho YS, Rimbach G, Packer L, Chung AS. Effect of bioflavonoids extracted from the bark of *Pinus maritima* on proinflammatory cytokine interleukin-1 production in lipopolysaccharide-stimulated RAW 264.7. Toxicol Appl Pharmacol 2000;168(1):64–71. https://doi.org/10.1006/taap.2000.9001.

[10] Comhaire FH, Mahmoud A. The role of food supplements in the treatment of the infertile man. Reprod Biomed Online 2003;7(4):385–91.

[11] Peng Q, Wei Z, Lau BH. Pycnogenol inhibits tumor necrosis factor-alpha-induced nuclear factor kappa B activation and adhesion molecule expression in human vascular endothelial cells. Cell Mol Life Sci 2000;57(5):834–41.

[12] Kim S-H, Lee I-C, Baek H-S, Moon C, Bae C-S, Kim S-H, et al. Ameliorative effects of pine bark extract on spermatotoxicity by alpha-chlorohydrin in rats. Phytother Res 2014;28(3):451–7. https://doi.org/10.1002/ptr.5016.

[13] Stanislavov R, Rohdewald P. Sperm quality in men is improved by supplementation with a combination of L-arginine, L-citrullin, roburins and Pycnogenol(R). Minerva Urologica e Nefrologica = Ital J Urol Nephrol 2014;66(4):217–23.

[14] Stanislavov R, Rohdewald P. Improvement of erectile function by a combination of French maritime pine bark and roburins with aminoacids. Minerva Urologica e Nefrologica = Ital J Urol Nephrol 2015;67(1):27–32.

[15] Ledda A, Belcaro G, Cesarone MR, Dugall M, Schönlau F. Parallel-Arm Study; 2010. p. 1030–3.

[16] Stanislavov R, Nikolova V, Rohdewald P. Improvement of erectile function with Prelox: a randomized, double-blind, placebo-controlled, crossover trial. Int J Impot Res 2008;20:173–80. https://doi.org/10.1038/sj.ijir.3901597.

[17] Stanislavov R, Nikolova V. Treatment of erectile dysfunction with pycnogenol and L-arginine. J Sex Marital Ther 2003;29(3):207–13. https://doi.org/10.1080/00926230390155104.

[18] Aoki H, Nagao J, Ueda T, Strong JM, Schonlau F, Yu-Jing S, et al. Clinical assessment of a supplement of Pycnogenol(R) and L-arginine in Japanese patients with mild to moderate erectile dysfunction. Phytother Res 2012;26(2):204–7. https://doi.org/10.1002/ptr.3462.

[19] Asgarpanah J, Mohajerani R. Phytochemistry and pharmacologic properties of *Urtica dioica* L. J Med Plants Res 2012;6(46):5714–9. https://doi.org/10.5897/JMPR12.540.

[20] Azimi H, Khakshur A-A, Aghdasi I, Fallah-Tafti M, Abdollahi M. A review of animal and human studies for management of benign prostatic hyperplasia with natural products: perspective of new pharmacological agents. Inflamm Allergy Drug Targets 2012;11(3):207–21.

[21] Dhouibi R, Affes H, Ben Salem M, Hammami S, Sahnoun Z, Zeghal KM, Ksouda K. Screening of pharmacological uses of *Urtica dioica* and others benefits. Prog Biophys Mol Biol 2019. https://doi.org/10.1016/j.pbiomolbio.2019.05.008.

[22] El Haouari M, Rosado JA. Phytochemical, anti-diabetic and cardiovascular properties of *Urtica dioica* L. (Urticaceae): a review. Mini Rev Med Chem 2019;19(1):63–71. https://doi.org/10.2174/1389557518666180924121528.

[23] Ibrahim M, Rehman K, Razzaq A, Hussain I, Farooq T, Hussain A, Akash MSH. Investigations of phytochemical constituents and their pharmacological properties isolated from the genus *Urtica*: critical review and analysis. Crit Rev Eukaryot Gene Expr 2018;28(1):25–66. https://doi.org/10.1615/CritRevEukaryotGeneExpr.2018020389.

[24] Kregiel D, Pawlikowska E, Antolak H. *Urtica* spp.: ordinary plants with extraordinary properties. Molecules 2018;23(7):1664. https://doi.org/10.3390/molecules23071664.

[25] Esposito S, Bianco A, Russo R, Di Maro A, Isernia C, Pedone PV. Therapeutic perspectives of molecules from *Urtica dioica* extracts for cancer treatment. Molecules 2019;24(15):2753. https://doi.org/10.3390/molecules24152753.

[26] Dar SA, Ganai FA, Yousuf AR, Balkhi M-U-H, Bhat TM, Sharma P. Pharmacological and toxicological evaluation of *Urtica dioica*. Pharm Biol 2013;51(2):170–80. https://doi.org/10.3109/13880209.2012.715172.

[27] Golalipour MJ, Balajadeh BK, Ghafari S, Azarhosh R, Khori V. Protective effect of *Urtica dioica* L. (Urticaceae) on morphometric and morphologic alterations of seminiferous tubules in STZ diabetic rats. Iran J Basic Med Sci 2011;14.

[28] Jalilip C, Salahshoorp MR, Naserip A, Salahshoor MR. Protective effect of *Urtica dioica* L. against nicotine-induced damage on sperm parameters, testosterone and testis tissue in mice. Iran J Reprod Med 2014;12.

[29] Hartmann RW, Mark M, Soldati F. Inhibition of 5 alpha-reductase and aromatase by PHL-00801 (Prostatonin(R)), a combination of PY102 (*Pygeum africanum*) and UR102 (*Urtica dioica*) extracts. Phytomed: Int J Phytother Phytopharmacol 1996;3(2):121–8. https://doi.org/10.1016/S0944-7113(96)80025-0.

[30] Konrad L, Muller HH, Lenz C, Laubinger H, Aumuller G, Lichius JJ. Antiproliferative effect on human prostate cancer cells by a stinging nettle root (*Urtica dioica*) extract. Planta Med 2000;66(1):44–7. https://doi.org/10.1055/s-2000-11117.

[31] Lichius JJ, Lenz C, Lindemann P, Muller HH, Aumuller G, Konrad L. Antiproliferative effect of a polysaccharide fraction of a 20% methanolic extract of stinging nettle roots upon epithelial cells of the human prostate (LNCaP). Pharmazie 1999;54(10):768–71.

[32] Lichius JJ, Muth C. The inhibiting effects of *Urtica dioica* root extracts on experimentally induced prostatic hyperplasia in the mouse. Planta Med 1997;63(4):307–10. https://doi.org/10.1055/s-2006-957688.

[33] Asadi-Samani M, Rafieian-Kopaei M, Lorigooini Z, Shirzad H. A screening of growth inhibitory activity of Iranian medicinal plants on prostate cancer cell lines. Biomedicine 2018;8(2):8. https://doi.org/10.1051/bmdcn/2018080208.

[34] Mohammadi A, Mansoori B, Aghapour M, Baradaran B. *Urtica dioica* dichloromethane extract induce apoptosis from intrinsic pathway on human prostate cancer cells (PC3). Cell Mol Biol (Noisy-le-Grand) 2016;62(3):78–83.

[35] Durak I, Biri H, Devrim E, Sozen S, Avci A. Aqueous extract of *Urtica dioica* makes significant inhibition on adenosine deaminase activity in prostate tissue from patients with prostate cancer. Cancer Biol Ther 2004;3(9):855–7. https://doi.org/10.4161/cbt.3.9.1038.

[36] Hirano T, Homma M, Oka K. Effects of stinging nettle root extracts and their steroidal components on the Na+,K(+)-ATPase of the benign prostatic hyperplasia. Planta Med 1994;60(1):30–3. https://doi.org/10.1055/s-2006-959402.

[37] Nahata A, Dixit VK. Ameliorative effects of stinging nettle (*Urtica dioica*) on testosterone-induced prostatic hyperplasia in rats. Andrologia 2012;44(Suppl. 1):396–409. https://doi.org/10.1111/j.1439-0272.2011.01197.x.

[38] Lombardo F, Sansone A, Romanelli F, Paoli D, Gandini L, Lenzi A. The role of antioxidant therapy in the treatment of male infertility: an overview. Asian J Androl 2011;13:690–7. https://doi.org/10.1038/aja.2010.183.

[39] Reza Moradi H, Erfani Majd N, Esmaeilzadeh S, Reza Fatemi Tabatabaei S. The histological and histometrical effects of *Urtica dioica* extract on rat's prostate hyperplasia. Vet Res Forum 2015;6.

[40] Ghafari S, Balajadeh BK, Golalipour MJ. Effect of *Urtica dioica* L. (Urticaceae) on testicular tissue in STZ-induced diabetic rats. Pak J Biol Sci 2011;14(16):798–804. https://doi.org/10.3923/pjbs.2011.798.804.

[41] Aktas C, Erboga M, Fidanol Erboga Z, Bozdemir Donmez Y, Topcu B, Gurel A. Protective effects of *Urtica dioica* L. on experimental testicular ischaemia reperfusion injury in rats. Andrologia 2017;49(4). https://doi.org/10.1111/and.12636.

[42] Pigat N, Reyes-Gomez E, Boutillon F, Palea S, Delongchamps NB, Koch E, Goffin V. Combined *Sabal* and *Urtica* extracts (WS R 1541) exert antiproliferative and anti-inflammatory effects in a mouse model of benign prostate hyperplasia. Front Pharmacol 2019;10:311. https://doi.org/10.3389/fphar.2019.00311.

[43] Santos HO, Howell S, Teixeira FJ. Beyond tribulus (*Tribulus terrestris* L.): The effects of phytotherapics on testosterone, sperm and prostate parameters. J Ethnopharmacol 2019;235:392–405. https://doi.org/10.1016/j.jep.2019.02.033.

[44] Pavone C, Abbadessa D, Tarantino ML, Oxenius I, Lagana A, Lupo A, Rinella M. Associating *Serenoa repens*, *Urtica dioica* and *Pinus pinaster*. Safety and efficacy in the treatment of lower urinary tract symptoms. Prospective study on 320 patients. Urologia 2010;77(1):43–51.

[45] Berges RR, Windeler J, Trampisch HJ, Senge T. Randomised, placebo-controlled, double-blind clinical trial of beta-sitosterol in patients with benign prostatic hyperplasia. Beta-sitosterol study group. Lancet (London, England) 1995;345(8964):1529–32. https://doi.org/10.1016/s0140-6736(95)91085-9.

[46] Wilt T, Ishani A, MacDonald R, Stark G, Mulrow C, Lau J. Beta-sitosterols for benign prostatic hyperplasia. Cochrane Database Syst Rev 2000;2. https://doi.org/10.1002/14651858.CD001043.

[47] Wilt TJ, MacDonald R, Ishani A. Beta-sitosterol for the treatment of benign prostatic hyperplasia: a systematic review. BJU Int 1999;83(9):976–83. https://doi.org/10.1046/j.1464-410x.1999.00026.x.

[48] Safarinejad MR. *Urtica dioica* for treatment of benign prostatic hyperplasia: a prospective, randomized, double-blind, placebo-controlled, crossover study. J Herb Pharmacother 2005;5(4):1–11.

[49] Lopatkin N, Sivkov A, Schlafke S, Funk P, Medvedev A, Engelmann U. Efficacy and safety of a combination of Sabal and Urtica extract in lower urinary tract symptoms—long-term follow-up of a placebo-controlled, double-blind, multicenter trial. Int Urol Nephrol 2007;39(4):1137–46. https://doi.org/10.1007/s11255-006-9173-7.

[50] Lopatkin N, Sivkov A, Walther C, Schlafke S, Medvedev A, Avdeichuk J, et al. Long-term efficacy and safety of a combination of sabal and urtica extract for lower urinary tract symptoms—a placebo-controlled, double-blind, multicenter trial. World J Urol 2005;23(2):139–46. https://doi.org/10.1007/s00345-005-0501-9.

[51] Sokeland J. Combined *Sabal* and *Urtica* extract compared with finasteride in men with benign prostatic hyperplasia: analysis of prostate volume and therapeutic outcome. BJU Int 2000;86(4):439–42. https://doi.org/10.1046/j.1464-410x.2000.00776.x.

[52] Bercovich E, Saccomanni M. Analysis of the results obtained with a new phytotherapeutic association for LUTS versus control [corrected]. Urologia 2010;77(3):180–6.

Chapter 6

Quality control, extraction methods, and standardization: Interface between traditional use and scientific investigation

Srinivas Patnala[a] and Isadore Kanfer[a,b]

[a]Faculty of Pharmacy, Rhodes University, Grahamstown, South Africa, [b]Leslie Dan Faculty of Pharmacy, University of Toronto, Canada

1 Introduction

Numerous therapies available as complementary and alternative medicines (CAMs) and herbal medicines are included and distinguished by established training and professional standards. Among the five discrete clinical disciplines such as chiropractic, homeopathy, osteopathy, acupuncture, and herbal medicines, the two latter are the most widely-used CAM therapies in the world [1, 2].

The use of phytomedicines, natural products as well as complementary and alternate medicines (CAMs) in general, is now a global phenomenon, which has gained tremendous popularity. Herbal medicines have been used as primary health care among the poor in many developing countries and have also gained much acceptance even in countries where conventional medicines (allopathic) are the predominant form of medical care. However, the use of herbal medicines varies depending on specific regions and cultures around the world, which makes this form of treatment inconsistent [2]. Quality, safety, and efficacy are major concerns due to poor regulatory control and a dearth of scientific research and associated data on this subject [2].

Herbal medicines are considered an integral part of medical treatment and 25% of modern medicines are reported to be derived from herbal origin and are extensively used today [3]. The World Health Organization (WHO) notes that of the 119 plant-derived pharmaceutical medicines, about 74% are used in modern medicine in ways that correlate directly with their traditional use as herbal medicines [4]. Major pharmaceutical companies have and are currently conducting extensive research on various species of plants for their potential medicinal value.

The accumulated knowledge of herbal traditions lack vital information relating to quality, safety, and efficacy and are generally without modern scientific controls, which are important to distinguish between the placebo effect, natural ability of the body to heal itself, and the inherent benefits of the herbal medicine per se [5]. Traditional use of herbal medicines refers to the long historical use of these medicines. Their use has been well established and widely acknowledged to be safe and effective and is generally accepted by most global regulatory/health authorities [6]. However, it has been observed that in some instances modern medicine may sometimes not be a realistic treatment option. In contrast to allopathic medicines, herbal medicines are generally readily available, accessible, and more affordable, even in remote areas. Herbal medicines play an important role in health care in both developed and developing countries. The United Nations Conference on Trade and Development (UNCTAD) document states that many activities and products based on traditional knowledge are important sources of income, food, and health care for large parts of populations in various developing countries [7].

The herbal industry has expanded from a small market segment to a major industry globally, with total access of herbal medicines available in health food stores as well as in drug stores and supermarkets, which serve as channels of distribution [8]. One of the major reasons for the increased interest in herbal medicine is the perception by consumers that conventional pharmaceutical products are expensive and of high risk in contrast to herbal remedies that are perceived to be natural, cheaper, and safe. Other factors that have contributed to an exponential increase in the use of herbal products include an increase in public knowledge as a result of access to information through a variety of sources such as the media, journals, and the internet. Among the major types of herbal medicines that have evolved, Asian, European, Indigenous, and Neo-Western have topped the list. The first two types have been used for thousands of years and appear in pharmacopeias and are now better understood [9]. As a consequence of the increased popularity of herbal medicines, the role of traditionally

Herbal Medicine in Andrology. https://doi.org/10.1016/B978-0-12-815565-3.00006-0

trained practitioners who identified ingredients, harvested plants at specific times, prepared remedies under strict rules, and prescribed appropriately, has been replaced by mass production of herbal medicines providing increased access of these medicines to consumers [8].

2 Quality of herbal medicines

The quality of herbal medicines is a major concern worldwide. Lucrative markets for herbal medicines are fueled by heightened consumer interest. Unfortunately, however, herbal preparations are not governed by the same quality, safety, and efficacy criteria as prescription and over-the-counter (OTC) products. The absence of quality control (QC) requirements for potency and purity as well as lenient labeling standards results in questionable standards and quality. Generally, product quality and integrity are not established because of the lack of safety and efficacy testing and purity between batches and manufacturers [10]. The amount of active ingredients can vary greatly between different brands and some may not even contain the assumed active ingredients [11]. The factors that affect active constituents of herbal plants include age of the plant, temperature, daylight length, atmosphere, sampling, toxic residues, manufacture and preparation, rainfall, altitude, soil, microbial contamination, deterioration, and heavy metal(s) contamination, among others [6]. Variation in the activity of phytopharmaceuticals is largely due to the presence of numerous constituents. Illegal contamination or spiking with prescription ingredients and impurities is quite frequent because potency and purity are not appropriately monitored by regulatory agencies. When the raw materials for herbal medicines are collected from the wild or cultivated fields, toxic contaminants can arise from conditions where the plants are grown or collected and where they are dried, processed, stored, and transported before and during manufacture [1, 10]. Other problems specific to the quality of herbal medicines are that they are usually complex mixtures of many constituents and many, if not all, of the active principles are often unknown. Selective analytical methods and monographs may not yet exist. When several relevant constituents have to be considered, standardization is even more complicated because of the variation in ratios of those relevant constituents in different batches [11].

Since, different growing, harvest, drying, and storage conditions can result in variation in the quality of raw materials, it is important to cultivate plants under standardized conditions. Phytopharmaceuticals intended for use as medicines must be standardized and the pharmaceutical quality approved, since the efficacy and safety are based on reproducible quality [12].

3 Extraction of herbal medicines

Natural products are known to contain mixtures of complex chemical components and it is thus essential that any active components in such products are identified and analyzed by validated methods to ensure product quality. The development and validation of the requisite analytical method and procedures for QC can only be achieved by testing the product using qualified reference standards. Since reference standards are generally not available for many herbal medicines, chemical components from the plant materials need to be extracted, isolated, identified, and characterized to serve as such reference standards. In order to achieve the latter, optimized extraction procedures [13] primarily for analysis and for separation and characterization to qualify the relevant markers to identify medicinally important species are required. A further consideration is that extraction methodologies become important for commercial purposes to obtain the desired yields and to maintain the quality of the product and thereby, its safety and efficacy for the intended clinical use.

An important aspect of extraction is to assure that potential active constituents are not altered or destroyed during the process. Furthermore, if the choice of the selected plant was based on ethnopharmacological evidence or its traditional use, the extraction procedure or the preparation should preferably closely match the process used by traditional healers [14].

Since extraction is based on relative solubilities of the required chemical components, which are usually secondary metabolites present in the plant material at the time of processing, the optimization depends on the solvents used and the technique in which the specific chemical components are enriched. The polarity of the extraction solvent, mode of extraction, and instability of constituents can therefore influence the composition and the quality of herbal extracts.

Two specific examples of extraction processes of selected herbal medicines are described and discussed in detail to provide insight into

- what is reported and how an extraction process can yield certain phytochemical(s);
- how the components alter based on species or the extraction procedure;
- cases where traditional methods of extraction can affect the purported "pharmacologically active" component(s).

Furthermore, and importantly, the application of scientific analytical procedures such as basic chromatographic separations involving thin-layer chromatography (TLC) to more complex spectroscopic methods such as mass spectroscopic techniques, to ensure identities of the extracted components is necessary.

Example 1 *Sceletium* plant species

The medicinal use of the *Sceletium* plant has been reported using a traditional method of preparation, where it is purported that fermented material is claimed to have higher pharmacological activity than the unfermented material [15]. It is interesting, however, that one of the purported important alkaloidal components, Δ^7mesembrenone, whose pharmacological activity as an antianxiety moiety had not been previously established results from exposure of the main alkaloid, mesembrine, to sunlight under aqueous conditions [16]. Moreover, from the studies conducted [16], the amount of Δ^7mesembrenone that is transformed from mesembrine is extremely low, and importantly, chemical transformation can only result if mesembrine was initially present as the major alkaloid in the plant in sufficient amounts [17].

It is important to note that the specific plant, *Sceletium,* as with many other plants, occurs in various *"types"* and species. Of the eight known different species of *Sceletium* [18], five are of the *tortuosum type* and three are of the *emarcidum type.* It has been established that all *emarcidum-type* species (*S. emarcidum, S. exalatum, S. rigidum*) are devoid of *mesembrine-type* alkaloids. The five species in the *tortuosum type,* however, do possess *mesembrine-type* alkaloids (not necessarily as a putative alkaloid) along with other different alkaloids [17]. Identification of the specific *"type"* is based on the differences in venation pattern observed in the skeletonized leaves, which distinctly differentiate the various plant types [18]. Another important issue that needs to be understood is the chemotaxonomic variations that the *Sceletium* plant species exhibit, whereby different *mesembrine-type* alkaloids exist in each particular species [19]. These issues make it difficult in selecting a particular *Sceletium* species for commercial propagation and present a challenging process to keep the cultivated plants and the collection of seeds to continue the genotype and maintain the phenotype.

During our studies on various *Sceletium* plant species and interaction with local cultivators at various locations in South Africa and neighboring Namibia, it was observed that some farmers were inadvertently cultivating the *emarcidum type,* which, as previously explained, is of no value for use as a medicine due to the absence of pharmacologically active alkaloids. Furthermore, farmers who were cultivating *tortuosum-type* species were unaware that these *Sceletium* plants varied in both genotype and phenotype. In addition, the putative alkaloid mesembrine varied in concentration and in some of the plant specimens was present in extremely low quantities and even negligible in some cases [19]. The above clearly indicates that claiming or conducting a traditional (fermentation) method of extraction and processing of *Sceletium* plants could be misleading if mesembrine in the cultivator's *Sceletium* plants was absent as the major *mesembrine-type* alkaloid since the resulting Δ^7mesembrenone cannot be formed.

Several reports on the extraction and isolation of alkaloids [15, 20–26] from *Sceletium* species are depicted in Table 1. Although the reported methods above provided an insight into specific extraction methods and isolation of relevant alkaloids, issues regarding the quality control of herbal medicines require consideration as follows.

TABLE 1 Selected literature on extraction and isolation of alkaloids from *Sceletium* species.

Year	Authors	Alkaloids reported/extracted	Reference
1937	Rimington and Roets	"*mesembrine*" with the reassigned molecular formula of $C_{17}H_{23}NO_3$ was based on combustion analysis	[20]
1957	Bodendorf and Krieger	Preparation of crystals of mesembrine hydrochloride	[21]
1967	Popelak and Lettenbauer	Isolation of some alkaloid bases including the preparation hydrochloride salts of mesembrine and mesembrine	[22]
1970	Arndt and Kruger	The extraction of alkaloidal components from *Sceletium joubertii*	[23]
1990	Herbert and Kattah	"*non-mesembrine*-type" alkaloid, joubertiamine from *Sceletium subvelutinum*	[24]
1982	Jeffs et al.	Putative alkaloids—mesembrine, mesembrenone, and Δ^7mesembrenone. Nonmesemebrine type alkaloids - SceletiumA4, N-formyltortuosamine, tortuosamine and some unidentified alkaloids from *Sceletium namaquence*	[25]
1998	Smith et al.	extraction of three previously reported mesembrine alkaloids, mesembrenone, mesembrine and 4-*O*-demethylmesembrenol	[15]
2006	Gericke et al	extraction process, patented for the medicinal use and pharmacological application of mesembrine-type *Sceletium* alkaloids	[26]

First, all the reported methods were developed in academic research laboratories, where those objectives were mainly for analytical requirements/estimations and not intended for subsequent commercial purposes. Second, extraction processes and purification methods vary quite considerably between the various reports and descriptions published in the literature. Third, the plant species used also varied and depend on the collection and correct taxonomical identification and, therefore, the associated extracted compounds were often misidentified. Thus, there are two important aspects that need to be carefully considered, as follows:

- How is the commercial production of the *Sceletium* plant material carried out between various suppliers who commercialize such products?
- Which is the correct *Sceletium* species for commercial propagation?
- If traditional methods of preparation are used, what impact will that have on the subsequent constituent content in commercial dosage forms?

The standard alkaloids (Fig. 1) are depicted where the chromatographic separation of various components, Δ^7mesembrenone, mesembrenol, mesembranol, mesembrenone, mesembrine, Sceletium A4 and epimesembranol are shown using the HPLC method [27]. The reference substances (Table 2) were extracted/synthesized, purified, and characterized by various spectral methods [17]. Fig. 2 depicts the chromatogram of the extract from a sample collected from a farm located near Ceres, Western Cape, South Africa. This plant shown in Fig. 3 (encircled in gray) was identified as a *tortuosum-type* species and was found to contain "mesembrenol" as the major alkaloid along with small proportions of dimethyl mesembranol (based on mass spectrometric analysis [28]) and mesembrenone. Fig. 3 shows another Sceletium plant (encircled in yellow) that has slightly larger stems growing adjacent to the other plant whose leaves were leaner and smaller. This observation prompted the authors to collect a separate sample for analysis in order to verify the possibility of a difference in phenotype. Extraction of the long-stemmed plant and subsequent analysis indicated that it was also a *tortuosum-type* species but contained different alkaloidal components (Fig. 4), and did not contain mesembrenol, but rather mesembranol as the major alkaloid along with small proportions of dimethyl mesembranol, mesembrenone, and mesembrine. This observation clearly indicates the difficulty of collecting an exclusive batch of the same plant. Consequently, a high probability exists of collecting a mixture of different plants in spite of belonging to the same species. Hence, necessary propagation precautions and strict adherence to proper species identity are essential to maintain the selectivity of a specific genotype and subsequent proper cultivation to ensure the consistency of the alkaloidal components for use as an herbal medicine.

Further important issues include variations in secondary metabolites, which are dependent on factors such as age, geography, time of harvest, and inevitably impact on the method of extraction to standardize a batch process. In order to explain

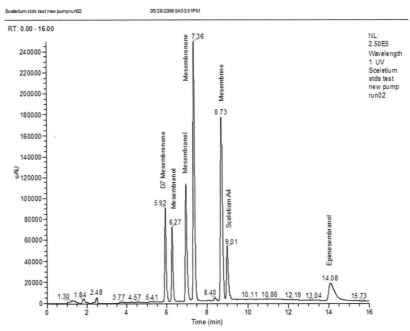

FIG. 1 HPLC chromatogram of mesembrine-type reference alkaloids and *Sceletium* A4.

TABLE 2 Selected structures of alkaloids from *Sceletium* species.

Structures						
Name	Mesembrine	Mesembrenone	Δ7Mesembrenone	Mesembrenol	Mesembranol	Epimesembranol	Sceletium A4
Molecular weight	289	287	287	289	291	291	324

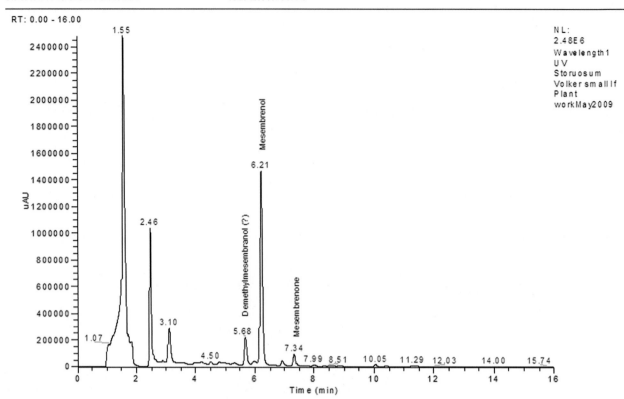

FIG. 2 HPLC chromatogram of *Sceletium tortuosum* mother plant (Ceres, RSA).

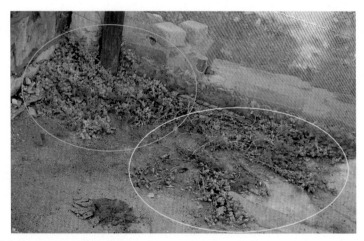

FIG. 3 Photograph of the *Sceletium tortuosum* mother plants.

this issue, a good example is the interesting evidence, which shows how alkaloids in *Sceletium crassicaule* varied within the species and the effect of years of growth on alkaloid content. This plant sample was collected from a farm located in Van Wyksdorp, Western Cape, South Africa, grown in a greenhouse and identified as *Sceletium crassicaule*. The alkaloidal profile (Fig. 5A) showed mesembrenone as the major alkaloid along with mesembrine and a lower proportion of mesembranol. Incidentally, this was the first plant that showed the presence of a non-*mesembrine-type* alkaloid, Sceletium A4, first reported in *Sceletium namaquence* by Jeffs et al. [25]. Subsequently, another sample of the plant, *S. crassicaule*, which was about 3 years old and apparently propagated from the above-mentioned *S. crassicaule* plants, was investigated. The latter plants showed an interesting profile, vastly different from the initial sample of *S. crassicaule*. The major alkaloid was mesembrine with lower proportions of mesembranol and mesembrenone. The non-*mesembrine-type* alkaloid Sceletium

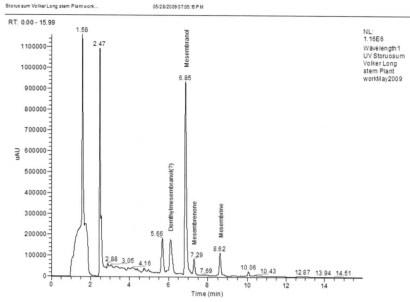

FIG. 4 HPLC chromatogram of *Sceletium tortuosum* mother plant—long stem (Ceres, RSA).

A4 was also present but in a considerably higher proportion (Fig. 5B). A further investigation was undertaken on plants collected from the same area where these plants were grown in the wild and purported to have been used for propagating the *S. crassicaule* plant. However, these samples showed a completely different profile (Fig. 6) contrary to the other two cultivated *S. crassicaule* plants. The *Crassicaule* plants collected from the wild were shown to contain mesembrenol and mesembrenone (Fig. 6), albeit in somewhat lower quantities, but interestingly void of any non-*mesembrine-type* alkaloid, Sceletium A4. More *Sceletium* plants were collected from a source where *Sceletium tortuosum* was cultivated and these plants contained the highest content of mesembrine along with lower proportions of mesembrenone (Fig. 7). These plants clearly represent the best source of mesembrine and genotype. This is an important observation in terms of the traditional fermentation method since only such a genotype can produce Δ^7mesembrenone, when fermented.

Many marketed products containing *Sceletium*, based on the labels, indicate that the unprocessed plant material is incorporated as powder. However, other marketed products containing *Sceletium* such as capsules and powder describe the content as containing powdered extract. A further product marketed as a solution describes the content as a "mother tincture" (Min 64% EtOH Extract) on its label. These are examples of the varied content of *Sceletium* in marketed products, with some products containing unprocessed powdered plant whereas others contain dry powdered extracts or solutions, which contain extracts of *Sceletium* plants [17]. Interestingly, that although claims that Δ^7mesembrenone resulting from fermentation is the main active therapeutic component in *Sceletium*, analysis of the marketed product containing the powder extract confirmed its absence.

In general, extraction procedures should start by using simple techniques to screen for the presence or absence of required components. Importantly, an initial qualitative analysis is necessary to establish the presence of specific expected compounds. For example, since *Sceletium* plants (*tortuosum type*) are expected to contain alkaloids, it is prudent to first establish such content in specific plant material. Thin-layer chromatography (TLC) could be the method of choice as it is rapid and relatively simple to detect the alkaloids using Dragendorff's reagent [29]. However, one disadvantage using TLC maybe inadequate resolution, hence a suitable TLC method should be developed that can resolve relevant components [17].

When preparing plant material to manufacture dosage forms for commercial purposes two basic options need to be considered:

- Using dried powdered plant material without further processing to include in the final product, or
- Using extracted material from a specific plant.

In considering the above options, the following issues need to be emphasized. Plant material per se not only includes the intended therapeutic components, but also contains numerous associated materials including impurities and possible microbial contamination. Furthermore, standardization and QC of the plant material is extremely difficult and often not possible. Hence, variability of the final product is highly likely from batch to batch. On the other hand, a purified extract

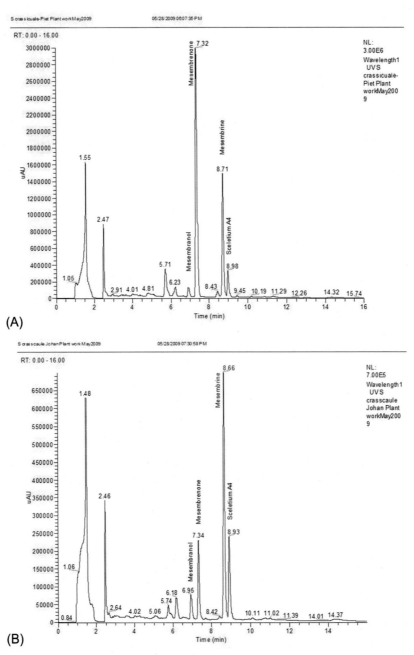

FIG. 5 (A) HPLC chromatogram of *Sceletium crassicaule* plant (Van Wyksdorp, RSA). (b) HPLC chromatogram of *Sceletium crassicaule*—wild plant (Van Wyksdorp, RSA).

is readily accessible to standardization and QC whereby the quality and quantity of specific components can be assured including product purity. These are important advantages, which are essential to ensure product performance.

The following is an example of a procedure to extract alkaloids from alkaloid-containing plants.

Dried plant material is roughly powdered and extracted with a solvent such as ethanol (95%), which is a Class 3 solvent associated with useful properties and, in particular, regarded as safe with low toxic potential [30]. The ethanolic extract is then evaporated under vacuum with an added advantage of permitting recycling of the distilled ethanol for further use. The subsequent steps will require specific treatment depending on the nature and chemistry of the targeted components. If the intent is to extract alkaloids, then treatment with dilute hydrochloric acid (or other suitable acid) to form salt derivatives, which render them soluble in aqueous media, is necessary. A cleanup step is then necessary to remove unwanted lipid-soluble material from the crude acidic extract, which can be done by treatment with an appropriate nonpolar solvent such as

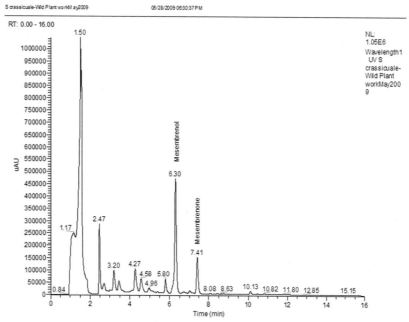

FIG. 6 HPLC chromatogram of *Sceletium tortuosum* (Gouda, RSA).

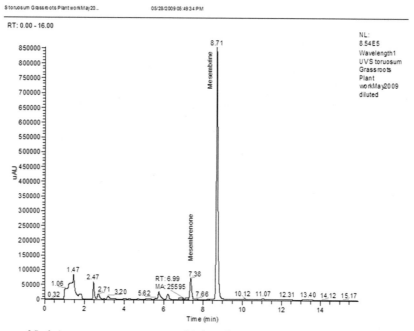

FIG. 7 HPLC chromatogram of *Sceletium tortuosum* extract—spray dried powder.

n-hexane. The enriched acidic solution is then treated with a basic solvent such as ammonium hydroxide solution to release the alkaloids as free bases. The alkaline liquid layer is then further treated with an immiscible solvent such as ethyl acetate (Class 1) and/or methylene dichloride (Class 2), which have lower and higher densities, respectively, than water and then further extracted to ensure that these basic components have been completely extracted into the organic layer. Finally, the organic layer is evaporated under vacuum and this extract is then tested for the presence of required components using TLC.

If a specific component is required to be isolated from a mixture of similar components a fractionation step is necessary. This is usually performed using column chromatography assisted with appropriate further separation and detection procedures such as TLC, HPLC, and LC-MS [17]. The following is an example of an TLC system, which shows the separation and identification of individual alkaloidal components using an appropriate visualization technique by spraying with

Dragendorff's reagent [29]. Visualization under UV light as shown in the second plate (UV 254) is useful to detect other components such as those which absorb UV light which may be present in the extract (Fig. 8).

Example 2 Sutherlandia.

Sutherlandia frutescens (SF), (family: Fabaceae/Leguminosae), is another traditional African medicinal plant indigenous to South Africa, which has been used to treat symptoms of stress and anxiety [31] and also claimed for use as cancer therapy [32].

Traditionally, *Sutherlandia* extracts are prepared by an infusion method by placing 2.5–5 g of dry plant material in boiling water and used as a medicine, which is administered orally [33]. Sutherlandia has also been promoted as an "adaptogenic tonic," which is based on anecdotal claims that aqueous extracts are useful for alleviating the condition, cachexia (muscle wasting) [34], commonly observed in HIV/AIDS patients in the end stages of the disease. Pharmaceutical dosage forms containing unprocessed dried and powdered leaves are available as tablets and capsules in local pharmacies.

Avula et al. in 2010 reported the presence of triterpenoid glycosides known as Sutherlandiosides A–D [35] and another group, Fu et al. reported the presence of some flavonol glycosides, kaempferol and quercetin glycosides known as Sutherlandins A–D [36], which were isolated from SF plant material. In addition, Prevoo et al. identified components, which included L-canavanine, pinitol, gamma-aminobutyric acid (GABA), some flavonoids, and triterpenoid glucosides [37]. A recent report on *Sutherlandia* extracts described the chemical profiling of components in three different extracts of plant material [38]. Numerous compounds from these extracts were detected by TLC and time-of-flight (ToF) electrospray ionization (ESI) methods, but claims relating to the identity of some components were unsubstantiated based on the described spectral data and simply presumed to correspond to previously published information [36]. The traditional infusion using water will only result in the presence of extracted water-soluble compounds (Fig. 9), mainly the soluble flavonoid components whereas the more nonpolar cycloartane glycosides are unlikely to be present. Hence, using a traditional

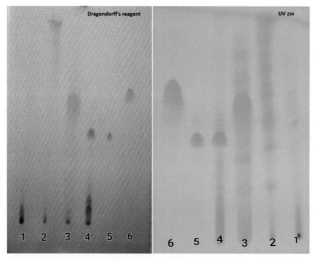

FIG. 8 TLC of Sceletium alkaloids—Left plate visualization using Dragendorff's reagent and Right plate visualization under UV 254. 1. DCM fraction; 2. Acetone-1 fraction; 3. Acetone-2 fraction; 4. ACN fraction; 5. ACN fraction purified; 6. Acetone-2 purified.

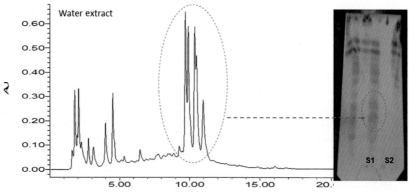

FIG. 9 HPLC of water extract and TLC profile of *Sutherlandia frutescens*.

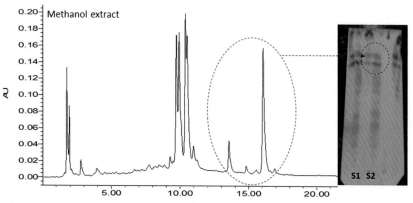

FIG. 10 HPLC of methanol extract and TLC profile of *Sutherlandia frutescens*.

aqueous extract as medicine, would exclude any possible therapeutic activity purported to be associated with glycosidic components such as the cycloartanes. Clearly, a systematic approach to extract all relevant components associated with therapeutic activity requires an appropriate preparative technique [39]. On the other hand, a methanol extract of the same SF sample showed the same flavonoid cluster and, in addition, terpenoid glycosides (encircled in the chromatogram) eluting in 13–18 min and TLC provided information on other likely nonpolar components (Fig. 10).

The above are only two examples showing some extraction procedures, whereas herbal medicines include myriads of different plants the components of which include a variety of different chemical components. Hence, extraction procedures must be tailored for specific components and clearly could be quite different from those described above.

4 Conclusions

Since herbal medicines consist of plant material containing various constituents, evidence of quality, efficacy, and safety is an important consideration yet generally not required by most regulatory agencies before marketing. Furthermore, quality control and production standards provide a huge challenge in view of the complexity of the purported active constituents as well as methods to exclude toxic components [40]. It is important to note that quality is highly dependent on the source of plants and related materials, which in turn are dependent on numerous intrinsic (genotype) and extrinsic factors such as taxonomy, selection, and cultivation including environmental conditions and geography. Hence, correct identification of species, careful collection, and appropriate storage are additional essential requirements for the quality control of raw materials to ensure that products containing plant material or extracts are of the requisite quality.

Standardizing herbal extract is a process that depends on various factors and requires logical, stepwise preparation of the sample. It is well understood that commercial processing of herbals is a highly technological process involving large volumes of solvents and optimized controls for best yields. As mentioned above, the QC of such herbal extracts depends on the consistency and efficiency of the extraction process, which in turn also depends on the source and correct identity of the herbal plant in order to ensure a consistent profile of pharmacologically active components.

Standardization of extracts using alcohol and/or hydro-alcoholic solvents is the preferred procedure from both regulatory and use perspectives. As previously indicated, an initial crude extraction is extremely useful to screen multiple components and is subsequently used for further processing to standardize the composition of an intended dosage form for commercialization as a product.

Unlike for allopathic medicines, QC of herbal medicines remains largely unregulated resulting in high variability in specific content and potency between batches and questionable control of impurities and presence of possible toxic contaminants. However, appropriate extraction procedures and the use of qualified reference standards in conjunction with GMP to produce high-quality products remain an important objective to ensure appropriate clinical performance of such products.

References

[1] Chan K. Some toxic contaminants in herbal medicines. Chemosphere 2003;52:1361–71.

[2] WHO. General guidelines for methodologies on research and evaluation of traditional medicine. WHO/EDM/TRM/2000.1. Geneva: WHO; 2006. p. 1–74.

[3] WHO Traditional Medicine Strategy 2014–2023. World Health Organization, Available from: http://www.searo.who.int/entity/health_situation_trends/who_trm_strategy_2014-2023.pdf?ua=1 [Accessed 14 June 2019].WHO Traditional Medicine Strategy 2014–2023. World Health Organization, Available from: http://www.searo.who.int/entity/health_situation_trends/who_trm_strategy_2014-2023.pdf?ua=1 [Accessed 14 June 2019].

[4] UNCTAD. Background note by the UNCTAD secretariat. Systems and National Experiences for protecting traditional knowledge, innovations and practices. TD/B/COM.1/EM/13/2. UNCTAD; 2000. p. 1–35.

[5] Herbalism. Available from: https://en.wikipedia.org/wiki/Herbalism. Accessed 9 May 2019.

[6] Ekor M. The growing use of herbal medicines: issues relating to adverse reactions and challenges in monitoring safety. Front Pharmacol 2014;4(177):1–10.

[7] Zhang X. Traditional medicines and its knowledge. World Health Organization; 2000. p. 1–5. UNCTAD expert meeting on systems and national experiences for protecting traditional knowledge, innovations and practices.

[8] Stroube WB, Rainey C, Tanner JT. Regulatory environment in the advertising of dietary supplements. Clin Res Regul Aff 2002;19(1):109–14.

[9] Elvin-Lewis M. Should we be concerned about herbal remedies. J Ethnopharmacol 2001;75:141–64.

[10] Marrone CM. Safety issues with herbal products. Ann Pharmacother 1999;33:1359–61.

[11] Zhang J, Wider B, Shang H, Li X, Ernst E. Quality of herbal medicines: challenges and solutions. Complement Ther Med 2012;20(1–2):100–6.

[12] Essential medicines and health products information portal – a World Health Organization resource. Available from https://apps.who.int/medicinedocs/en/d/Js4928e/4.4.html#Js4928e.4.4 Accessed 18 May 2019.

[13] Azwanida NN. A review on the extraction methods use in medicinal plants, principle, strength and limitation. Med Aromatic Plants 2015;4:196.

[14] O'Malley P, Trimble N, Browning M. Are herbal therapies worth the risks? Nurse Pract 2004;29(10):71–5.

[15] Smith MT, Field CR, Crouch NR, Hirst M. The distribution of mesembrine alkaloids in selected TAXA of the mesembryanthemaceae and their modification in the Sceletium derived 'Kougoed'. Pharm Biol 1998;36(3):173–9.

[16] Patnala S, Kanfer I. Investigations of phytochemical content of *Sceletium tortuosum* following the preparation of "kougoed" by fermentation of plant material. J Ethnopharmacol 2009;12(1):86–91.

[17] Patnala S. Pharmaceutical analysis and quality control of Sceletium plant species and associated products [PhD thesis]. Grahamstown, South Africa: Rhodes University; 2007.

[18] Gerbaulet M. Revision of the genus Sceletium N.E. Br (Aizoaceae). Botanishce Jarhbücher 1996;118(1):9–24.

[19] Patnala S, Kanfer I. Chemotaxonomic studies of mesembrine-type alkaloids in Sceletium plant species. S Afr J Sci 2013;109(3/4):1–5. Art. #882.

[20] Rimington C, Roets GCS. Notes upon the isolation of the alkaloidal constituent of the drug "Channa" or "Kougoed" (Mesebryanthemumanatomicum and M. tortuosum). Ondersteproot J Vet Sci Anim Ind 1937;9:187–91.

[21] Bodendorf K, Krieger W. Über die alkaloide von Mesembryanthemumtortuosum L. Arch Pharm 1957;290/62(10):441–8.

[22] Popelak A, Lattenbauer G. The mesembrine alkaloids. In: Manske RHF, editor. The alkaloids. New York: Academic Press; 1967. p. 467–81.

[23] Arndt RR, Kruger PEJ. Alkaloids from *Sceletium joubertii* Bol. The structure of joubertiamine and dehydrojoubertiamine. Tetrahedron Lett 1970;37:3237–40.

[24] Herbert RB, Kattah AE. The biosynthesis of Sceletium alkaloids in *Sceletium subvelutinum* L. Bolus. Tetrahedron Lett 1990;46(20):7105–18.

[25] Jeffs PW, Capps T, Redfearn R. Sceletium alkaloids. Structures of five new bases from *Sceletium namaquense*. J Org Chem 1982;47:3611–7.

[26] Gericke, N.P., Van Wyk, B-E. (2006). N.P. Gericke and B-E Van Wyk. Pharmaceutical compositions containing mesembrine and related compounds. 09/194,836 [US6,288,104B1] 9-11-2006. South Africa. 3-22-1997 [Patent].

[27] Patnala S, Kanfer I. HPLC analysis of mesembrine-type alkaloids in Sceletium plant material. J Pharm Pharmaceut Sci 2010;13(4):558–70.

[28] Patnala S, Kanfer I. Medicinal use of *Sceletium*: characterization of phytochemical components of *Sceletium* plant species using HPLC with UV and electrospray ionization–tandem mass spectroscopy. J Pharm Pharmaceut Sci 2015;18(4):414–23.

[29] Recipes for chemical test reagents. Available from: https://link.springer.com/content/pdf/bbm%3A978-1-4615-5809-5%2F1.pdf [Accessed 6 May 2019].Recipes for chemical test reagents. Available from: https://link.springer.com/content/pdf/bbm%3A978-1-4615-5809-5%2F1.pdf [Accessed 6 May 2019].

[30] International Council for Harmonisation of technical requirements for pharmaceuticals for human use. Impurities: guideline for residual solvents Q3C(R6); Current *Step 4* Version (2016). https://www.ich.org/fileadmin/Public_Web_Site/ICH_Products/Guidelines/Quality/Q3C/Q3C__R6___Step_4.pdf [Accessed 6 May 2019].International Council for Harmonisation of technical requirements for pharmaceuticals for human use. Impurities: guideline for residual solvents Q3C(R6); Current *Step 4* Version (2016). https://www.ich.org/fileadmin/Public_Web_Site/ICH_Products/Guidelines/Quality/Q3C/Q3C__R6___Step_4.pdf [Accessed 6 May 2019].

[31] Van Wyk B-E, Wink M. Medicinal plants of the world. Pretoria, South Africa: Briza Publications; 2004. pp. 7–26, 313, 356, 364, 367, 428.

[32] Gericke N, Albrecht CF, Van Wyk B, Mayeng B, Mutwa C, Hutchings A. Sutherlandia frutescens. Aust J Med Herb 2001;13:9–15.

[33] van Wyk B-E, Albrecht C. A review of the taxonomy, ethnobotany, chemistry and pharmacology of *Sutherlandia frutescens* (Fabaceae). J Ethnopharmacol 2008;119:620–9.

[34] Van Wyk BE, Gericke N. In: Smit J, editor. People's plants: A guide to useful plants of southern Africa. Pretoria, South Africa: Briza Publications; 2000. p. 139–54.

[35] Avula B, Wang Y-H, Smillie TJ, Fu X, Li XC, Mabusela W, Syce J, Johnson Q, Folk W, Khan IA. Quantitative determination of flavonoids and cycloartanol glycosides from aerial parts of *Sutherlandia frutescens* (L.) R. BR. by using LCUV/ELSD methods and confirmation by using LC-MS method. J Pharm Biomed Anal 2010;52:173–80.

[36] Fu X, Li X-C, Wang Y-H, Avula B, Smillie TJ, Mabusela W, Syce J, Johnson Q, Folk W, Khan IA. Flavonol glycosides from the South African medicinal plant *Sutherlandia frutescens*. Planta Med 2010;76:178–81.

[37] Prevoo D, Swart P, Swart AC. The influence of *Sutherlandia frutescens* adrenal steroidogenic cytochrome P450 enzymes. J Ethnopharmacol 2007;118(1):118–26.

[38] Mabusa IH, Howard R, Masoko P. *Sutherlandia frutescens* (Fabaceae) extracts used for treating tuberculosis do not have high activity against *Mycobacterium smegmatis*. Suid-Afrikaanse Tydskrif vir Natuurwetenskapen Tegnologie 2017;36(1):a1486.

[39] Müller AC, Patnala S, Kis O, Bendayan R, Kanfer I. Effects of extracts and phytochemical components of *Sutherlandia frutescens* on the absorption and metabolism of the antiretroviral, atazanavir, in-vitro. J Pharm Pharmaceut Sci 2012;15(1):221–33.
[40] Kasilo OMJ, Trapsida JM. Decade of African traditional medicine, 2001–2010. Afr Health Monitor (Special Issue) 2011;14:25–31.

Chapter 7

Regulations for the use of herbal remedies

Isadore Kanfer[1] and Srinivas Patnala

Faculty of Pharmacy, Rhodes University, Grahamstown, South Africa

1 Introduction

Herbal remedies used as traditional medicine are currently considered as components of complementary or alternative medicines (CAMs). Depending on their use and nature of treatment, these are sometimes referred to as natural medicines, nonconventional medicines, or holistic medicines. These medications, in whichever form they are intended and used, have always maintained good popularity worldwide. Over the last decade, there has been a remarkable increase in the use of herbal medicines in many developed and developing countries. In some countries such as China and India, such medicines, mostly touted as traditional medicines or herbal medicines, can be prescribed by doctors but are only recommended as dietary supplements in certain other countries, such as in the United States [1].

The major difference between orthodox medicine and herbal medicines is that in the former case, mainly synthetic compounds are used, whereas in the latter instance, such products are mainly composed of naturally occurring biosynthesized complex compounds and their associated chemistries. Although the main compound(s) in herbal medicines may be identified, other components are generally left unidentified and any related pharmacological implications are usually unknown [2]. Furthermore, since a particular compound may commonly exist in a number of different species, especially those of the same genus, other similar components present in those different species may result in unwanted consequences if the correct species was not used to provide only the requisite particular compound [3]. Therefore, implementing a system of identification and chemical analysis to establish quality control (QC) systems for herbal extracts is not adequate since the current requirements to establish relevant quality criteria should include bioinformatics as well [4]. Currently, either most herbal extracts are sold as dried powders or the same plant may be extracted using a solvent and then formulated using the extract. However, often, many specific reference standards/markers for analysis of such herbal products may be unavailable resulting in challenging efforts to set specifications. As a result, the quality standards or specifications are arbitrarily self-established by manufacturers [5].

2 Classification of herbal medicines

The Guidelines for the regulation of herbal medicines in the South-East Asian Region [6] prescribes, for practical purposes, as follows: "…..*herbal medicines* are *classified into four categories, based on their origin, evolution and the forms of current usage. While these are not always mutually exclusive, these categories have sufficient distinguishing features for a constructive examination of the ways in which safety, efficacy and quality can be determined and improved.*"

This guideline provides the following definitions:

Category 1: Indigenous herbal medicines.

This category of herbal medicines is historically used in a local community or region and is very well known through long use by the local population in terms of its composition, treatment, and dosage. Detailed information on this category of TM, which also includes folk medicines, may or may not be available. It can be used freely by the local community or in the local region. However, if the medicines in this category enter the market or go beyond the local community or region in the country, they must meet the requirements of safety and efficacy laid down in the national regulations for herbal medicines.

Category 2: Herbal medicines in systems.

Medicines in this category have been used for a long time and are documented with their special theories and concepts, and accepted by the countries. For example, disciplines such as Ayurveda, Unani, and Siddha would fall into this category of TM.

Category 3: Modified herbal medicines.

---

1 Current Address: Leslie Dan Faculty of Pharmacy, University of Toronto, Canada.

Herbal Medicine in Andrology. https://doi.org/10.1016/B978-0-12-815565-3.00007-2

These are herbal medicines as described above in categories 1 and 2, except that they have been modified in some way—either shape, or form including dose, dosage form, mode of administration, herbal medicinal ingredients, methods of preparation, and medical indications. They have to meet the national regulatory requirements of safety and efficacy of herbal medicines.

Category 4: Imported products with an herbal medicine base.

This category covers all imported herbal medicines including raw materials and products. Imported herbal medicines must be registered and marketed in the countries of origin. The safety and efficacy data have to be submitted to the national authority of the importing country and need to meet the requirements of safety and efficacy of regulation of herbal medicines in the recipient country.

The classification of herbal medicines, however, may differ in various different global jurisdictions. For example, in South Africa [7] herbal medicines are included as a complementary medicine where:

"Complementary medicine" means any substance or mixture of substances that

(a) *originates from plants, fungi, algae, seaweeds, lichens, minerals, animals or other substance as determined by Council, and*

(b) *is used or purporting to be suitable for use or manufactured or sold for use (i) in maintaining, complementing, or assisting the innate healing power or physical or mental state, or (ii) to diagnose, treat, mitigate, modify, alleviate or prevent disease or illness or the symptoms or signs thereof or abnormal physical or mental state, of a human being or animal, and*

(c) *is used(i) as a health supplement, or (ii) in accordance with those disciplines as determined by the regulatory authority*

In 2005 in the United States, CAMs was defined as—*"a group of diverse medical and health care systems, practices, and products that are not presently considered to be part of conventional medicine"* [8]. Subsequently, the words complementary, alternative, and integrative are now used [9]. The FDA regulates dietary supplements under a different set of regulations than those covering *"conventional"* foods and drug products. Under the Dietary Supplement Health and Education Act (DSHEA) of 1994 and the Federal Food, Drug, and Cosmetic Act a dietary ingredient is defined as *"a vitamin; mineral; herb or other botanical; amino acid; dietary substance for use by man to supplement the diet by increasing the total dietary intake; or a concentrate, metabolite, constituent, extract, or combination of the preceding substances"* [10].

In Europe, the EU Directive defines phytomedicines under the following headings [11]:

- *"Herbal medicinal products: any medicinal product, exclusively containing as active ingredients one or more herbal substances or one or more herbal preparations, or one or more such herbal substances in combination with one or more such herbal preparations"*
- *"Herbal substances: all mainly whole, fragmented or cut plants, plant parts, algae, fungi, lichen in an unprocessed, usually dried form but sometimes fresh. Certain exudates that have not been subjected to a specific treatment are also considered to be herbal substances. Herbal substances are precisely defined by the plant part used and the botanical name according to the binomial system (genus, species, variety and author)."*
- *"Herbal preparations: preparations obtained by subjecting herbal substances to treatments such as extraction, distillation, expression, fractionation, purification, concentration or fermentation. These include comminuted or powdered herbal substances, tinctures, extracts, essential oils, expressed juices and processed exudates."*

The WHO, in its recent report on Traditional and Complementary Medicine 2019 [12], includes the following definition of herbal medicines:

"Herbal medicines include herbs, herbal materials, herbal preparations and finished herbal products that contain, as active ingredients, parts of plants, other plant materials or combinations thereof. In some countries, herbal medicines may contain, by tradition, natural organic or inorganic active ingredients that are not of plant origin (e.g. animal and mineral materials)."

The above examples and apparent variations in description, categorization, and classification of phytomedicines, botanicals, and/or herbal drugs, clearly indicate a farrago of information available for manufacturers, users, and practitioners.

3   Standardization of herbal extracts

The quality of herbal medicines is a major concern worldwide. Lucrative markets for herbal medicines are fueled by heightened consumer interest. The major factor(s) that hamper herbal medicines from fully utilizing its intended therapeutic potential are:

- First, the fundamental disconnect between the description of traditional use and the modern pharmacological mechanisms of drug disposition.
- Second, issues with QC of raw materials and the production process of herbal extracts, thereby resulting in inconsistent batch-to-batch quality.

Additionally, one more major concern is the issue of controlling toxic contaminants that may be inherent or added during the collection and/or manufacturing process [13]. These factor(s), indeed, raise major safety concerns that are either being studied or not fully understood [14]. Although quality testing by utilizing a specific marker or various components is one parameter that provides a rough estimate to standardize herbal preparations, it is not a clear indication of product consistency and safety. Herbal preparations are not governed by the same safety criteria as prescription and over-the-counter (OTC) products. Absence of QC requirements for potency and purity as well as lenient labeling standards results in standards and quality of herbal medicines not being maintained. Product integrity is not established because of lack of safety testing and purity between batches and manufacturers. The amount of active ingredient can vary greatly between brands and some may not even contain the assumed active ingredients [3].

3.1 Adulteration and contamination of herbal medicines

Quality, safety, and efficacy (QSE) issues relating to herbal medicines are not only due to the lack of testing procedures but also, since being "natural," they are mistakenly presumed to be safe and can be consumed with or without proper medical advice. There are several reports regarding herbal products being contaminated or spiked with synthetic drugs [15] and with heavy metals such as lead, mercury, cadmium, thallium, and arsenic [16]. The other adulterants could be due to contamination with pesticides and/or microbial growth due to improper storage and processing [13]. It is also reported that misidentification of certain plants, such as *Digitalis purpurea*, *Atropa belladonna*, and *Scutellaria lateriflora*, have had serious medical implications [17]. Substitution of herbal medicines with cheaper plants of unknown potency can also lead to substandard products [18].

A publication issued by the European Medicines Agency (EMA) on markers used for quantitative and qualitative analysis of herbal and traditional medicinal products [5] clearly indicates the problem by identifying the issues with respect to substances in herbal products that are in two forms. One group of substances is defined as *"constituents with known therapeutic activity"* and the other as *"active/analytical markers"* that are solely used for identification and quantification. This paper [5] suggests the following problems relating to the selection and quality requirements for markers:

- *"It is not always clear which constituents are characteristic of the herbal substance or characteristic constituents can be present in very low amounts.*
- *Markers can be unstable or difficult to define chemically.*
- *Markers are not always single compounds."*

Hence, specific monographs need to be developed to ensure that QSE issues are addressed adequately and to provide the intended therapeutic activity if the indications are only due to the natural constituents of the herbal product.

4 Regulatory challenges of herbal medicines

Differences in quality, variation between batches, and current lenient/flexible regulatory control on herbal medicines exert pressure on consumers to take onus regarding the purchase and use of herbal medicines [19]. As discussed in the previous section, among the most common problems with the use of herbal medicines are adulteration, substitution, contamination, misidentification, lack of standardization, nonadherence to GMPs and inappropriate labeling [13]. Substitution or adulteration with other herbs or synthetic medicines done intentionally or erroneously is also quite prevalent [18]. A direct consequence of the lack of an enforceable regulatory system on the practitioners and formulators of herbal medicines results in the use of such remedies not being bound by labeling requirements. Hence, the regulatory challenges of requiring claims of content and the QSE of herbal remedies are often not satisfied.

In 1991, the WHO developed a policy of traditional medicine in collaboration with its member states in the review of national policies, legislation, and decisions on the nature and extent of the use of traditional medicine in their health systems. It also notes that there are differences that exist between its member states, in defining and categorizing herbal medicines. Depending on the regulations that apply to foods and medicines in each specific country, a medicinal plant may be defined as a food, a dietary supplement, or an herbal medicine. This situation makes it difficult to define the concept of herbal medicines for the purpose of national drug regulations, which also confuses patients and consumers [20].

The main objective of the WHO is to facilitate the integration of traditional medicine into national health-care systems, to promote the rational use of traditional medicine through the development of technical guidelines for international standards of herbal medicines and related therapies and to provide information on various forms of traditional medicine. The guidelines developed in this regard define the basic criteria for the evaluation of safety, efficacy, and quality of herbal medicines to assist in developing documentation for national regulatory authorities and manufacturers. Accordingly, the

World Health Assembly adopted a resolution in May 2003 [20] on traditional medicine. The resolution requested the WHO to support member states by providing internationally acceptable guidelines and technical standards and also evidence-based information to assist member states in formulating policy and regulations to control the QSE of traditional medicines.

The recent 2019 report on Traditional and Complementary medicines (T&CM) released by the WHO indicates a substantial improvement of regulations and implementation among its member states and 109 of them reported the inclusion of a legal or regulatory framework for T&CM [12].

4.1 Regulations for herbal medicines

4.1.1 World Health Organization (WHO)

The WHO defines the regulation of herbal medicines as "a principle, rule or law designed to control or govern manufacturers and producers of herbal medicines" and proposes that "regulations should state that herbal medicines must have been proven to be safe, effective and of good quality [12]."

Interestingly, based on their survey, the WHO report also indicates several descriptions for regulatory categories for herbal medicines: *prescription medicines, nonprescription medicines (includes OTC/self-medication), dietary supplements and health foods (includes functional foods), and general food products.* Based on these descriptions the regulatory claims made about herbal medicines include *"medical claims; health claims; nutrient content claims"* [12].

4.2 Regulatory requirements for herbal medicines—Some selected countries

4.2.1 Australia

In Australia, medicinal products containing ingredients such as herbs, vitamins, minerals, nutritional supplements, homeopathic, and certain aromatherapy preparations are referred to as "complementary medicines" and are regulated as medicines under the Therapeutic Goods Act 1989 (the Act) [21]. The Australian regulatory guidelines for complementary medicines (ARGCM), Version 8.0, April 2018, defines herbal medicines under types of complementary medicines, viz.:

"Herbal medicines are therapeutic goods that are, or contain as the major active ingredient(s), herbal substances. Herbal substances are preparations of plants, and other organisms that are treated as plants in the International Code of Botanical Nomenclature, such as fungi, algae and yeast."

The ARGCM provides detailed guidance for the regulation of complementary medicines in Part A of the guidance [22]. Australia has a risk-based approach with a two-tiered system for the regulation of all medicines, including complementary medicines, i.e., A Listing System and a Registration System, viz.:

- Lower risk medicines can be **listed** on the Australian Register of Therapeutic Goods (ARTG).
- Higher risk medicines must be **registered** on the ARTG.

The listed medicines should comply with the following:

- *can only contain certain low-risk ingredients in acceptable amounts that are permitted for use in listed medicines by the TGA;*
- *must be manufactured in accordance with the principles of Good Manufacturing Practice (GMP); and*
- *can only make indications (for therapeutic use) for health maintenance and health enhancement or certain indications for nonserious, self-limiting conditions.*

When submitting a **Listed medicine** application, the sponsor must certify that the goods in the application meet all of the legislative requirements of Section 26A (Part 3-2, Division 2) of the Therapeutic Goods Act 1989 (the Act) [21]. Medicines listed on the ARTG are assigned a unique AUST L number, which must be displayed on the medicine label [23].

Registration of complementary medicines is required when such CMs *"are considered to be of relatively higher risk than listed medicines, based on their ingredients or the indications made for the medicine."* Registered medicines are fully evaluated by the TGA for QSE before being accepted on the Australian Register of Therapeutic Goods (ARTG) and obtaining permission for marketing. Medicines registered on the ARTG are assigned a unique AUST R number, which must be displayed on the medicine label [24].

4.2.2 Brazil

In Brazil, the current guidelines for herbal medicine registration is provided in the Ministério daSaúde Agência Nacional de Vigilância Sanitária, Resolution of The Board of Directors—RDC No. 26, of May 13, 2014 [25]. Under Section I,

Objective, Art. 1, *"Resolution defines the categories of herbal medicine and traditional herbal medicine and establishes the minimum requirements for the registration and registration of herbal medicine, and for registration, renewal of registration and notification of traditional herbal product."* The *"Scope of Article 2"* continues as follows: *"Resolution applies to industrialized products that fall under the categories of herbal medicines and traditional herbal products."* The Resolution describes various definitions under

- Paragraph 1: *"Medicinal products considered as herbal medicines of plant active raw materials whose safety and clinical evidences and that are characterized by the constancy of their quality."*
- Paragraph 2: *"Traditional herbal products are those obtained with employment of active plant raw materials whose safety and effectiveness are based on the in safe and effective use data published in the technical-scientific literature and that are designed to be used without the supervision of a doctor for diagnostic purposes, prescription or monitoring."*
- Paragraph 5:*"Herbal medicinal products may be registered, and the products traditional herbal medicines are subject to registration or notification."*

The National Policy on Medicinal Plants and Herbal Medicines (PNPMF) further differentiates herbal medicine (HM) and traditional herbal preparation (THP) where the registration of HMs [26] have to include data on safety and efficacy based on nonclinical and clinical data, whereas submission of a THP has to provide data to prove safe human use for a period of at least 30 years for minor indications. Quality control criteria, however, are similar for both HM and THP [27].

A report by Carvalho et al. indicates that *"ANVISA recognizes, within those herbal medicines with the greatest number of scientific studies, the "List of simplified registration of herbal medicines" containing 34 (thirty four), the majority of exotic species, allowed to obtain the simplified registration by industry"*; there is no need to validate the therapeutic indications and safety of use. If the herbal medicine does not incorporate the *"list of simplified registration of herbal medicines"* to obtain registration and renewal, the company must petition with ANVISA, a dossier with technical and administrative product information according to specific regulations [28].

4.2.3 Canada

In Canada, Natural Health Products (NHP) are regulated by the Natural Health Products Directorate (NHPD) under a Canada Gazette for NHP regulations as per the Food and Drugs Act [29]. These regulations apply to the sale, manufacture, packaging, labeling, importation, distribution, and storage of natural products in Canada. In accordance with the annexed Natural Health Products Regulations [30] *"a natural health product means a substance or a combination of substances in which all the medicinal ingredients are, a homeopathic medicine or a traditional medicine, that is manufactured, sold or represented for use in*

(a) *the diagnosis, treatment, mitigation or prevention of a disease, disorder or abnormal physical state or its symptoms in humans;*
(b) *restoring or correcting organic functions in humans; or*
(c) *modifying organic functions in humans, such as modifying those functions in a manner that maintains or promotes health."*

The sale of natural products requires a product license based on the following submitted information for each medicinal ingredient contained in the product:

(i) *its proper name and its common name;*
(ii) *its quantity per dosage unit;*
(iii) *its potency, if a representation relating to its potency is to be shown on any label of the natural health product;*
(iv) *a description of its source material and.*
(v) *a statement indicating whether it is synthetically manufactured;*

(d) *a qualitative list of the nonmedicinal ingredients that are proposed for the natural health product and for each ingredient listed, a statement that indicates the purpose of the ingredient;*
(e) *each brand name under which the natural health product is proposed to be sold;*
(f) *the recommended conditions of use for the natural health product;*
(g) *information that demonstrates the safety and efficacy of the natural health product when it is used in accordance with the recommended conditions of use;*
(h) *the text of each label, that is, proposed to be used in conjunction with the natural health product;*
(i) *a copy of the specifications to which the natural health product will comply;* and

Part 3 of the regulations require that natural health products comply with Good Manufacturing Practices (GMPs). The following specifications are required:

(a) *"detailed information respecting the purity of the natural health product, including statements indicating its purity tolerances;*
(b) *for each medicinal ingredient of the natural health product, detailed information respecting its quantity per dosage unit and its identity, including statements indicating its quantity and identity tolerances;*
(c) *if a representation relating to the potency of a medicinal ingredient is to be shown on a label of the natural health product, detailed information respecting the potency of the medicinal ingredient, including statements indicating its potency tolerances; and*
(d) *a description of the methods used for testing or examining the natural health product."*

Importantly, *Section 103.3 of the regulations specifies that a natural health product cannot be sold as a treatment or cure, for any of the diseases, disorders or abnormal physical states referred to in Schedule A (Section 3) to the Act* [29].

4.2.4 Chile

In Chile, there is a list of traditional herbal medicines containing 103 different plant species provided in Resolution No. 548, which are exempt from formal registration, as published in the Official Gazette of 08.09.09. Through the Supreme Decree No. 286/2001, published in the Official Gazette on 02/18/02 and officially introduced in the Regulation of the National System of Control of Pharmaceutical Products [31], phytodrugs or herbal medicines *"are finished and labeled pharmaceutical products, whose principles assets are exclusively plant drugs or plant preparations."* A second category relates to plants or parts of plants used in Chilean cultural traditions that meet the following requirements:

- *"must be in a list approved by resolution of the Ministry of Health, issued in use of its power's legal technical regulations;*
- *be hand-packed as isolated plant species, not mixed, and consign in their labels only those properties recognized in the aforementioned resolution."*

From these provisions, it is understood that the Chilean authority has initiated the normalization of the rational use of medicinal plants and industrially produced pharmaceutical specialty (phytopharmaceutical), as well as its popular rustic use (traditional herbal medicine).

4.2.5 China

The following is an excerpt from the WHO report [12]:

"In the People's Republic of China, herbal products are categorized as prescription medicines, non-prescription medicines, health foods and general food products. Traditional Chinese medicines (TCMs) are sold with medical claims. The drug administration law (revised in 2001) provides the national regulatory system on traditional Chinese medicines and natural medicines (herbal medicines). Regulatory requirements for herbal medicines include adherence to information contained in pharmacopoeias and monographs and the same GMP rules that apply to conventional pharmaceuticals. The selection criteria for herbal medicines is based on traditional use, clinical data and long-term historical use."

4.2.6 Egypt

The 2015 Egyptian guidelines [32] provide information for the registration of herbal medicines. The guideline describes herbal medicines as follows: *"medicinal products that contain active ingredients aerial or underground parts of plants, or other plant materials, or combinations thereof, whether in the crude state or as plant preparations."* Definitions include the following:

- Herbal medicines: *"Any finished, labeled medicinal product (for oral, external or inhalation uses), exclusively containing as active substances one or more herbal substances or one or more herbal preparations, or one or more such herbal substances in combination with one or more such herbal preparations; Herbal medicines may contain conventional excipients in addition to the plant-based active ingredients. In some cases, they may also contain, by tradition, natural organic or inorganic ingredients that are not of plant origin. However, products to which chemically defined active substances have been added, including for example, synthetic compounds and/or isolated constituents from herbal materials, are not considered to be herbal medicinal products."*
- Herbal substances: *"All mainly whole, fragmented or cut plants, plant parts, algae, fungi, lichen in an unprocessed, usually dried, form, but sometimes fresh. Certain exudates that have not been subjected to a specific treatment are also*

considered herbal substances. Herbal substances are precisely defined by the plant part used and the botanical name according to the binomial system (genus, species, variety and author)."

- Herbal preparations: *"They are obtained by subjecting herbal substances to treatments such as extraction, distillation, expression, fractionation, purification, concentration or fermentation. These include comminuted or powdered herbal substances, tinctures, extracts, essential oils, expressed juices and processed exudates."*

Safety requirements are considered in three categories, viz.,

Category 1: *safety established by use over long time (more than 30 years in Egypt).*
Category 2: *safe under specific conditions of use (such herbal medicines should be covered by well-established documentation).*
Category 3: *herbal medicines of uncertain safety (the safety data required for this class of drugs will be identical to that of any new substance). Furthermore, "acute toxicity and long-term toxicity data may also be necessary on the following: Organ-targeted toxicity; Immunotoxicity; Embryo/fetal and prenatal toxicity; Mutagenicity/genotoxicity; Carcinogenicity" and are required for submission.*

4.2.7   European Union

The EU member countries include Austria (AT), Belgium (BE), Cyprus (CY); Czech Republic (CZ), Denmark (DK), Germany (DE), Estonia (EE), Spain (ES), Finland (FI), France (FR), Greece (GR), Hungary (HU), Ireland (IE), Iceland (IS), Italy (IT), Lithuania (LT), Luxembourg (LU), Latvia (LV), Malta (MT), Netherlands (NL), Norway (NO), Poland (PL), Portugal (PT), Sweden (SE), Slovenia (SI); Slovakia (SK), United Kingdom (UK), Croatia (HR)*, Romania (RO)*, and Bulgaria (BG)* (*Candidate Member State Dir: Directive 2004/24/EC).

In 2004, the EU issued a Directive (2004/24/EU) [33] regarding traditional herbal medicinal products as follows:

"to provide a high level of health protection and consumer access to medicines of their choice, and also provide QSE of such products. In their efforts to ensure a single market, the EMEA introduced new legislation and procedures for traditional herbal medicines, which also encourages trade between member states. According to the directive, herbal preparations are expected to meet the quality requirements similar to medicines approved officially."

Current regulations according to the amended *Directive 2004/24/EC*, a new pathway for marketing traditional herbal medicinal products was introduced as follows: *"simplified registration" and lays down specific provisions applicable to traditional herbal medicinal products*. These are introduced in Chapter 2a in Title III of Directive 2001/83/EC1 as amended by Directive 2004/24/EC [11]. The legal basis for the simplified registration procedure is laid down in Article *16a of Directive 2001/83/EC as amended* [34]. It further states that *"Only traditionally used herbal medicinal products are eligible for this procedure and only if certain criteria are fulfilled*, viz.:

"In order to obtain traditional-use registration, the applicant shall submit an application to the competent authority of the Member State concerned. The registration is a national procedure and there are no provisions for a centralized registration procedure. However, mutual recognition and decentralized procedures for traditional-use registration will be applicable as long as a Community herbal monograph or Community list entry has been established. The Member State, where the application for traditional-use registration has been submitted, can request the HMPC to draw up an opinion on the adequacy of the evidence of the long-standing use of the product, or of the corresponding product. For further information on this and other referral procedures involving the HMPC, cf. Section II.7." Further requirements on safety and efficacy under Traditional use registration Article 16a (1) of the directive 2001/83/EC in a publication entitled *"Questions & Answers on the EU framework for (traditional) herbal medicinal products, including those from a 'non-European' tradition"* includes the following [34]:

- *"No clinical tests and trials on safety and efficacy are required as long as sufficient safety data and plausible efficacy are demonstrated.*
- *Involves assessment of mostly bibliographic safety and efficacy data.*
- *Must have been used for at least 30 years, including at least 15 years within the EU.*
- *Are intended to be used without the supervision of a medical practitioner and are not administered by injection."*

The Committee on Herbal Products (HMPC) Directive 2003/63/EC (Annex I; CTD criteria) requires submission of the dossier in accordance with the presentation and format requirements of a Common Technical Document (CTD) [35] for traditional herbal medicinal products. This document is a revision of pharmaceutical legislation for a simplified registration procedure for traditional herbal medicinal products and refers to the data requirements for such applications as follows:

"In order to streamline the legislative provisions on the data requirements, it recommends the introduction of explanatory notes in the existing CTD format for submission of applications for registrations. The anticipated impact of this guideline is to improve the understanding on how applications for traditional herbal medicinal products should be presented. This is expected to help reduce problems with assessment of applications, the resources needed and also facilitate the reduction of the inconsistencies in expectations of the designated authorities with respect to documentation." [35]. It should be noted that apart from the above EU regulations, some countries such as Germany, Ireland, and the United Kingdom, for instance, include additional requirements based on their domestic regulatory jurisdictions.

4.2.8 Germany

CAM and Traditional Medicinal Products are described under German Medicines Act or Arzneimittelgesetz (AMG). According to § 109a AMG, traditional medicinal products *"may also include medicinal products which do not belong to the so-called "particular therapeutic systems"* [36]. AMG—Division 4 peruses the scientific evaluation pertaining to efficacy, safety, and pharmaceutical quality of such products relevant to particular therapeutic systems and of traditional medicinal products. Division 4 is further responsible for the preparation and assessment in conjunction with the administrative work that includes issuing of marketing authorization. Additionally, *"the Division 4 develops scientific principles and guidelines relating to the evaluation of medicinal products of the particular therapeutic systems and traditional medicinal products. Members of Division 4 participate in national and international expert committees (e.g. Herbal Medicinal Products Committee (HMPC) of the European Medicines Agency (EMA), Homeopathic Medicinal Products Working Group (HMPWG) of the EU Heads of Agencies) and are thus essentially involved in transferring current scientific knowledge into European and WHO guidelines"* [36].

Regulatory requirements for the manufacture of herbal medicines include adherence to EU requirements and also to the information in relevant pharmacopeias and, in the absence of pharmacopeias, monographs, other monographs, the GMP rules for conventional pharmaceuticals and special GMP rules, the German Medicines Act, and Eudralex (the European Union rules relating to medicinal products) [11].

4.2.9 India

Regulations for herbal medicines were updated in 2017, by the Ministry of Ayurveda, Yoga and Naturopathy, Unani, Siddha, and Homeopathy (AYUSH) that falls under the Drug and Cosmetic Act (D and C) 1940 and Rules 1945 in India [37]. Herbal medicines are also included under Schedule E of the Drugs and Cosmetics Rules. Good Manufacturing Practice (GMP) has also been implemented through schedule "T" in 2016. The regulatory provisions for Ayurveda, Unani, and Siddha (ASU) medicine are clearly laid down in Chapter IV-A, which includes a list of 18 sections (33C to 33O). The Regulation of manufacture for sale of medicines in the disciplines of Ayurvedic, Siddha, and Unani drugs is discussed under Section 33EEB [38].

4.2.10 Ireland

The Guide to Traditional Herbal Medicinal Products by Health Products Regulatory Authority in Ireland (HPRA)—AUT-G0029, dated October 2018 [39], provides registration information according to the Directive 2004/24/EC, which was transposed into Irish law with the implementation of the Medicinal Products (Control of Placing on the Market) Regulations 2007 (S.I. No. 540 of 2007) on July 23, 2007. The intention of such legislation is to provide an appropriate legal framework for marketing traditional herbal medicinal products (THMPs) within the EU that involves a "simplified" registration procedure as described in the EU regulations [11]. In 2007, the Department of Health and Children designated the HPRA as the competent authority for the implementation of this legislation; on the basis of this, the traditional herbal medicinal products registration scheme was established. Accordingly, an applicant can apply for a certificate of traditional-use registration for their THMP, and a THMP registration is known as a traditional-use registration, where each registered THMP is allocated a TR number. Hence, all THMPs currently on the market in Ireland must be registered with the HPRA and have a TR number. In terms of the Irish requirements for herbal medicines, all traditional herbal medicinal products, as defined in Article 16(a)(1) of Directive 2004/24/EC [33] and the scientific guidelines for human medicinal products and specific herbal guidelines published by the EMA, are available on their website [40].

4.2.11 Japan

In Japan [41], two categories of traditional herbal medicines coexist, namely, *Kampo* and *non-Kampo* products. The *Kampo* products are based on *Kampo* medicinal principles and *non-Kampo* products comprise one or more crude drugs based on folk medicines.

In general, the regulation of herbal medicines (indicated as Western traditional herbal medicines) requires submission of an application that includes the following:

- Origin of discovery, conditions of use in foreign countries, therapeutic indication, and relevant information
- Manufacturing process—chemistry, standards, and testing methods
- Stability—long-term and accelerated stability studies
- Pharmacology—primary and secondary pharmacodynamics and related actions; safety
- Absorption, distribution, metabolism, and excretion profile
- Toxicological studies that includes single/multiple dose studies, genotoxicity, carcinogenicity, and reproductive toxicity
- Clinical studies that are scientifically designed

4.2.12 New Zealand

Dietary supplements are regulated under the Dietary Supplements Regulations [42] of the Food Act 2014 [43] and Medsafe published under New Zealand Medicines and Medical Devices Safety Authority [44] is the body for administering the dietary supplement regulations. Accordingly, the following describes products containing herbs, which are categorized under 2A of the Act.

"Dietary supplements must comply with the Dietary Supplements Regulations that describe a number of requirements including, but not limited to, labeling and maximum permitted daily doses for several vitamins and minerals. There is no preapproval process for dietary supplements and it remains the responsibility of the sponsor (the person legally responsible for placing the product on the market) to ensure that such products are manufactured to an acceptable quality, is safe to use and complies with the law."

The New Zealand requirements state the following [42]:

"Dietary supplements cannot:

- *contain controlled drugs—dietary supplements cannot contain ingredients scheduled as controlled drugs under the Misuse of Drugs Act 1975*
- *contain substances listed in the First Schedule to the Medicines Regulations 1984—dietary supplements cannot contain ingredients that are scheduled as prescription medicines, restricted (pharmacist-only) medicines or pharmacy-only medicines under the Medicines Act 1981*
- *have a stated or implied therapeutic purpose—the definition of a therapeutic purpose is given in the Medicines Act 1981."*

4.2.13 Nigeria

In Nigeria, the trade of herbal products is regulated by the National Agency for Food and Drug Administration and Control (NAFDAC) [45]. The 2019 Regulations classify such products as *Herbal Medicines and Related Products* as follows:

"(a) finished medicinal product containing plant and their preparation presented with therapeutic or prophylactic claim and includes all preparations containing a plant material in part or wholly. (b) preparation or admixture of herbal medicinal products presented with prophylactic or therapeutic claim; and (c) preparation or admixture used for restoring, correcting or modifying organic functions in man or in animal."

Regulatory requirements for herbal medicines require adherence to the following controls:

- Methods used and facilities and controls for the manufacture, processing, and packing of herbal medicines must ensure identity, strength, quality, and purity.
- An appropriate laboratory report must be provided.
- Acceptable GMP requirements and appropriate product handling.

4.2.14 Russia

Herbal medicine preparations (HMP) are handled as official medicines in Russia. A summary of the quality control and standardization requirements are provided in an abstract published in Planta Medica in 2012 [46]. In that publication, an HMP is considered as the finished product and is classified into the following categories:

- *medicinal plant material*
- *galenic formulations*

- *novo-galenic formulations*
- *active pharmaceutical ingredients and combined phyto-preparations.*

The regulatory control of HMPs include the following requirements:

- *safety and efficacy and approval of permission for clinical trials*
- *description of proposed methods for quality control of the drug and the quality of the drug samples*
- *evaluation of the relationship between expected benefit and possible risk of drug application after its clinical study.*

In accordance with the Russian State Duma of April 12, 2010 №. 61-FZ [47] relating to *"On Circulation of Medicines,"* Chapter 1. General Provisions, Article 4 (Basic terms 13 and 14 used in this Federal Law) provides the following definitions:

- *herbal medicinal raw material is fresh or dried plants or parts thereof used for manufacturing of medicines by institutions producing medicines, or for compounding of medicinal products by pharmacy institutions, veterinary pharmacy institutions, and individual entrepreneurs holding pharmaceutical licenses;*
- *herbal medicinal product is a medicinal product manufactured or compounded of one type of herbal medicinal raw material or several types of such raw materials and being distributed as packed in the secondary (retail) packaging.*

4.2.15 South Africa

In SA, currently six major disciplines have been identified and preparations associated therewith, namely, Homeopathy, Western Herbal Medicine, Traditional Chinese Medicine, Ayurveda, Unani Medicine (Unani-Tibb), and Aromatherapy. Evidence required to substantiate the claims made for products falling under any of the above is divided into high-risk or low-risk categories [7].

Registration requirements for such products include provision of bibliographical evidence or expert evidence to the effect that the medicinal product in question, or its ingredients or a corresponding product, has a history of traditional medicinal use within the Republic of South Africa or within a particular country.

The following definition of complementary medicine (CM) in South Africa is provided by the SAHPRA (South African Health Products Regulatory Authority), formerly the Medicines Control Council (MCC) [7].

Complementary medicine means "any substance or mixture of substances that

(a) originates from plants, fungi, algae, seaweeds, lichens, minerals, animals, or other substances as determined by Council, and

(b) is used or purporting to be suitable for use or manufactured or sold for use: (i) in maintaining, complementing, or assisting the innate healing power or physical or mental state, or (ii) to diagnose, treat, mitigate, modify, alleviate or prevent disease or illness or the symptoms or signs thereof or abnormal physical or mental state, of a human being or animal, and (c) is used as a health supplement."

A **Health supplement** means "any substance, extract or mixture of substances that may supplement the diet, have a nutritional physiological effect or include pre- and probiotics and are sold in pharmaceutical dosage forms not usually associated with a foodstuff and excludes injectables or substances schedule 1 or higher."

In the case of herbal remedies, "A herbal substance/preparation in any discipline, means all or part of a plant, fungus, alga, seaweed or lichen, or other substance:

(a) that is obtained only by drying, crushing, distilling, freezing, fermentation, lyophilisation, extracting, expressing, comminuting, mixing with an inert diluent substance or another herbal substance or mixing with water, ethanol, glycerol, oil or aqueous ethanol; or other permitted solvents; with or without the addition of heat;

(b) that is not subjected to any other treatment or process other than a treatment or process that is necessary for its presentation in a pharmaceutical form, and

(c) where part of a plant, fungus, seaweed or lichen refers to a structure such as a root, root bark, rhizome, mycelium, fruiting body, bulb, corm, tuber, stem, inner, or outer bark, wood, meristematic tissue, shoot, bud, thallus, resin, oleoresin, gum, natural exudate or secretion, gall, leaf, frond, flower (or its parts), inflorescence, pollen, fruit, seed, cone, spores or other whole plant part, and

(d) that does not include:

    (i) a pure chemical or isolated constituent unless the isolated herbal constituent is formulated with the herbal substance from which it arises and is demonstrated to have "essentially the same" 3 action as the whole herbal substance, or

    (ii) a substance of mineral, animal or bacterial origin."

For all CMs, the following QSE information is required.

Quality

Registration of a CM, including herbal preparations requires the demonstration of the quality of the product, including the identity, impurities, and stability of the ingredients and details of the quality control measures as well as information on the manufacturing processes and standards of good manufacturing practice (GMP). In addition, stability data are required to determine a shelf life for the product.

The following pharmacopeial methods and international standards are considered acceptable:

United States Pharmacopeia (USP) including Dietary Supplements Compendium
British Pharmacopeia (BP)
European Pharmacopeia (Ph. Eur.)
Pharmacopée Française (Ph.F.)
Pharmacopeia Internationalis (Ph.I.)
Japanese Pharmacopeia (JP)
Food Chemicals Codex (FCC)
Deutsches Arzneibuch (DAB)
Deutsches Homöopathisches Arzneibuch (HAB)

Other pharmacopeias or monographs may be used provided a suitable motivation of its/their equivalence in standing and quality to any of those listed above is given. Alternate methods that meet the pharmacopeial requirements are also acceptable under certain conditions.

Nomenclature

Herbal names must be stated in the Latin binomial format, which must include the genus, species, subspecies, variety, subvariety, form, subform or chemotype and author where appropriate. Reference must be made to the internationally accepted name for the plant, fungus, or alga, e.g.,

"*Olea europaea* subsp. *africana (Mill.) P.S. Green*
Crataegus curvisepala Lindm.
Thymus zygis subsp. *gracilis (Boiss.) R. Morales ct. thymol*"

The following also refers to:

Herbal Component Name (HCN)

"*HCNs are names for classes of constituents that are found in herbal ingredients. The need for a HCN most often arises when a herbal extract is standardised to a particular class of constituents, or where particular classes of constituents are restricted (e.g. hydroxyanthracene derivatives). Where a herbal extract is standardised to a single constituent, the single constituent should have a chemical name. The HCN is not a stand-alone name and should be used only when expressing a herbal substance.*"

The following structural information is required:

"*Where appropriate the chemical structure (graphic), molecular formula, molecular mass and Chemical Abstracts Service Registry (CAS) number for the substance should be provided, unless provided in the relevant monograph or standard.*

For herbal substance/s and preparation/s the physical form and a description of the constituents with known therapeutic activity or markers (molecular formula, relative molecular mass, structural formula, including relative and absolute stereochemistry, the molecular formula, and the relative molecular mass) should be provided. Other constituents, if relevant, should be stated."

The following quality information relating to general properties must be included:

"*Physico-chemical information relevant to the characterisation of the substance and may be required for the manufacture, performance or stability of its intended final dosage form that is not covered by the relevant monograph or standard (e.g. solubility or particle size) in order to adequately characterise/describe the active ingredient(s), determine the shelf life and demonstrate that the active ingredient(s) will be of appropriate and consistent quality.*"

Other general quality information such as description of the manufacturing process, process controls, control of materials, process validation and/or evaluation, impurities, control of active pharmaceutical ingredients including specifications, minimum tests and limits included in specifications for an active ingredient, analytical and validation of analytical procedures are required.

Safety

"*Appropriate data must be provided that demonstrate the safety of the product. Safety may be established by detailed reference to the published literature and/or the submission of original study data. If the product has been traditionally used without demonstrated harm, a review of the relevant literature should be provided with original articles or references to the original articles. If official monograph/review results exist, reference should be made to them. Toxicological studies, if available, should be part of the assessment. If a toxicological risk is known, relevant toxicity data must be submitted. The assessment of risk, whether independent of dose or related to dose, should be documented."*

The following aspects of safety are required:

- the nature of the patient population and the extent of patient exposure/worldwide marketing experience to date
- common and nonserious adverse events
- serious adverse events
- methods to prevent, mitigate, or manage adverse events
- reactions due to overdose
- long-term safety if relevant data is available
- special patient populations, e.g., children and pregnant or lactating women
- relevant animal toxicology and product quality information
- If risks have been identified, the report must explain why a positive benefit/risk-balance for a traditional use is justified. For example, if there are reports of serious adverse events, this must be balanced by sufficient evidence of appropriate benefit.

Five pivotal pieces of information must be included, viz.,

- traditional use
- therapeutic indication and associated clinical evidence where necessary
- strength/type of substance
- posology
- specific information on safe use and evidence of safety

Efficacy

Information relating to the evaluation of efficacy *"may include established traditional use, pre-clinical data and evidence from clinical trials in animals and human beings as well as those references specified below appropriate for the risk level of associated claim. Evidence (data) must be provided to support the product's efficacy for the proposed indication(s) and claims for inclusion in the product labeling. Proof of efficacy, including the documentation required to support the indicated claims, should depend on the nature and level of the indications. For the treatment of minor disorders, for nonspecific indications, or for limited prophylactic uses, less stringent requirements (e.g. observational studies) may be adequate to prove efficacy, especially when the extent of traditional use and the experience with a particular herbal medicine and supportive pharmacological data are taken into account. Where traditional use has not been established, appropriate preclinical and/or clinical evidence will be required, dependent on level of claim. Where an active ingredient is well described in standard sources, it is possible to use these descriptions as the basis of the efficacy and safety information."*

The following statement relates to the quality of the requisite data:

- *"When more than one active ingredient is included in a product, the rationale for the inclusion of each active ingredient must be stated and justified. The inclusion of each active ingredient and the intended use of the product as a whole should be justified in terms of each ingredient's and the product as a whole's efficacy and safety."*

The South African Health Products Regulatory Authority (SAHPRA) regulations [7] require CAMs to comply with the following practices:

- *Good Manufacturing Practice (GMP)*
- *Good Laboratory Practice (GLP)*
- *Good Agricultural and Collection Practices (GACP) as well*
- *as the WHO Guidelines on Good Agricultural and Collection Practices (GACP) for Medicinal Plants, if applicable.*

4.2.16 Switzerland

In Switzerland, the legal and regulatory status of CAM and CAM practices [48] is controlled by Swissmedic [49]. The Swiss health-care system is decentralized, and the legislative authority is a unicameral parliament where each Canton has its own regulations for health practice in addition to some federal regulations. Since 2009, complementary medicine has been included under Swiss Federal Law, Article. 118a 52 of the Federal Constitution of the Swiss Confederation [50].

The practice and use of Swiss CAM is divided as follows:

Complementary medicine (CM) described as Komplementär Arzneimittel (KA) is reserved for Medical Doctors (MDs), whereas the use of alternative medicine (AM) can be practiced by nonmedically trained practitioners' CM associations.

The approval of CM products includes requirements for herbal medicines where herbal products are considered together with homeopathic, anthroposophical, and spagyric KA [49]. A decision tree for the type of application for the approval of complementary medicinal products is provided in Appendix 8 of Swissmedic [49]. Authorization requirements for such products are separated into two classes, products with indications and those without indications.

Chapter 5 of the Federal Constitution of the Swiss Confederation [50] provides information on the general requirements and assessment principles and selection of the appropriate approval procedures, viz.:

"For the authorization of homeopathic and anthroposophic medicines as well as other complementary medicines, different approval procedures are possible depending on the composition of the medicine and the intended use. The appendix to this guidance provides an overview of these procedures and also serves as a decision tree on which procedure to use for a particular drug." The requirements for herbal substances and preparations are provided in the guidelines for the authorization of phytochemicals [49]. Quality requirements include the following: *"The raw materials used must comply with the pharmacopoeia monographs for homeopathic and anthroposophic medicinal products and the general requirements for pharmacopoeia raw materials (HAB-Deutsches homöopathisches Arzneibuch, PhF–Pharmacopée Française and the BHomP—British Homeopathic Pharmacopoeia)* [49]. *If a single monograph exists for a source substance in a recognized pharmacopoeia, the requirements documented there must be met. If a corresponding monograph for a starting material is missing, an in-house monograph must be prepared. Taking into account the nature of the source substance concerned (for example of plant, animal, mineral or human origin), quality criteria as specified in analogous monographs of recognized pharmacopoeias must be specified. The chosen tests must be justified and the methods validated. In the case of vegetable raw materials, moreover, it is generally necessary to give precise details of the parent plant (s) and the plant parts used.*

For active ingredients, both the quality of the starting materials used and the quality of the active substances themselves must be documented." Details of the documentation required for the quality of the finished product, validation requirements for manufacture and control of the finished product with indications are described in Chapter 6 of the Swissmedic [49], whereas substances and products without indications are described in Chapter 7.

Chapter 6 also contains information relating to safety and efficacy requirements. The clinical documentation for these products, as in most global jurisdictions, require only bibliographic references and information of use and associated safety/toxicity reports, as follows:

Section 6.5.1 states that bibliographic documents should prove that:

(a) the composition can be sufficiently substantiated by the application in the respective therapeutic direction for the claimed field of application.
(b) there is sufficient knowledge about possible side effects.

The literature must be evaluated and referenced. Clinical studies may be submitted and the author should be a knowledgeable and technically qualified expert. For the approval of medicines without indication, documents to be submitted regarding quality and safety are described under Art. 24 KPAV (Komplementär- und Phytoarzneimittelverordnung) [49].

4.2.17   United Kingdom

The Traditional Herbal Medicines Directive (Directive 2004/24/EC) was published on April 30, 2004 and implemented by the Medicines (Traditional Herbal Medicinal Products for Human Use) [51]. According to The British Herbal Medicine Association (BHMA), *"Manufactured herbal medicines placed on the UK market since April 2011 are required to have either a Traditional Herbal Registration (THR) or a Marketing Authorisation (MA). In due course, therefore, all herbal medicines on the market will meet the same stringent criteria, satisfying EU requirements applicable to any medicine: a consistently high standard of quality, regular monitoring of safety, and full information for safe and beneficial use of the product provided by in-pack leaflets"* [52].

In the guidance entitled, *Apply for a Traditional Herbal Registration (THR)* issued by the MHRA [53], herbal medicines can be registered under the THR scheme. According to the Human Medicines Regulation (2012), *"a product is a herbal medicine if the active ingredients are herbal substances and or herbal preparations only."*

The following definition relates to herbal preparations, viz.: *"A herbal preparation is when herbal substances are put through specific processes, which include: extraction; distillation; expression; fractionation; purification; concentration; fermentation. The herbal substance being processed can be: reduced or powdered; a tincture; an extract; an essential oil; an expressed juice; a processed exudate (rich protein oozed out of its source)."*

The suitability of registered herbal medicines for general sale is described in the document issued by the MHRA as follows *"Under the provisions of Part III of the Medicines Act 1968 General Sale List classification is appropriate for medicines which can, with reasonable safety, be sold or supplied otherwise than by or under the supervision of a pharmacist. When considering the suitability of a product for GSL status it is necessary to confirm firstly that the hazard to health and the risk of misuse is small and that significant special precautions in handling are not required. If there are no safety, impediments it is then necessary to consider whether the convenience to the purchaser outweighs the benefit of availability of professional advice at the point of sale. As indicated above, the MHRA anticipates that the majority of registered products will be suitable for GSL status, with only a minority requiring restriction to pharmacy sale"* [54].

Regarding the eligibility for THRs, the indication of the herbal medicine must ensure that its indication is agreed under legislation and which is indicated for the medical condition that the product has traditionally been used to treat [53]. Stability studies for herbal products are required to be conducted as per Directive 2003/83EEC [11] and the EMA 2018 Directive EMA/HMPC/162241/20051 Rev. 3 [55] stipulates that a comprehensive study program based on validated analytical methods and appropriate fingerprinting of the herbal constituents in the product is required. In addition to the EU regulations, provisions for herbal medicinal products are laid down in Directive 2004/24/EC49 (the Traditional Herbal Medicinal Products Directive, THMPD) amending Directive 2001/83/EC [56].

4.2.18 The United States of America

Since the Food Drug and Cosmetic Act (FD&C Act) was published in the late 1930s, the United States Food and Drug Administration (FDA) introduced regulatory requirements for dietary supplements, nutraceuticals, and other related herbal products. Natural products have been considered under "generally recognized as safe" (GRAS) status when confirmed by qualified experts and without any further contradictions by other experts [57]. The Dietary Supplement Health and Education Act (DSHEA) was signed into law in October 1994, and it amended the FD & C Act by prescribing GMPs for dietary supplements [58].

A Dietary Supplement, according to DSHEA [59], is defined as *"a product (other than tobacco) intended to supplement the diet that bears or contains one or more of the following dietary ingredients:*

- *(A) a vitamin;*
- *(B) a mineral;*
- *(C) an herb or other botanicals;*
- *(D) an amino acid;*
- *(E) a dietary substance for use by man to supplement the diet by increasing the total dietary intake; or*
- *(F) a concentrate, metabolite, constituent, extract, or combination of any ingredient described in clause (A), (B), (C), (D), or (E)."*

The FDA regulates both finished dietary supplement products and dietary ingredients and dietary supplements are regulated under a different set of regulations than those covering "conventional" foods and drug products. The FDA also provides further definitions and descriptions as follows [60]:

"Dietary supplements are regulated by the FDA as food, not as drugs" and the definitions according to the FDA 101: Dietary Supplements [61] are as follows:

"Dietary supplements in part are products taken by mouth that contain a "dietary ingredient."

Dietary ingredients include vitamins, minerals, amino acids, and herbs or botanicals, as well as other substances that can be used to supplement the diet." In terms of regulations—*"the Federal law requires that every dietary supplement be labeled as such, either with the term "dietary supplement" or with a term that substitutes a description of the product's dietary ingredient(s) for the word "dietary" (e.g., "herbal supplement" or "calcium supplement"). The FDA further states that the "Federal law does not require dietary supplements to be proven safe to FDA's satisfaction before they are marketed."*

The *Dietary* Supplement Health and Education Act of 1994 (DSHEA) [59] makes the following provisions:

- *"Manufacturers and distributors of dietary supplements and dietary ingredients are prohibited from marketing products that are adulterated or misbranded. That means that these firms are responsible for evaluating the safety and labeling of their products before marketing to ensure that they meet all the requirements of DSHEA and FDA regulations.*
- *FDA is responsible for taking action against any adulterated or misbranded dietary supplement product after it reaches the market."*

Recently, the FDA published a draft guideline (December 2016) [62] entitled ***"Botanical Drug Development"*** which is denoted as *"non-binding recommendations."* The guidance focuses *"on appropriate development plans for botanical drugs* *to be submitted in new drug applications (NDAs) and specific recommendations on submitting investigational new drug applications (INDs) in support of future NDA submissions for botanical drugs. In addition, this guidance provides general information on the over-the-counter (OTC) drug monograph system for botanical drugs."*

The guidance contains the following definition: *"the term botanicals means products that include plant materials, algae, macroscopic fungi, and combinations thereof..."* which is comprehensive and covers topics including

- regulatory requirements for botanical drug products that could be marketed as over the counter (OTC) and those that would require New Drug Application (NDA).
- Investigational New Drugs for phase 1–3 clinical trials and NDAs for herbal medicinal products

The definition of a botanical product under this draft guidance is equivalent to a drug and is described as follows: *A botanical product intended to prevent disease would also generally meet the definition of a drug under Section 201(g)(1)(B) and be regulated as a drug.*

However, currently, there is no preapproval process for dietary supplements; it remains the responsibility of the sponsor (the person legally responsible for placing the product on the market) to ensure that such products are manufactured to an acceptable quality, is safe to use, and complies with the law. However, once the draft guideline [62] has become official, registration of herbal medicines will need to comply with the following requirements: *"Any person who wishes to market a new drug in the United States must submit an NDA and obtain Agency approval prior to marketing the new drug product for the proposed use (see Sections 201(p) and 505 of the FD&C Act). FDA may approve a drug product containing such a drug substance for OTC sale pursuant to an application submitted under Section 505 of the FD&C Act. Accordingly, an applicant could seek marketing approval for a botanical drug under Section 505 of the FD&C Act for either prescription or OTC use."* The above requirements are based on the following statement in the draft guidance [62], *"A botanical product may be classified as a food (including a dietary supplement), drug (including a biological drug), medical device, or cosmetic under the Federal Food, Drug, and Cosmetic Act (FD&C Act)."*

5 Conclusions

Undoubtedly, the popularity and commercialization of herbal products has been increasing exponentially over the past few years. In the present scenario with rapid globalization, herbal products play a vital role in the economies of countries around the world. Many herbals are being incorporated into various medicinal products due to presumed inherent pharmacological effects or sometimes even due to unsubstantiated claims by dubious manufacturers. Herbal product adulteration, substitution of active principles, formulation as inappropriate dosage forms, and manufacturing and processing under non-cGMP conditions (i.e., improper QC and quality assurance) are some of the major issues associated with herbal products. This has prompted implementation of revised regulations in an effort to ensure the QSE of herbal products in numerous countries around the world.

In many instances, patients are reported to take prescription medicine together with OTCs and herbal medicines, leading to possible adverse reactions. The pharmacist is well equipped to provide effective counseling in this area and appropriate regulations should be considered to enhance the consultations between patients and health practitioners to ensure continued safety and awareness.

Regulations are essential to ensure the QSE of herbal products, especially when marketed with specific claims and indications. However, in many global jurisdictions, appropriate regulations and control of herbal products appear to be lacking. Since herbal medicines are natural products, they are generally considered safe and many such remedies are available over the counter. However, such misconceptions of their inherent safety have resulted in serious, sometimes disastrous, ramifications. Appropriate criteria are currently being developed and implemented in an effort to improve the situation and to harmonize regulations between international regulatory bodies. The challenge for most regulatory bodies is to strike a balance between maintaining availability of herbal products for consumers at an affordable price and ensuring the best possible levels of QSE. While methods and related procedures for the control of allopathic medicines have been well established over many years, suitable and appropriate methods and procedures for the control of herbal medicines remain unresolved. Although, in many instances, similar methods used to control the quality of allopathic medicines may well be applicable to herbal medicines, some of these may not be appropriate and or practical for the regulation of the latter. In such instances, different and innovative approaches for the QC of herbal medicines present a daunting challenge to ensure the SQE of these medicines. Furthermore, since procedures for the assessment of safety and efficacy of allopathic medicines are generally not appropriate to regulate herbal medicines, relevant alternative approaches need to be investigated.

References

[1] IARC. Some traditional herbal medicines, some mycotoxins, naphthalene and styrene. In: IARC monographs on evaluation of carcinogenic risks to humans, vol. 82. Lyon: International Agency for Research on Cancer, WHO. IARC Press; 2002. p. 43. https://www.ncbi.nlm.nih.gov/books/NBK326619/pdf/Bookshelf_NBK326619.pdf. [Accessed 05 September 2019].

[2] Firenzuoli F, Gori L. Clinical and research issues evidence based complementary and alternative medicine. Herb Med Today 2007;4(Suppl. 1):37–40.

[3] Patnala S, Kanfer I. Chemotaxonomic studies of mesembrine-type alkaloids in Sceletium plant species. S Afr J Sci 2013;109(3/4):1–5.

[4] Pandey R, Tiwari RK, Shukla SS. Omics: a newer technique in herbal drug standardization and quantification. J Young Pharm 2016;8(2):76–81.

[5] Reflection paper on markers used for quantitative and qualitative analysis of herbal medicinal products and traditional medicinal products. Doc. Ref. EMEA/HMPC/253629/2007. European Medicines Agency (EMEA), London, England, UK. Available from: https://www.ema.europa.eu/en/documents/scientific-guideline/draft-reflection-paper-markers-used-quantitative-qualitative-analysis-herbal-medicinal-products_en.pdf. [Accessed 05 September 2019].

[6] Regional Office for South-East Asia. Guidelines for the regulation of herbal medicines in the South-East Asia region-World Health Organization. SEA-Trad. Med.-82, New Delhi: Regional Office for South-East Asia; 2003.

[7] Medicines Control Council. Complementary medicines—Health supplements safety and efficacy. Republic of South Africa: South African Health Products Regulatory Authority (Medicines Control Council), Department of Health; 2016. 7.04_SE_Health_Supplements_Jun16_v2. Available from https://www.sahpra.org.za/documents/d0f3f80c7.04_SE_Health_Supplements_Jun16_v2.pdf. [Accessed 05 September 2019].

[8] Medical Library Association. Electronic resources reviews. J Med Libr Assoc 2005;93(3). Available from: https://www.ncbi.nlm.nih.gov/pmc/articles/PMC1176230/pdf/i0025-7338-093-03-0410.pdf. [Accessed 05 September 2019].

[9] U.S. Department of Health and Human Services, National Institutes of Health, National Center for Complementary and Integrative Health. Available from: https://nccih.nih.gov/. [Accessed 05 September 2019].

[10] Dietary Supplement Products & Ingredients, U.S. Food Drug Administration. Available from: https://www.fda.gov/food/dietary-supplements/dietary-supplement-products-ingredients. [Accessed 05 September 2019].

[11] Directive 2004/24/EC of the European Parliament and of the Council of 31 March 2004 – Amending, as regards traditional herbal medicinal products, Directive 2001/83/EC on the Community code relating to medicinal products for human use. Off J Eur Union L 136/85. Available from: https://eur-lex.europa.eu/LexUriServ/LexUriServ.do?uri=OJ:L:2004:136:0085:0090:en:PDF. [Accessed 05 September 2019].

[12] WHO global report on traditional and complementary medicine 2019. Available from: https://apps.who.int/iris/bitstream/handle/10665/312342/9789241515436-eng.pdf?ua=1. [Accessed 05 September 2019].

[13] Chan K. Some toxic contaminants in herbal medicines. Chemosphere 2003;52:1361–71.

[14] Marrone CM. Safety issues with herbal products. Ann Pharmacother 1999;33:1359–61.

[15] Ernst E. Adulteration of Chinese herbal medicines with synthetic drugs: a systematic review. J Intern Med 2002;252:107–13. Available from: https://onlinelibrary.wiley.com/doi/epdf/10.1046/j.1365-2796.2002.00999.x. [Accessed 05 September 2019].

[16] Saper RB, Phillips SR, Sehgal A, Khouri N, Davis RB, Paquin J, Thuppil V, Kales SN. Lead, mercury, and arsenic in US- and Indian-manufactured ayurvedic medicines sold via the internet. J Am Med Assoc 2008;300(8):915–23.

[17] Elvin-Lewis M. Should we be concerned about herbal remedies. J Ethnopharmacol 2001;75:141–64.

[18] Ang HH. Quality assessment of herbal preparations—an overview. Int J Risk Saf Med 2004;16:239–45.

[19] O'Malley P, Trimble N, Browning M. Are herbal therapies worth the risks? Nurse Pract 2004;29(10):71–5.

[20] World Health Organization. National policy on traditional medicine and regulation of herbal medicines. France: WHO; 2005. p. 1–168.

[21] An overview of the regulation of complementary medicines in Australia. Department of Health, Therapeutic Goods Administration. Available from: https://www.tga.gov.au/overview-regulation-complementary-medicines-australia#how. [Accessed 05 September 2019].

[22] Australian regulatory guidelines for complementary medicines (ARGCM), Version 8.0, April 2018. Available from: https://www.tga.gov.au/sites/default/files/australian-regulatory-guidelines-complementary-medicines-argcm-v8.0.pdf. [Accessed 05 September 2019].

[23] Listed complementary medicines, Therapeutic good Administration, Department of health, Australian government. Available from: https://www.tga.gov.au/listed-complementary-medicines. [Accessed 05 September 2019].

[24] Registered complementary medicines, therapeutic good Administration, Department of Health, Australian government. Available from: https://www.tga.gov.au/registered-complementary-medicines. [Accessed 05 September 2019].

[25] Ministério daSaúde Agência Nacional de Vigilância Sanitária Resolution of The Board of Directors—RDC N° 26, of May 13 2014. Available from: http://bvsms.saude.gov.br/bvs/saudelegis/anvisa/2014/rdc0026_13_05_2014.pdf. [Accessed 05 September 2019].

[26] Ministry of Health of Brazil, Office of Health Care Department of Primary Care, National Policy on Integrative and Complementary Practices of the SUS, 2008. Available from: http://bvsms.saude.gov.br/bvs/publicacoes/pnpic_access_expansion_initiative.pdf. [Accessed 05 September 2019].

[27] Carvalho ACB, Ramalho LS, Marques RFO, Perfeito JP. Regulation of herbal medicines in Brazil. J Ethnopharmacol 2014;158:503–6.

[28] Carvalho ACB, Balbino EE, Maciel A, Perfeito JPS. Situação do registro de medicamentos fitoterápicos no Brasil. Rev Bras Farmacogn 2008;18(2):314–9.

[29] Canada, Food and Drugs Act, Current to June 20, 2019. Available from: https://laws.justice.gc.ca/PDF/F-27.pdf. [Accessed 05 September 2019].

[30] Natural Health Products Regulations SOR/2003-196 (Current to June 20, 2019) Last amended on October 17, 2018 https://laws-lois.justice.gc.ca/PDF/SOR-2003-196.pdf. [Accessed 05 September 2019].

[31] Regulation of the National System of Control of Pharmaceutical Products, the phyto drug and drug categories traditional herbarium. Available from: https://www.minsal.cl/wp-content/uploads/2018/02/Libro-MHT-2010.pdf. [Accessed 05 September 2019].

[32] The Egyptian Guidelines for Registration of Herbal Medicines 2015. Available from: http://www.eda.mohp.gov.eg/images/News/F_53.pdf. [Accessed 05 September 2019].

[33] Directive, 2004/24/EU. Available from: http://ec.europa.eu/health/files/eudralex/vol-1/dir_2004_24/dir_2004_24_de.pdf. [Accessed 05 September 2019].

[34] Questions & Answers on the EU framework for (traditional) herbal medicinal products, including those from a 'non-European' tradition. European Medicines Agency. Available from: https://www.ema.europa.eu/en/documents/regulatory-procedural-guideline/questions-answers-european-union-framework-traditional-herbal-medicinal-products-including-those-non_en.pdf. [Accessed 05 September 2019].

[35] Volume 2B Notice to Applicants Medicinal products for human use. Available from: https://ec.europa.eu/health/sites/health/files/files/eudralex/vol-2/b/update_200805/ctd_05-2008_en.pdf. [Accessed 05 September 2019].

[36] Complementary and Alternative Medicines (CAM) and Traditional Medicinal, Federal Institute for Drugs and Medical Devices. Available form https://www.bfarm.de/EN/Drugs/licensing/zulassungsarten/pts/_node.html. [Accessed 05 September 2019].

[37] Guidelines for Inspection of GMP Compliance by Ayurveda, Siddha and Unani Drug industry, Department of AYUSH, Ministry of health and Family Welfare, Government of India, February 2014. Available from: http://ayush.gov.in/sites/default/files/File779%20%20%204.pdf. [Accessed 05 September 2019].

[38] The Drugs and Cosmetics Rules, 1945. Government of India. https://www.cdsco.gov.in/opencms/export/sites/CDSCO_WEB/Pdf-documents/acts_rules/2016DrugsandCosmeticsAct1940Rules1945.pdf. [Accessed 05 September 2019].

[39] Guide to Traditional Herbal Medicinal Products Registration Scheme, Health Products Regulatory Authority, Ireland. Available from: https://www.hpra.ie/docs/default-source/publications-forms/guidance-documents/aut-g0029-guide-to-traditional-herbal-medicinal-products-registration-scheme-v3.pdf?sfvrsn=8. [Accessed 05 September 2019].

[40] Regulation (EC) No 726/2004 of The European Parliament and of The Council of 31 March 2004. Available from: https://ec.europa.eu/health//sites/health/files/files/eudralex/vol-1/reg_2004_726/reg_2004_726_en.pdf. [Accessed 05 September 2019].

[41] Maegawa H, Nakamura T, Saito K. Regulation of traditional herbal medicinal products in Japan. J Ethnopharmacol 2014;158:511–5.

[42] Dietary Supplements Regulations 1985 (SR 1985/208). Reprint as at March 2016. Available from: http://www.legislation.govt.nz/regulation/public/1985/0208/latest/DLM102109.html?src=qs. [Accessed 05 September 2019].

[43] Food Act 2014, New Zealand Legislation, Available from: http://www.legislation.govt.nz/act/public/2014/0032/75.0/DLM2995811.html. [Accessed 05 September 2019].

[44] Regulation of Dietary Supplements – MEDSAFE. New Zealand Medicines and Medical Devices and Safety Authority. Available from: https://www.medsafe.govt.nz/regulatory/DietarySupplements/Regulation.asp. [Accessed 05 September 2019].

[45] Herbal medicines and related products registration regulations 2019, National Agency for Food and Drug Administration and Control (NAFDAC). Available from: https://www.nafdac.gov.ng/wp-content/uploads/Files/Resources/Regulations/HERBAL_REGULATIONS/Herbal-Medicines-and-Related-Products-Registration-2019.pdf. [Accessed 05 September 2019].

[46] Shikov AN, Pozharitskaya ON, Makarov VG. Regulation of herbal medicinal products in Russia. Planta Med 2012;78–OP10. Available from: https://www.thieme-connect.com/products/ejournals/abstract/10.1055/s-0032-1307488. [Accessed 05 September 2019].

[47] On Circulation of Medicines. Available from: https://www.wipo.int/edocs/lexdocs/laws/en/ru/ru239en.pdf. [Accessed 05 September 2019].On Circulation of Medicines. Available from: https://www.wipo.int/edocs/lexdocs/laws/en/ru/ru239en.pdf. [Accessed 05 September 2019].

[48] CAM regulations in Switzerland. Available from: http://cam-regulation.org/en/switzerland. [Accessed 05 September 2019].CAM regulations in Switzerland. Available from: http://cam-regulation.org/en/switzerland. [Accessed 05 September 2019].

[49] HD—Help Document. Guidance Approval Homeopathic, Anthroposophic and other complementary drugs HMV4, SwissMedic. Available from: https://www.swissmedic.ch/dam/swissmedic/de/dokumente/zulassung/zl_hmv_iv/zl101_00_016d_wlzulassungsverfahrenfuerhomoeopathischeundanthroposophi.pdf.download.pdf/zl101_00_016d_wlzulassungsverfahrenfuerhomoeopathischeundanthroposophi.pdf. [Accessed 05 September 2019].

[50] Federal Constitution of the Swiss Confederation. Available from: https://www.admin.ch/opc/en/classified-compilation/19995395/index.html. [Accessed 05 September 2019].

[51] A guide to what is a medicinal product, MHRA Guidance Note No. 8, revised 2012. Available from: https://assets.publishing.service.gov.uk/government/uploads/system/uploads/attachment_data/file/380280/guide_8_what_is_a_medicinal_product.pdf. [Accessed 05 September 2019].

[52] The British Herbal Medicine Association (BHMA), Available from: https://bhma.info/index.php/legislation-on-herbal-medicines/ [Accessed 05 September 2019].

[53] Guidance to apply for a traditional herbal registration, MHRA. Available from: https://www.gov.uk/guidance/apply-for-a-traditional-herbal-registration-thr#herbal-medicine-definition. [Accessed 05 September 2019].

[54] Permitted indications under the Directive on Traditional Herbal Medicinal Products, MHRA. Available from: http://ehtpa.eu/pdf/medicines_legislation/MHRA-examples-of-permitted-indications-under-THMPD.pdf. [Accessed 05 September 2019].

[55] Guideline on specifications: test procedures and acceptance criteria for herbal substances, herbal preparations and herbal medicinal products/traditional herbal medicinal products, EMA, June 2018. Available from: https://www.ema.europa.eu/en/documents/scientific-guideline/draft-guideline-specifications-test-procedures-acceptance-criteria-herbal-substances-herbal/traditional-herbal-medicinal-products-revision-3_en.pdf. [Accessed 05 September 2019].

[56] Medicinal products in the European Union – Legal framework for medicines for human use. Regulatory rule 3.5. European Parliament. Available from: http://www.europarl.europa.eu/RegData/etudes/IDAN/2015/554174/EPRS_IDA(2015)554174_EN.pdf. [Accessed 05 September 2019].

[57] Stroube WB, Rainey C, Tanner JT. Regulatory environment in the advertising of dietary supplements. Clin Res Regul Aff 2002;19(1):109–14.

[58] Wechsler J. Standards for supplements. Pharm Technol 2003;28–36.

[59] National Institutes of Health, Office of Dietary Supplements. Available from: https://ods.od.nih.gov/About/DSHEA_Wording.aspx#sec3. [Accessed 05 September 2019].

[60] Dietary Supplements, U.S. Food and Drug Administration. Available from: https://www.fda.gov/food/dietary-supplements. [Accessed 05 September 2019].

[61] FDA 101: Dietary Supplements https://www.fda.gov/consumers/consumer-updates/fda 101-dietary-supplements. [Accessed 05 September 2019].

[62] Botanical Drug Development Guidance for Industry, U.S. Department of Health and Human Services Food and Drug Administration Center for Drug Evaluation and Research (CDER), December 2016 Pharmaceutical Quality/CMC Revision 1. Available from: https://www.fda.gov/media/93113/download. [Accessed 05 September 2019].

Chapter 8

Herbal medicines used for andrological problems and drug interactions

Paul Moundipa Fewou

Laboratory of Pharmacology and Toxicology, Department of Biochemistry, University of Yaounde I, Yaounde, Cameroon

1 Introduction

According to a recent review study, the prevalence of erectile dysfunction is 3%–76.5% worldwide [1]. Its occurrence increases with age and is frequent in some metabolic conditions (diabetes, hypertension, obesity) [2]. Therefore, the use of herbal remedies for sexual dysfunction in these conditions may lead to an interaction between the herbal products and conventional drugs administered in these diseases.

Herbal remedies are used for sexual dysfunction, many of which are sold in health food centers or over the counter in different formulations for specific cases [3]. A review of some of these herbal drugs that have been formulated in some clinical trials and used to treat andrological problems brings out some observations on the type and the age of patients, the dosage used, and the duration of administration, varied from one study to another (see Table 1). Many of the herbal drugs are mixtures of more than one plant [3, 20]. In a review of herbal agents sold in the United States for the treatment of sexual dysfunction, Rowland and Tai [3] described many of the herbal supplements as mixture of more than one component. As example, Cobra which is used only for men contains six different herbs (*Panax ginseng*, damiana, yohimbine, saw palmetto, muira puama, Siberian ginseng). These different plants are highly cited in food supplements for sexual problems. In VigRX Plus a multi-ingredient supplement containing 10 plant extracts [21], catuaba, puncture vine, and dodder are found in addition to the 6 previously named herbs. All these ingredients are used for sexual dysfunction purposes.

The efficacy of some of these plants is yet to be proven and studies investigating the efficacy of *Tribulus terrestris* in erectile dysfunction are still controversial [4, 5]. The plant is claimed for its aphrodisiac properties and is not active in some types of infertility and does not ameliorate athletes condition [6]. In a review reporting some studies on this herb, the efficacy was proven in animal studies, and combination with other components increases testosterone levels in human trials [7]. However, the bioactive compounds of the mixture that contribute to this effect are yet to be discovered. Aerial parts and fruits of *T. terrestris* contain mainly flavonoids (tribuloside, kaempferol, kaempferol-3-glucoside, kaempferol-3-rutinoside, caffeoyl derivatives, quercetin glycosides), saponins (furostanol and spirostanol saponins of tigogenin), alkaloids in minor quantities (β-carboline alkaloid, tribulusterine), and steroidal glycosides whose pharmacological actions in humans is not yet completely explained [8]. However, it is suggested that protodioscin and protogracillin are responsible for the claimed activities.

The clinical efficacy of herbal medicines used in andrological problems was reviewed in a recent publication by Santos et al. [9]. In this study, the uses of *Tribulus terrestris* and Maca (*Lepidium meyenii*) to improve serum testosterone levels in men were not scientifically supported. Some reports support the use of *Tongkat ali* (*Eurycoma longifolia* Jack), mucuna (*Mucuna pruriens*), ashwagandha (*Withania somnifera*), Fenugreek (*Trigonella foenum-graceum*), and black seeds (*Nigella sativa*) to increase total testosterone levels and improve seminal parameters [10–13]. The use of powdered mucuna seed over a 12-week period in patients with oligozoospermia improved sperm concentration [11]. While evidence supporting the use of saw palmetto (*Serenoa repens*) to improve prostate health remains equivocal [14], evidence supporting the use of *Pygeum africanum*, *Urtica dioica*, beta-sitosterols, pollen extract, onion, garlic, and tomato appears favorable and promising [9, 15].

The active principles of many of these herbal drugs are not very precisely known. The roots of *E. longifolia* plant are reported to be rich in various classes of bioactive compounds such as quassinoids, canthin-6-one alkaloids, β-carboline alkaloids, triterpene tirucallane type, squalene derivatives, biphenyl neolignan, eurycolactone, laurycolactone, and eurycomalactone, and bioactive steroids [16]. Alcohol extract of *M. pruriens* seeds is rich in cyclitols, oligosaccharides, and phenols [17]. Many herbal products contain flavonoids among which quercetin is a potent antioxidant molecule [8, 9, 18].

Herbal Medicine in Andrology. https://doi.org/10.1016/B978-0-12-815565-3.00008-4

TABLE 1 Some reported clinical trials on herbal medicines used in andrology.

Study	Dosage	Effects	Reference
Lepidium meyenii (Maca)			
1. Healthy men	1.5 or 3 g/d for 4 months	Increased sperm count and volume	[4]
2. Healthy men	« » for 12 weeks	Improved sexual desire	[5]
3. Caucasian mild ED	2.4 g/d for 12 weeks	Improvement of erectile function and sexual well-being	[6]
A review of safety studies		Normal liver, kidney, and spleen	[4]
Panax ginseng			
1. Patients with ED		60% increase in penile rigidity, libido, and patient satisfaction	[7]
2. Patients with ED	0.9 g or 1 g 3 times/d Korean ginseng	No sign of toxicity	[8]
3. Patients with ED	Tablets 0.35 g ginseng berry extract for 8 w	Improvement of erectile function	[9]
Eurycoma longifolia (Tongkat ali)			
1. Men with Idiopathic infertility of 5.3 yrs	200 mg for 3–9 months	Increased sperm concentration and normal sperm morphology	[10]
2. Healthy men and men with stable chronic medical illness	300 mg for 6–12 weeks	Improved sperm quality and quantity	[11]
3. Healthy men	400 mg for 5 weeks	Increase in total and free testosterone	[12]
4. Late onset Hypogonadism	200 mg for 1 month	Increased testosterone concentration and ageing-male symptom score	[13]
Tribulus terrestris			
Idiopathic infertility	750 mg for 3 months	No change	[14]
Partial Androgen Deficiency	750 mg for 3 months	Slight increase in testosterone and LH	[15]
Human trial	20, 450, 750 mg sole or plus androgen	Increase in testosterone in androgen supplemented groups	[16]
Mucuna pruriens			
Healthy and infertile men	5 g/d for 3 months	Improved testosterone, LH, dopamine, adrenaline, and noradrenaline Reduction of FSH and PRL. Sperm count and motility recovered in infertile men after treatment.	[17]
Cordyceps sinensis			
Human trial	8 weeks	Increase in sperm count, decreased sperm malformations, and 79% increase in sperm survival rate	[18,19]

This flavonoid also found in onion has many health benefits [18] and is known to increase blood testosterone in animal and human trials [15]. Table 2 lists some herbal drugs, their active principles and targets.

Clinical trials on drug-herbal medicine interactions are the gold standard and are usually carried out when indicated by unexpected consumer side effects or preferably by predictive preclinical studies. Unfortunately, most of these herbal products lack standardization as conventional drugs; the active principles or fractions, though not precisely known, are not always supplied at the same concentration. However, a review published by Sprouse and van Breemen [19] contributes to fill the gaps in knowledge of the potential of some popular herbal supplements to interact with therapeutic agents with respect to absorption, transport, and metabolism.

TABLE 2 Some herbal drugs, their active principles and targets.

Species	Active principles	Targets	References
Lepidium meyenii	Glucosinolates (1%) Alcaloids: macaridine Sterol	Antioxidant	[22]
Panax ginseng	Ginsenosides (steroid glycosides, triterpene saponins)	Endothelial NO release, agonist of Estrogen receptor alpha	[23,24]
Eurycoma longifolia	Dichloromethane fraction Eurycomanone eurypepetides	Inhibition of ACE, angiotensin II, and relaxation of aortic ring Increased testosterone	[25–27]
Tribulus terrestris	Ethanol extract	Nitric oxide/nitric oxide synthase pathway and inhibition of endothelium of the CC	[28].
Cordyceps sinensis	Cordycepin (3-deoxyadenosine)	Adenosine receptors	[18]
Mucuna pruriens	L-dopa, tetrahydroisoquinolines compounds, some alkaloids as mucunine, prurienine, etc. gpMUC protein		[29,30]
Custuta chinensis	Quercetin 3-O-beta-D-galactoside-7-O-beta-D-glucoside, quercetin 3-O-beta-D-apiofuranosyl-(1 → 2)-beta-D-galactoside, hyperoside, isorhamnetin, kaempferol, quercetin , D-sesamin, 9(R)-hydroxy-D-sesamin	Antioxidant	[31]
Allium cepa	Quercetin	Antioxidant, lueinizing hormone, nitric oxide	[15]

2 Study of drug interactions

The popular and worldwide use of herbal medicines in andrology makes the study of drug interactions particularly urgent. Very few studies have been undertaken on the interactions between herbal medicines and drugs. Due to their reliance on natural supplements, herbal products are often taken by consumers without prescription, at the same time with conventional drugs. Such therapy may lead to an unintended effect when the herbal supplement alters the drug-metabolizing enzyme system. The study of such interactions, though now generally recognized as important in pharmacology, is not well established. This is mainly due to the uncertainty in constituents of the herbal products. For a review see Ref. [32]. Drug-herbal medicine interactions include effect on drug-metabolizing enzymes (inhibition or induction), cytochrome P-450, phase I and phase II enzymes, drug transporters, and drug-efflux proteins (Fig. 1). Herbal constituents might inhibit or induce enzymes responsible for the metabolism of therapeutic agents or their transporters and cause drug-herbal medicine interactions. Inhibitors will slow down

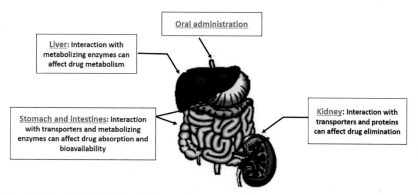

FIG. 1 Pharmacokinetic drug-herbal medicine. Herbal medicine constituents can cause drug interactions by interfering with drug-metabolizing enzymes (cytochrome P-450 and conjugation enzymes); drug transporters in the liver, kidneys, stomach, and intestines (particularly P-glycoprotein, an excretion protein that transport xenobiotics out of the body) will alter absorption, bioavailability, and drug elimination in the blood, which can alter drug distribution.

substrate drug metabolism and increase drug effect while inducers will increase substrate drug metabolism and decrease drug effect. A typical example comes from of St. John's Wort (*Hypericum perforatum*) medical herb used in mild depression, which is a potent inducer of cytochrome P-450 enzymes (CYP) and P-glycoprotein (P-gp), a transporter that excrete xenobiotics from the body [33]. When St. John Wort is taken concomitantly with nifedipine, a drug used in cardiovascular disorder, the induced cytochrome P-450 3A4 metabolizes the drug nifedipine into inactive compound, reducing its blood concentration thus its effectiveness in illness. When these interactions occur, the pharmacokinetics of therapeutic agents can be altered.

3 Some herbal-drug interactions

3.1 *Panax ginseng*

It is also known as Korean ginseng. A review has been published on the effect of *P. ginseng* on cytochrome P-450 when taken by human volunteers in clinical studies [32]. It was shown that its administration to healthy volunteers had no effect on CYP3A4, CYP1A2, CYP2E1, and CYP2D6 when midazolam, caffeine, chlorzoxazone, and debrisoquine were used. Let us recall that 50 CYP subfamilies are known and among them, CYP1A2, CYP2C9, CYP2C19, CYP2D6, CYP3A4, and CYP3A5 are subfamilies that metabolize about 90% of drugs [34]. In addition to other studies, these observations from the available clinical evidence suggested that the potential for ginseng-drug interactions was low. In another study conducted to determine the influence of *P. ginseng* (1000 mg/day) on CYP3A and P-gp function, midazolam and fexofenadine pharmacokinetic parameter values were calculated and compared before and after its administration. The area under the concentration-time curve was significantly reduced for Midozolam, implicating a low bioavailability of the benzodiazepine, while fexofenadine pharmacokinetics were unaltered by its administration [35]. Based on these results, *P. ginseng* appears to induce CYP3A activity in the liver and possibly the gastrointestinal tract. Therefore, it appears to lower the bioavailability of CYP3A substrates. Coadministration of *P. ginseng* and lopinavir/ritonavir (LVP-r), an HIV drug, did not alter their steady-state pharmacokinetics. Thus, a clinically significant interaction between the herbal drug and LPV-r is unlikely to occur in HIV-infected patients who choose to take these agents concurrently [36]. In a study using rats, Zhang et al. [37] reported that a mixture of a standard Chinese preparation (Sailuotong) containing *P. ginseng* (ginseng), *Ginkgo biloba* (ginkgo), and *Crocus sativus* (saffron) induced CYP1A2 and CYP2C11, and inhibited CYP3A (Table 3).

TABLE 3 Multiherbal composition of herbal supplement VigRX and some interaction between ingredients.

Species	Common name	Activity	Interactions	References
Serenoa repens	Saw palmetto	Prostatic hyperplasia	CYP2D6 and CYP3A4 (no effect)	[34]
Crategus rivularis	Hawthorn	Hypotensive	β-blockers, digoxin, Ca²⁺ channel blockers, PD5I	[35]
Ginkgo biloba	Ginkgo	Brain activity enhancer	CYP2C19 (induction)	[36]
Turnera diffusa	Damiana	Increase sexual desire	Hypoglyceamic properties	[37,38]
Tribulus terrestris	Puncture vine	Smooth muscle relaxation, sexual enhancer	Lower blood sugar, docking compound to ERα and ERβ, modulator of multidrug resistant protein	[28,39,40]
Erythroxylum catuaba	Catuaba	Aphrodisiac, fatigue, insomnia	Not documented	[22]
Ptychopetalum olacoides	Muira puama	Nerve tonic, aphrodisiac	interaction with dopaminergic and/or noradrenergic systems docking compound to ERα and ERβ	[40,41]
Cuscuta chinensis	Dodder	Increase sexual function, cardiovascular diseases, osteoporosis, senescence	A relaxing effect on penile cavernous tissue	[42]
Epimedium sagittatum	Barrenwort, bishop's hat, horny goat weed	Antiinflammatory, antiproliferative, and antitumor effects, erectile dysfunction	Modulation of CYP1A2, CYP3A4, and CYP2E1, lower AUC of Sidenafil	[43]
Bioperine	*Extract from Piper nigrum*	Added as bioavailability enhancer	Modulate the activity of DME	[23]

AUC, area under the curve; *CYP*, cytochrome P450; *DME*, drug-metabolizing enzymes; *ER*, estrogen receptor.

3.2 *Eurycoma longifolia* (Tongkat ali)

The pharmacokinetics of propranolol was studied when Tongkat ali was consumed by human volunteers. When propranolol was administered with *E. longifolia*, parameters such as bioavailability of propranolol has decreased, the time for the maximum peak concentration has prolonged, but the terminal elimination half-life, however, was not significantly affected. The study concluded that an interaction was due to a reduction in absorption rather than an increase in propranolol metabolism [38,39].

In vitro studies reported by Han et al. [28] evaluated the effects on cytochrome P450 (CYP) enzyme-mediated drug metabolism to predict the potential for herb-drug interactions using human liver microsomes or individual recombinant CYP isozymes. It was shown that *E. longifolia* slightly inhibited the metabolic activities of CYP1A2, CYP2A6, and CYP2C19 [28] and CYP2C9; however, the inhibitory action on CYP2D6 was not effective [40] at 1000 μg/mL [28]. It should be recalled that propranolol is mainly metabolized through CYP2D6 [33]. In male rat hepatocytes, an increase in the phase 1 metabolism of the antidiabetic drug rosiglitazone was reported [22]. From these studies it appears that dietary supplements containing *E. longifolia* extracts need more studies on drug-herbal interaction particularly in patients taking drugs for chronic diseases such as diabetes mellitus, hypertension, and other cardiovascular diseases.

3.3 *Lepidium meyenii* (maca)

A review published by Shin et al. [41] reported randomized clinical trials that are available for the study of maca efficacy in improving sexual function. The clinical trials did assess neither adverse effects of maca, nor its interaction with drugs. In a review by Gonzales [42], this herb significantly inhibited the hypertension relevant angiotensin I-converting enzyme (ACE) in vitro. In animal studies, maca significantly improved glucose tolerance and antioxidant status [43].

3.4 *Tribulus terrestris*

Also known as puncture vine, *T. terrestris* is a component of several supplements that are available over the counter and widely recommended generally as enhancer of human vitality. Tribulus standardized extract is obtained from the aerial parts of the plant that contain mainly saponins of the furostanol type (not less than 45%, calculated as protodioscin). Hence, a typical dose of 750 mg/day contains around 300 mg of protodioscin and prototribestin. These compounds have been found to interact with doxorubicin in multidrug-resistant cancer cells [23]. *T. terrestris* has also a diuretic effect which is less compared to hydrochlorothiazide [44]. In a report, *T. terrestris* herbal preparations was shown to be adulterated with banned steroid, and an herbal preparation was toxic at high dose [6].

3.5 Quercetin containing herbs

Many dietary supplements contain the flavonoid quercetin and its derivatives that are potent antioxidant molecules having a wide range of biological activities including enhancement of testosterone production in Leydig cells [15, 29, 45]. Quercetin is also known to modulate drug metabolizing enzymes in animal studies. When the preparation was given at 6 and 12 mg/kg per day, CYP3A and glutathione-S-tranferase were induced while CYP2C9 was inhibited. Higher doses (25–100 mg/kg) given to rats altered the bioavailability of cyclosporine, an immunosuppressive drug, and also inhibited expression of CYP3A P-gp [30]. Clarification on the coadministration of herbal medicines containing this compound and drug in chronic diseases is needed on clinical aspect.

4 Conclusion

Very few herbal medicines popularly used to treat andrological problems have been studied for drug interactions. For many, the active ingredients are not well characterized; some herbal products contain different compounds in the same chemical class that may act synergistically. Many formulations are mixtures of different herbs, and the dosage used varies from one study to another. The use of these dietary supplements may be popular in patients with chronic diseases as they usually face erectile dysfunction. Little knowledge of their effects on absorption, transport, and metabolism is documented. A few are known as inhibitors of some cytochrome P450 isoenzymes. Much still needs to be done to fill gaps in the knowledge of the potential interactions of herbal drugs used in andrology disorders with therapeutic agents with respect to absorption, transport, and metabolism. The flowchart of drug-herbal medicine interaction investigation suggested by Sprouse and van Breemen [17] may be used.

References

[1] Kessler A, Sollie S, Challacombe B, Briggs K, Van Hemelrijck M. The global prevalence of erectile dysfunction: a review: global prevalence of erectile dysfunction. BJU Int 2019;124(4):587–99.

[2] Kaminetsky J. Epidemiology and pathophysiology of male sexual dysfunction. Int J Impot Res 2008;20(S1):S3–10.

[3] Rowland DL, Tai W. A review of plant-derived and herbal approaches to the treatment of sexual dysfunctions. J Sex Marital Ther 2003;29(3):185–205.

[4] Kamenov Z, Fileva S, Kalinov K, Jannini EA. Evaluation of the efficacy and safety of *Tribulus terrestris* in male sexual dysfunction—a prospective, randomized, double-blind, placebo-controlled clinical trial. Maturitas 2017;99:20–6.

[5] Sanagoo S, Sadeghzadeh Oskouei B, Gassab Abdollahi N, Salehi-Pourmehr H, Hazhir N, Farshbaf-Khalili A. Effect of *Tribulus terrestris* L. on sperm parameters in men with idiopathic infertility: a systematic review. Complement Therap Med 2019;42:95–103.

[6] Pokrywka A, Obmiński Z, Malczewska-Lenczowska J, Fijatek Z, Turek-Lepa E, Grucza R. Insights into supplements with *Tribulus terrestris* used by athletes. J Human Kinet 2014;41(1):99–105.

[7] Qureshi A, Naughton DP, Petroczi A. A systematic review on the herbal extract *Tribulus terrestris* and the roots of its putative aphrodisiac and performance enhancing effect. J Diet Suppl 2014;11(1):64–79.

[8] Chhatre S, Nesari T, Kanchan D, Somani G, Sathaye S. Phytopharmacological overview of *Tribulus terrestris*. Phcog Rev 2014;8(15):45.

[9] Santos HO, Howell S, Teixeira FJ. Beyond tribulus (*Tribulus terrestris* L.): the effects of phytotherapics on testosterone, sperm and prostate parameters. J Ethnopharmacol 2019;235:392–405.

[10] Tambi MIBM, Imran MK, Henkel RR. Standardised water-soluble extract of *Eurycoma longifolia*, Tongkat ali, as testosterone booster for managing men with late-onset hypogonadism? Treatment of hypogonadism with *Tongkat ali*. Andrologia 2012;44:226–30.

[11] Shukla KK, Mahdi AA, Ahmad MK, Shankhwar SN, Rajender S, Jaiswar SP. *Mucuna pruriens* improves male fertility by its action on the hypothalamus–pituitary–gonadal axis. Fertil Steril 2009;92(6):1934–40.

[12] Ambiye VR, Langade D, Dongre S, Aptikar P, Kulkarni M, Dongre A. Clinical evaluation of the spermatogenic activity of the root extract of Ashwagandha (*Withania somnifera*) in oligospermic males: a pilot study. Evid Based Complement Alternat Med 2013;2013:1–6.

[13] Maheshwari A, Verma N, Swaroop A, Bagchi M, Preuss HG, Tiwari K, et al. Efficacy of Furosap™, a novel *Trigonella foenum-graecum* seed extract, in enhancing testosterone level and improving sperm profile in male volunteers. Int J Med Sci 2017;14(1):58–66.

[14] Tacklind J, MacDonald R, Rutks I, Stanke JU, Wilt TJ. Serenoa repens for benign prostatic hyperplasia. Cochrane Database Syst Rev 2012;87.

[15] Banihani SA. Testosterone in males as enhanced by onion (*Allium cepa* L.). Biomolecules 2019;9(2):75.

[16] Rehman S, Choe K, Yoo H. Review on a traditional herbal medicine, *Eurycoma longifolia* Jack (Tongkat Ali): its traditional uses, chemistry. Evid-Based Pharmacol Toxicol Mol 2016;21(3):331.

[17] Yadav MK, Upadhyay P, Purohit S, Pandey BL, Shah H. Phytochemistry and pharmacological activity of *Mucuna pruriens*: a review. IJGP 2017;11(2).

[18] Chen S, Jiang H, Wu X, Fang J. Therapeutic effects of quercetin on inflammation, obesity, and type 2 diabetes. Mediat Inflamm 2016;2016:1–5.

[19] Sprouse AA, van Breemen RB. Pharmacokinetic interactions between drugs and botanical dietary supplements. Drug Metab Dispos 2016;44(2):162–71.

[20] Jo J, Jerng UM. The effects of traditional Korean medicine in infertile male patients with poor semen quality: a retrospective study. Eur J Integr Med 2016;8(1):36–40.

[21] Shah GR, Chaudhari MV, Patankar SB, Pensalwar SV, Sabale VP, Sonawane NA. Evaluation of a multi-herb supplement for erectile dysfunction: a randomized double-blind, placebo-controlled study. BMC Complement Altern Med 2012;12(1):1083.

[22] Hussin AH, Chan KL. Herbdrug interaction studies of *Eurycoma longifolia* extract TAF273 on the metabolism of rosiglitazone, an antidiabetic drug. Asian J Pharmaceut Clin Res 2011;4(2):5.

[23] Ivanova A, Serly J, Dinchev D, Ocsovszki I, Kostova I, Molnar J. Screening of some saponins and phenolic components of *Tribulus terrestris* and *Smilax excelsa* as MDR modulators. In Vivo 2009;6.

[24] Leung KW, Wong AS. Ginseng and male reproductive function. Spermatogenesis 2013;3(3), e26391.

[25] George A, Henkel R. Phytoandrogenic properties of *Eurycoma longifolia* as natural alternative to testosterone replacement therapy. Andrologia 2014;46(7):708–21.

[26] Tee BH, Hoe SZ, Cheah SH, Lam SK. First report of *Eurycoma longifolia* jack root extract causing relaxation of aortic rings in rats. BioMed Res Int 2016;2016:1–9.

[27] Tee BH, Hoe SZ, Cheah SH, Lam SK. Effects of root extracts of *Eurycoma longifolia* jack on corpus cavernosum of rat. Med Princ Pract 2017;26(3):258–65.

[28] Han YM, Kim IS, Rehman SU, Choe K, Yoo HH. *In vitro* evaluation of the effects of *Eurycoma longifolia* extract on CYP-mediated drug metabolism. Evid Based Complement Alternat Med 2015;2015:1–6.

[29] Kim JK, Park SU. Quercetin and its role in biological functions: an updated review. EXCLI J 2018;17:856–63.

[30] Liu Y, Luo X, Yang C, Yang T, Zhou J, Shi S. Impact of quercetin-induced changes in drug-metabolizing enzyme and transporter expression on the pharmacokinetics of cyclosporine in rats. Mol Med Rep 2016;14(4):3073–85.

[31] Ye M, Yan Y, Qiao L, Ni X. Studies on chemical constituents of *Cuscuta chinensis*. Zhongguo Zhong Yao Za Zhi 2002;27(2):115–7.

[32] Shi S, Klotz U. Drug interactions with herbal medicines. Clin Pharmacokinet 2012;28.

[33] Soleymani S, Bahramsoltani R, Rahimi R, Abdollahi M. Clinical risks of St John's Wort (*Hypericum perforatum*) co-administration. Expert Opin Drug Metab Toxicol 2017;13(10):1047–62.

[34] Lynch T, Price A. The effect of cytochrome P450 metabolism on drug response, interactions, and adverse effects. Cytochrome P 2007;76(3):6.

[35] Malati CY, Robertson SM, Hunt JD, Chairez C, Alfaro RM, Kovacs JA, et al. Influence of *Panax ginseng* on Cytochrome P450 (CYP)3A and P-glycoprotein (P-gp) activity in healthy participants. J Clin Pharmacol 2012;52(6):932–9.

[36] Calderón MM, Chairez CL, Gordon LA, Alfaro RM, Kovacs JA, Penzak SR. Influence of *Panax ginseng* on the steady state pharmacokinetic profile of lopinavir-ritonavir in healthy volunteers. Pharmacotherapy 2014;34(11):1151–8.

[37] Zhang Y, Miao L, Lin L, Ren C-Y, Liu J-X, Cui Y-M. Repeated administration of Sailuotong, a fixed combination of *Panax ginseng*, *Ginkgo biloba*, and *Crocus sativus* extracts for vascular dementia, alters CYP450 activities in rats. Phytomedicine 2018;38:125–34.

[38] Salman SAB, Amrah S, Wahab MSA, Ismail Z, Ismail R, Yuen KH, et al. Modification of propranolol's bioavailability by *Eurycoma longifolia* water-based extract: propranolol's interaction with *E. longifolia*. J Clin Pharm Ther 2010;35(6):691–6.

[39] Ulbricht C, Conquer J, Flanagan K, Isaac R, Rusie E, Windsor RC. An evidence-based systematic review of Tongkat Ali (*Eurycoma longifolia*) by the natural standard research collaboration. J Diet Suppl 2013;10(1):54–83.

[40] Ismail S, Hussin AH, Chan KL. Inhibitory effect of *Eurycoma longifolia* extract and *Eurycomanone* on human cytochrome P450 isoforms. Int J Pharm Pharmaceut Sci. 6(6):4.

[41] Shin B-C, Lee MS, Yang EJ, Lim H-S, Ernst E. Maca (*L. meyenii*) for improving sexual function: a systematic review. BMC Complement Altern Med 2010;10(1):44.

[42] Gonzales GF. Ethnobiology and ethnopharmacology of *Lepidium meyenii* (Maca), a plant from the Peruvian Highlands. Evid Based Complement Alternat Med 2012;2012:1–10.

[43] Večeřa R, Orolin J, Škottová N, Kazdová L, Oliyarnik O, Ulrichová J, et al. The influence of Maca (*Lepidium meyenii*) on antioxidant status, lipid and glucose metabolism in rat. Plant Foods Hum Nutr 2007;62(2):59–63.

[44] Jabbar A, Nazir A, Khalil J, Ansari NI, Janjua KM, Javed F. To compare the effects of *Tribulus terristris* with hydrochlorothiazide on urine volume and electrolytes. Annals 2015;21(3):149–54.

[45] Khaki A, Khaki AA, Rajabzadeh A. The effects of Permethrin and antioxidant properties of *Allium cepa* (onion) on testicles parameters of male rats. Toxin Rev 2017;36(1):1–6.

Chapter 9

Acceptance of herbal medicines in andrology

Annie George[a] and Eckehard Liske[b]

[a]Biotropics Malaysia Berhad, Shah Alam, Selangor Darul Ehsan, Malaysia, [b]Department of Life Sciences, Technical University of Braunschweig, Braunschweig, Germany

1 Economic perspectives of herbal medicine and supplement markets

Complementary and alternative medicine has had a long history of use especially among ancient civilizations like China, India, South America, and Egypt [1, 2]. There is a renewed interest in alternative medicine as it is believed to be safe and efficacious compared to modern medicine, which is sometimes associated with adverse effects. It is also sought as a last remedial treatment for several chronic diseases, microbial resistance, and when new drugs are costly.

In China, over 90% of traditional Chinese medicine is focused on herbal remedies [3]. In 2017, the nation's medicinal herb-growing industry generated about $25 billion [4]. In India, the traditional medicinal systems used are Ayurveda, Siddha, and Unani. The Ayurvedic concept is the most popular among the three concepts, which existed between AD 2500 and 500 BC in India [5]. In the case of Egypt, the first recorded prescriptions were found in the ancient tombs, where the herbal drugs were of either animal, herbal, or mineral origin. In 2008, botanical exports from the African continent were the highest for Egypt at 77,850,312 kg with a reported value of $174,227,384 [6]. In South America, much of the knowledge of traditional medicine includes the Maya and Aztec traditions [7].

The world market value of the herbal industry has gradually increased over the period 2010–15 with an annual return of $29.5–35.7 million. Meanwhile, the sales of herbal products in the United States have reached $4.6 million, in Eastern Europe $1.2 million, and in the Asia Pacific region $21.1 million [8]. In 2017, US herbal supplement sales topped $8 billion, which is a 68% increase since 2008 [4]. Since many people prefer herbals over drugs due to safety and cost, the global herbal medicine market is expected to reach $117.02 billion by 2024. Europe is expected to be the largest market for traditional medicines, contributing to 40.8% of the market share, and by increasing awareness for herbals it is anticipated to generate maximum revenue over the forecast period [9]. In the Asia Pacific region, growth is expected to record the fastest compound annual growth rate (the measure of growth over multiple time periods) of 6.8% over the forecast period, and in Malaysia the value of sales of herbal and traditional dietary supplements grew from RM424.2 million in 2010 to RM532.7 million in 2015 [8].

2 Men's sexual health and its related issues

In the decade 1990–99, 52 empirical studies providing epidemiological data on sexual dysfunction have been published compared to 47 studies in a 50-year time period from 1940 to 1989 [10]. An international survey, *The Global Study of Sexual Attitudes and Behaviors* (GSSAB), identified the prevalence of various sexual health problems among 40–80-year-old adults (13.882 women, 13.618 men) from 29 countries [11]. Twenty-three percent of European males reported at least one sexual dysfunction symptom, including early ejaculation, erection difficulties, lack of interest in sex, inability to achieve orgasm, pain during sex, and sex not pleasurable [12]. The most common sexual dysfunction of men in the United States was "early ejaculation" (26.2%) followed by "erectile difficulties" (22.5%), "lack of sexual interest" (18.1%), "inability to achieve orgasm" (12.4%), "sex not pleasurable" (11.2%), and "pain during sex" (3.1%) [13]. The GSSAB subgroup study for 10 Asian countries reported "early ejaculation" and "erection difficulties" as the highest prevalence of sexual dysfunction with the highest frequencies in the Philippines (55% and 33%, respectively), followed by Malaysia (31% and 28%, respectively) and Thailand (23% and 29%, respectively) [14]. Collectively, other epidemiological studies in Asian countries show that the overall prevalence for erectile dysfunction (ED) in Asian men ranges widely from 2% to 88% [15], indicating widespread sexual disorders among men [16]. In 2025, it is estimated that approximately 322 million adult

Herbal Medicine in Andrology. https://doi.org/10.1016/B978-0-12-815565-3.00009-6

males worldwide will be diagnosed with ED (compared to approximately 152 million in 1995) with the highest predicted increase in Africa (169%), Asia (130%), and South America (150%) [17].

Sexual problems and ED are multifactorial and can have many causes, including increasing age, physical and mental health, stress, depression, anxiety, socioeconomic factors, smoking, obesity, diabetes mellitus, hypertension, heart disease, fatigue, hypothyroidism, prostate disorders, sexual hormones, and excessive alcohol consumption [11, 18, 19]. Epidemiological and clinical data indicate that men's sexual dysfunction is strongly associated with physical and psychological health [20] with the latter being responsible for problems in about 20% [18]. It was shown for an urban Malaysian male population that there is a strong correlation between ED and premature ejaculation (PE) and between PE and severe anxiety [21]. The management of sexual dysfunction, particularly erectile difficulties, can be treated successfully with phosphodiesterase-5 inhibitors, which are currently considered the first-line treatment for ED [22]. However, since caution is required regarding contraindications, side effects, and long-term risks, alternative natural therapy is preferred, particularly with herbs, which are traditionally known for their ergogenic, aphrodisiac, and adaptogenic properties for general well-being. However, adequate clinical evidence to support natural products as an effective treatment for sexual dysfunction is often not available or is of questionable quality [19, 23, 24].

3 Current clinical status of selected herbs with therapeutic value in andrology

Some herbs are reportedly popular in Asia as traditional remedies for ED, e.g., yohimbine (*Pausinystalia johimbe*), *Panax ginseng*, *Tribulus terrestris*, horny goat weed (*Epimedium* spp.), tongkat ali (*Eurycoma longifolia*), and *Ginkgo biloba* [25].

Fenugreek (*Trigonella foenum-graecum*), a traditional herb used for breast milk production, age-related symptoms of androgen decline [26], menopausal symptoms [27], and low sperm counts [28], is ranked 10th in the 2017 US "Mainstream Multi-Outlet Channel" with an increase in sales of 33.5% from 2016 [29]. Sales of ashwagandha, a traditionally used Ayurvedic plant with andrological benefits, increased by 25.6% from the previous year and is ranked 6th in the 2017 US top-selling herbal supplements [29]. Maca and saw palmetto are two other plants known for andrological benefits gaining traction in US sales, where saw palmetto ranked 11th in the US Natural Channel with an increase of 11.0%, and ranked 14th with an increase of 10.8% from 2016 to 2017 (Mainstream Multi-Outlet Channel); for maca no increase was noted [29].

In 2011, the three top-selling botanical products in Europe were identified as the traditionally well-known *G. biloba*, *Allium sativum* (garlic), and *P. ginseng* [30]. *Gingko* and *P. ginseng* are renowned for possessing andrological benefits [31]. The European Community, in spite of its strict regulatory requirements, is seen to be more welcoming of Asian herbs, where the root extract of a Malaysian plant (Physta, Biotropics Malaysia Berhad), *E. longifolia* was selected as the "Industry Success Story" in the Healthy-Aging category in its role as a natural alternative to testosterone replacement therapy at the leading conference for nutraceuticals, Vitafoods, in Europe in 2016. The acceptance of andrological herbals was obvious with the featuring of *E. longifolia* on the famous US talk show ("Dr. Oz") as a remedy for natural exhaustion. It was named as one of the herbs for vigor, through its ability to increase testosterone levels and reduce cortisol, which incidentally imbalances due to stress and overtraining [32]. Currently, a rigorous application for *E. longifolia* is being evaluated as a novel food in Europe [33].

The further acceptance of andrological herbs by the masses can be seen by the formulation of these herbs in the more accepted and widely used multivitamin supplementations as seen for *E. longifolia* [34] and ashwagandha [35]. None of this was observed for maca and fenugreek. Hence, there is a shift in the herbal portfolio to biologically functional food, addressing andrological issues for the broader consumer market for an all-in-one benefit for total maintenance.

Currently, research follows internationally accepted high scientific standards of pharmaceutical quality (Good Manufacturing Practice), as well as medical-scientific standards (Good Clinical Practice) applied in clinical trials contributing considerably to the efficacy and safety of herbal extracts. It is widely accepted that the best way to meet the principles of evidence-based medicine is to properly conduct randomized and controlled trials (RCTs). Therefore the clinical evidence from RCTs performed with well-known traditionally used herbs *E. longifolia* (tongkat ali), *Lepidium meyenii* (maca), *T. foenum-graecum* (Fenugreek), and *Withania somnifera* (ashwagandha) is reviewed.

Biomedical databases via the web were searched in PubMed with the following terms: botanical and vernacular names of the herbs (*Eurycoma* or tongkat ali, *Lepidium* or maca, *Trigonella* or fenugreek, *Withania* or ashwagandha) in combination with, e.g., "review" and/or "randomized" and/or "controlled." The search was then combined with more specific terms such as "sexual dysfunction," "stress," "mental health," "performance-enhancing," etc. Other literature databases and scientific information sources from well-known herbal institutions, e.g., the American Botanical Council (HerbMedPro, HerbClip, HerbalGram, HerbalEGram), were used. Since the causes for male's andrological issues are considered to be multifactorial, clinical data were included if outcome measures contained global (sexual) well-being issues, sexual dysfunction as well as ED, reproductive and anabolic hormone profiles, stress, psychological/physical/sexual health, and quality of life (QOL).

The randomized, double-blind, placebo-controlled trials with the plants ashwagandha, fenugreek, maca, and tongkat ali show many and quite promising evidence-based clinical qualities in managing men's health in the area of sexual health, physical strength (ergogenic), fertility, stress alleviation, and immunity, as discussed next.

4   *Trigonella foenum-graecum* (fenugreek; family Leguminosae)

Fenugreek is native to the southern Mediterranean regions, India, China, Northern Africa, and Ukraine. It is traditionally used for treating baldness, cancer, elevated cholesterol levels, diabetes, inflammations, microbial and fungal infections, stomach ulcers, and as an appetite stimulant [36, 37]. References also cite aphrodisiac, improving muscle strength, and male reproductive health [38].

The Commission E of the German Health Authorities [39], the Committee of Herbal Medicinal Products (HMPC) from the European Medicine Agency (EMA) [40], the World Health Organization (WHO) [41], and the European Scientific Cooperative on Phytotherapy [42] established a monograph of ripe, dried seeds of *T. foenum-graecum* L. (fenugreek). It was found to have a positive benefit–risk ratio for medicinal and traditional uses of "loss of appetite" and as "treatment for local/minor inflammation" [39, 40], as well as "adjuvant therapy in diabetes mellitus" and "management of hypercholesterolemia and hyperglycemia" [41, 42].

Due to its traditional nutritional properties, fenugreek can also be found in various foods [43]. The European Food Safety Authority sees no general risk for consumers [44] and the US Food and Drug Administration (US FDA) considers fenugreek seed extract Generally Recognized As Safe (GRAS) [45].

Evidence-based research concentrated mainly on the traditionally reported aphrodisiac and potential performance enhancing/anabolic effects of fenugreek seed extracts. Possible effects on resistance training [45–47] as well sexual function issues in healthy males [26, 48] were clinically investigated in placebo-controlled and double-blind RCTs.

The ergogenic benefit of fenugreek in subjects who underwent resistance training over a period of 8 weeks recorded a significant increase in lean body mass for the fenugreek group ($P = .004$), reduction in body fat (fenugreek: reduction $-2.3\% \pm 1.4\%$ vs placebo: $-0.39\% \pm 1.6\%$, $P < .001$), strength and muscular endurance accessed by leg press 1 repetition maximum (RM), i.e., the most weight one can lift once for an exercise (fenugreek: 84.6 ± 36.2 kg vs placebo: 48 ± 29.5 kg, $P < .001$), and bench press 1 RM (fenugreek: 9.1 ± 6.9 kg vs placebo: 4.3 ± 5.6 kg, $P = .01$) [46]. For free testosterone, a nonsignificant decrease over time by -10% was observed and for placebo a $+17.5\%$ increase. A second study with the same experimental setup as described in Poole et al. [46] demonstrated significant group × time interaction effects over the 8-week period for percent body fat (fenugreek: $-1.77\% \pm 1.52\%$, placebo: $-0.55\% \pm 1.72\%$, $P = .048$), total testosterone (fenugreek: 0.97 ± 2.67 ng/mL, placebo: -2.10 ± 3.75 ng/mL, $P = .018$), and bioavailable testosterone (fenugreek: 1.32 ± 3.45 ng/mL, placebo: -1.69 ± 3.94 ng/mL, $P = .049$) [47]. Significant effects over time were observed for bench- and leg-press 1 RM, lean body mass, and estradiol (E_2), where the increase in testosterone did not correspond with an increase in E_2 and 5-α-reductase. Fenugreek may potentially be an aromatase and 5-α-reductase inhibitor [47].

During a controlled resistance training program with 60 (18–35 years) healthy male subjects, no significant differences in 1-RM bench/leg press and repetitions to failure in bench/leg press could be demonstrated between groups [45]. In both groups, free testosterone increased (fenugreek $+98.7\%$ at end of study, $P < .001$ and placebo $+48.8\%$, $P < .01$) and was significantly different between the groups ($P < .05$). Total testosterone did not change significantly within and between groups. Significant body fat reduction was observed only in the fenugreek group in thigh ($P < .05$), triceps ($P < .01$), and chest ($P < .01$), but not in the placebo group. No serious adverse events occurred.

The effects of fenugreek on male libido, reflecting sexual drive, urge, and desire, were investigated in 60 healthy subjects (age 25–52 years) with low libido, but without ED in an RCT trial for 6 weeks [48]. There was a significant increase in total Derogatis Interview for Sexual Functioning-Self Report (DISF-SR) scores, which is a 21-item questionnaire, including the four domains: sexual cognition/fantasy, sexual arousal, sexual behavior/experience, and orgasm, designed to measure quality of sexual functioning, with fenugreek intake at 600 mg/day compared to placebo ($P < .01$) at end of trial. No changes were reported for the placebo group. The questionnaire for QOL for rating satisfaction for fenugreek showed an increase in libido ($+81.5\%$), recovery time ($+66.7\%$), and quality of sexual performance ($+63\%$). No changes were observed in the placebo group. Testosterone and prolactin levels did not change over time in either group (within normal reference range) and no correlations between different study parameters were identified.

The effects on possible androgen deficiency symptoms, sexual function, and androgenic hormone levels were investigated in 120 healthy aged males (43–70 years) for a treatment period of 12 weeks [26]. Fenugreek seed extract at 600 mg/day showed a significant decrease in total score of Aging Male Syndrome (AMS) over time and between groups ($P < .01$). Sexual function DISF-SR changed significantly over time with fenugreek intake ($P = .006$). The hormone levels for sex hormone binding globulin (SHBG), dehydroepiandrosterone sulfate (DHEA-S), androstenedione, E_2, and prolactin did not change over time and between groups. Small increases in total and free testosterone were observed after 12 weeks with fenugreek intake. In summary, the results showing the effects of fenugreek in conjunction with resistance training indicate a significant impact on body composition and an overall performance-enhancing benefit. However, the effects on reproductive hormones are inconsistent. Androgenic effects of fenugreek showed consistent findings in the clinical trials. Fenugreek is one of the top 20 selling herbs in the United States and the fact that it is officially monographed (Com. E [39], HMPC [40]) allows for market authorization in Europe. It has been demonstrated in a clinical study that fenugreek in combination with *Lespedeza cuneata* (Chinese bush clover) exhibits potential as an alternative to testosterone hormone therapy [49].

5   *Withania somnifera* (ashwagandha; family Solanaceae)

The traditional Ayurveda medicinal herb *W. somnifera* is native to India, parts of Africa, and the Mediterranean area and has already been in use for thousands of years in India for healing, alleviating, and preventing several ailments. It is commonly thought that ashwagandha exhibits various actions in males and females, including adaptogenic, antiarrthritic, antiepileptic, analgesic, antiinflammatory, anticancer, aphrodisiac, neuroprotective, antimicrobial, spermatogenic, hepatoprotective, astringent, hypoglycemic and hypolipidemic, ergogenic, and cardioactive effects [50–56].

The WHO monograph [53] of *Radix Withaniae* lists the plant's medical uses as an "antistress agent to improve reaction time and as a general tonic to increase energy, improve overall health and prevent diseases in athletes and the elderly." In 2013, the EMA finally announced that it was not possible to establish a Community Herbal Monograph for *W. somnifera* due to insufficient data for extract specifications that meet EU requirements [57]. In 2011, the evaluation process was rejected due to insufficient pharmaceutical quality data and lack of marketed ashwagandha products [58, 59]. However, the well-known Ayurvedic multiherb tonic formulation Chyawanprash is available in the European Union [52].

Throughout the last few years several clinical trials with ashwagandha focused primarily on the adaptogenic potential of this herb in the area of psychological stress and anxiety [60–65], followed by sexual dysfunction and spermatogenic effects [66, 67], as well as anabolic effects in sportsmen [68].

When analyzing effects of ashwagandha on sexual dysfunction, males (age 18–60 years, $N = 95$) with psychogenic ED, a serum testosterone level > 239 ng/dL, and supplemented with ashwagandha root powder at 6 g/day showed no significant difference between ashwagandha and placebo after 60 days ($P > .05$). However, significant changes were observed in the International Index of Erectile Function (IIEF)-item 4 ("maintenance of erection after penetration,", $P < .01$) and IIEF-item 8 ("enjoyable sexual intercourse," $P < .05$) [66]. The spermatogenic effects of ashwagandha in 46 male infertile patients with oligozoospermia (age 22–40 years) demonstrated increased sperm count (+ 167%), semen volume (+ 53%), and sperm motility (+ 57%) compared to baseline ($P < .0001$ for all), and hormone levels of testosterone (+ 17%, $P < .001$) and luteinizing hormone (+ 34%, $P < .002$) with 675 mg/day ashwagandha over 90 days. Only minimal and insignificant changes of the outcomes were observed with the placebo [67].

Anabolic effects of ashwagandha root extract (600 mg/day, KSM-66) were investigated in 57 healthy males aged 18–50 years with no experience in resistance training [69]. Over 8 weeks with the resistance training program, beneficial effects were observed in both groups; however, a greater significant increase for the herb in upper ($P = .001$) and lower body ($P = .04$) strength and better muscle recovery ($P = .03$) was seen compared to placebo. Also, a significantly greater increase in the muscle size of the arm ($P = .01$) and chest ($P < .001$) were observed. There were no group differences between *W. somnifera* and placebo, except for chest muscle size. Over time a greater increase in testosterone ($P = .004$) was observed in the *W. somnifera* group compared to placebo; however, this was not significant between groups ($P = .42$).

In summary, ashwagandha has demonstrated the ability to reduce anxiety and stress. It was not able to provide relief in psychogenic-related ED although semen quality and reproductive hormones improved significantly. The clinical use of ashwagandha in semen quality improvement has been shown in previous investigations with normozoospermic, oligozoospermic, and asthenozoospermic infertile males, and normozoospermic males with psychogenic stress-related infertility [70–72]. Treatment with the plant extract improved muscle strength and testosterone levels.

6   *Lepidium meyenii* (maca; family Brassicaceae)

Maca, an Andean plant, can be found in several South American countries but has been cultivated for more than 2000 years exclusively on the plateaus between 4000 and 4500 m in the Peruvian Central Andes as food and medicine [68, 73]. The traditional medical uses of maca dried root extract are mainly related to sexual dysfunction and lack of energy, and therefore it is well known for its adaptogenic and aphrodisiac as well as fertile-enhancing effects [73–75]. The monograph for Natural Health Products from Health Canada [76] lists the plant's uses or purpose: (1) "Helps to support emotional aspects of sexual health" (3–3.5 g/day), (2) "Helps to support healthy mood balance during menopause" (2–3.5 g/day), and (3)

"Provides antioxidants" (up to 3 g/day). A dietary supplement intake of 1–3 g/day maca extract is considered to be safe (USP-DS-EC) [77].

In 2014, Peruvian maca root powder exports grew by 111% due to the increase in demand from the United States, China, and Japan. The largest importer was the United States with US$9.7 million, followed by Hong Kong (US$5.3 million) and China (US$5 million) [78]. Due to the surge in demand, prices of maca increased. Maca then began to be planted in the high mountain region in Southwest China [79]. Eventually, an overproduction of domestically grown maca had caused a drastic price reduction in 2016. Since it is planted in very different regions, the phytochemistry and composition of the plant may vary considerably, and thus quality, safety, and efficacy of maca products cannot be ascertained [80]. However, it has not lost its allure and, according to the US Natural Channel, it was a top 20 selling herbal supplement in 2017 [29]. Through the last decade and until today, several clinical studies (randomized, double blind, placebo controlled) have been initiated to support the medicinal use of maca extract, analyzing the effects on sexual performance, reproductive hormones, semen quality, and anabolic and ergogenic effects [81–85].

With regard to sexual desire in healthy males (age 21–56 years, $n = 57$), the effects of maca (1500 mg/day or 3000 mg/day of gelatinized extract) over a 12-week period demonstrated a significant increase in self-perception at week 8 (+ 40%) and week 12 (+ 42.2%) with no between-group differences in testosterone. Reproductive hormones did not change over time in all maca and placebo groups [81].

Reproductive hormone profile and semen analysis were investigated in another study of 20 healthy males aged 20–40 years over 12 weeks, with 1.75 g/day dried powdered maca root [84]. There were no significant differences in any semen parameter between groups over time ($P > .05$). However, increasing trends could be observed in the maca group for sperm count (+ 20%), motile sperm count (+ 14%), sperm concentration (+ 14%), semen volume (+ 9%), and normal sperm morphology (+ 21%). No significant changes were observed in hormones (luteinizing hormone, follicle-stimulating hormone, prolactin, E_2, testosterone, thyroxin, and thyroid stimulating hormone).

The influence of maca root extract on well-being and sexual performance was investigated over 12 weeks in 50 males (age 36 ± 5 years) with mild ED supplemented with 1200 mg of dried pulverized maca root [82]. There was a significant increase in sexual well-being IIEF-5 score in both groups with a greater increase in the maca group ($+ 1.6 \pm 11; P < .001$) compared to placebo ($+ 0.5 \pm 0.6$). Similar results showed the Satisfaction Profile score for psychological performance, which improved significantly in the maca group ($+ 9 \pm 6$) than in the placebo group ($+ 6 \pm 5$). Hormones (follicle-stimulating hormone, luteinizing hormone, prolactin, total and free testosterone) did not change significantly in both groups.

The effect of maca on endurance performance and sexual desire was investigated (RCT crossover) with 2 g/day dried powdered maca root in eight trained cycling sportsmen over a 14-day supplementation [83]. There was a significant improvement ("faster") in time for subjects in the maca group ($P = .001$); however, neither significant differences in the placebo group, nor significant differences between groups ($P = .49$) were observed. Overall sexual desire increased in the maca group ($P = .01$) and the changes were significantly different compared to placebo ($P = .03$).

Based on a systematic review of five studies (three RCTs, two uncontrolled observational studies (UOSs)), published in 2016, favorable effects of maca were found for sperm motility in infertile men (one RCT) or showed positive effects of maca on several semen quality parameters (two RCTs, UOSs) [29]. However, judging by the total number of trials and small sample size, the risk of bias of the included studies prevented the drawing of firm conclusions. Hence, more rigorous studies were proposed by the author. An earlier published systematic review concluded that there was limited proof for maca's improvement of sexual function [86]. In summary, with recent advances the overall sexual desire and erectile function of males increased significantly during treatment with maca although the improvement was not linked to increase in testosterone.

7 *Eurycoma longifolia* (tongkat ali; family Simaroubaceae)

In Southeast Asia *E. longifolia* is one of the best-known plants in traditional herbal medicine and is indigenous to countries like Malaysia, Indonesia, and Vietnam and in some regions of Cambodia, Myanmar, and Thailand [87, 88]. *E. longifolia* is used traditionally as an aphrodisiac agent, and is well known for its ergogenic activity and ability to treat sexual dysfunction. It also has other effects such as antimalarial, antiproliferative/cytotoxic, antiinflammatory, antimicrobial, antianxiolytic, and antidiabetic properties, as well as prevention of osteoporosis and insecticidal activity [87–89]. The therapeutic importance of tongkat ali for the local population of Malaysia and Indonesia is expressed by the fact that more than 200 products with tongkat ali are available on the Malaysian market [90].

Tongkat ali has gained approval as a Natural Health Product ingredient by Health Canada, with self-affirmed US-FDA GRAS status [91]. Certification is granted for the standardized and patented tongkat ali root extract (LJ100/Physta, Phytes Biotek/Biotropics, Malaysia; US Patent No. 7,132,117, EU Patent No. 1313491) with the bioactive peptide fraction of a

4300-Da glycopeptide with 36 amino acids: standardized to 0.8%–1.5% eurycomanone, > 40% glycosaponin, > 30% polysaccharide, and > 22% protein [92]. The same extract is currently evaluated as a novel food in Europe [33].

In Asia, tongkat ali is known as Malaysian ginseng [93]. In Malaysia, due to regulatory categorization, products based on herbals and used traditionally must be registered as traditional medicine, which is akin to the dietary supplement category in the United States. Recent regulatory requirements have allowed tongkat ali to be combined with minerals and vitamins that fall under the health supplement category provided it is accompanied by clinical study that supports its safety and efficacy for the combination [34]. The expansion of herbs beyond andrology is an indication of acceptance from a narrow use in men to a wider use for men of all ages and also potentially in women albeit at a lower dose to address hormonal imbalance in aging women.

Several private medical practitioners in Malaysia, Vietnam, and China are beginning to dispense tongkat ali as an alternative treatment for testosterone replacement therapy. In Malaysia, Prof. Tambi was one of the first andrologists to administer tongkat ali in patients who were hypogonadic and suffering from idiopathic infertility [94]. It is prescribed as an alternative to testosterone replacement therapy in some clinics in Malaysia. It is also indexed in the Malaysian index for drugs, i.e., Monthly Index of Medical Specialties, a multichannel drug and resource portal providing drug information, medical education, and services connecting healthcare communities. It is also used as a supplement to enhance vigor, sexual and physical vitality, testosterone deficiency in hypogonadic males, various sexual and reproductive disorders, and idiopathic infertility, and to reduce symptoms of aging in males. In addition, it improves fatigue recovery and physical strength among sporting individuals, reduces mental stress by decreasing cortisol in both men and women, and boosts immunity in adults. Likewise, it is sold in Vietnam.

In the last few years, major efforts have been made within the scope of evidence-based clinical trials with tongkat ali extracts, namely Physta (PTA) (Physta, Biotropics Malaysia Berhad), investigating the overall effect on male sexual well-being, including infertility problems, anabolic properties, and performance-enhancing effects, as well as psychological stress issues. Primarily, randomized, double-blind, and placebo-controlled trials were conducted [94–103].

The ergogenic effect of PTA in andrology was investigated first in 14 volunteers taking 100 mg of PTA for 8 weeks. PTA significantly increased fat free mass, reduced body fat percentages, increased gross muscle power, increased significantly arm circumference, and reduced the mean sEMG reading [104]. The anabolic effect was further confirmed in a study by Talbot [105], where 30 volunteers taking 100 mg or a placebo had testosterone levels that were 16.4% higher and cortisol levels 32.3% lower in the PTA group compared to the placebo group at the end of 24-hour endurance cycling. In another study on 25 physically active elderly subjects, supplemented with 400 mg of PTA for 4 weeks, increased total testosterone (15.1% in men, 48.6% in women), free testosterone (61.1% in men, 122% in women), muscular force (16.6% in men, 13.7% in women), and decreased SHBG (20.8% in women, 5.6% men) were observed [106]. The findings provide potential evidence for treating age-related sarcopenia.

Possible immune-modulatory effects of PTA and its influences on mental states were observed with 200 mg/day of PTA extract over a period of 4 weeks [103]. The Scoring of Immunological Vigor and immunological grade/age were significantly higher with PTA compared to placebo ($P < .05$). The numbers of total, naïve, CD4$^+$ T cells were higher with PTA than in the placebo group ($P < .05$). The mental Profile of Mood States domain of anxiety and tension in the PTA group reached near significance ($P < .054$) compared to placebo.

The stress-alleviating effect of PTA was demonstrated during a 4-week supplementation with 200 mg/day of PTA [97] in both men and women. After PTA intake, "tension" (− 11%), "anger" (− 12%), and "confusion" (− 15%) were significantly reduced compared to placebo. Cortisol values significantly decreased by 16% and testosterone level increased by + 37% compared to placebo at the end of the study. This corresponds with an earlier preliminary investigation by Tambi [93] on andropause in 30 men, taking 100 mg of LJ100/PTA daily for 3 weeks, where DHEA-S, the precursor to testosterone, increased from 26% to 47% in 3 weeks, while SHBG reduced from 36% to 66% of the men. Improving trends were also observed in the AMS and Sexual Health Inventory Questionnaire score.

Effects of PTA on sexual well-being, QOL, and physical fitness were examined in 109 healthy males (30–55 years) for 12 weeks with 300 mg/day of PTA extract [96]. After 12 weeks there was no significant difference in the overall QOL measured with the 36-Item Short Form Health Survey (SF-36) for both groups. However, the domain "physical functioning" of SF-36 QOL improved significantly for PTA subjects ($P = .006$) and in between groups ($P = .028$). The overall ED score of the IIEF increased significantly from baseline to week 12 as compared to placebo ($P < .001$), indicating a meaningful improvement in erectile functioning in subjects on PTA. A higher score in the overall "Sexual Function" domain in IIEF ($P < .001$) was observed in the PTA group. PTA increased sexual libido by 14%. Hormonal profiles showed no significant changes or differences between both groups throughout the trial. There was a reduction in fat in subgroups of BMI > 35 in the PTA group.

The anabolic and doping effects of PTA were analyzed using the ratio testosterone to epitestosterone (T:E) in healthy nonathletic males [98]. The T:E ratio of urine samples remained in the "normal" range of < 1, without significant difference between both groups. The weight lifting force significantly increased with PTA over time (+ 14 kg, $P = .0166$) compared to placebo showing an improvement in muscle strength without doping effects. The nondoping effect was further confirmed by the National Sports Institute of Malaysia who tested selected national athletes who were on PTA supplementation at an accredited laboratory conforming to World Anti-Doping Code International Standard of Laboratories [107].

A herbal combination of PTA root extract (200 mg/day, Physta) and *Polygonum minus* aqueous leaves extract (100 mg/day), from Biotropics Malaysia Berhad (PTA-P), was investigated for sexual well-being and QOL in healthy males [100]. Thirty subjects with a testosterone level of ≤ 450 ng/dL, an index of erectile function score 17–25 (IIEF-5), and ages between 40 and 65 years were evaluated in an RCT over a period of 12 weeks. At 6 and 12 weeks, significant improvements were observed for Sexual Health Inventory in Men (SHIM) and Erection Hardness Scale (EHS) scores over time for the herbal combination compared to placebo (a difference of 39% and 26% for SHIM and EHS, respectively). The Sexual Intercourse Attempt improved in 7 of 11 items, and AMS showed significant reduction by 24% compared to placebo; total testosterone increased (PTA-P: 10.36%; placebo 4:28%).

Late-onset hypogonadism, which results in a severe drop of testosterone levels in men, can affect men. The standardized root extract of PTA was found to be an effective testosterone booster in managing men with late-onset hypogonadism [108]. In the study, where 76 patients took 200 mg of PTA per day for 4 weeks, normal testosterone levels rose from 35.5% to 90.8% of the men. Mean testosterone levels improved from 5.66 nmol (before study) to 8.31 nmol (after study), which represents an increase of 46% in 30 days.

There are several causes for infertility in men and a lack of functional sperm is one of them. In two separate clinical studies, the seminal volume increased with PTA supplementation. In the study by Ismail et al. [96], an increase in sperm motility (+ 44.4%) and semen volume (+ 18.2%) was observed in 22 subjects. When PTA was supplemented in men with idiopathic infertility for a period of 9 months in three cycles with each cycle totaling 3 months of treatment, improvements in semen parameters were observed. Sperm volume, concentration, and morphology improved from baseline to each of the three cycles, and by the third cycle an improvement of 19.3%, 65% ($P < .007$), and 94% ($P < .003$), respectively, was observed. The proprietary extract significantly improved the sperm quality in these patients, allowing for 11 (14.7%) spontaneous pregnancies [94]. *E. longifolia* has also been reported to improve bone density possibly preventing testosterone deficiency-associated osteoporosis as a result of aging [109].

8   Challenges in using herbals

Considering that the methods of preparation either do not meet regulatory standards or are not similar to the traditional preparation, the use of herbals is sometimes associated with a lack of safety and efficacy. In 2011, for example, a shipment of fenugreek seeds from Egypt was said to cause Shiga toxin-producing *Escherichia coli* outbreaks in Europe causing severe health problems after eating raw fenugreek sprouts harvested from contaminated seeds [110]. As a result, a robust regulatory system to check the quality of the product has been in place for most countries.

While many of the herbs are traditionally prepared as a decoction, the same herbs are also powdered by other manufacturers and then sold without meeting quality control standards. The concentration of bioactive compounds in such preparations is far less, therefore a physiological effect is not reached. In addition, the often nondigestible powdered material may pose a health risk causing damage particularly to kidneys and liver. The shift toward producing standardized extract is now the gold standard to ensure batch-to-batch consistency and safety, and the presence of bioactives in consistent and reproducible amounts follows worldwide accepted pharmaceutical manufacturing procedures.

9   Conclusion

The traditional belief that herbs possess aphrodisiac and performance-enhancing properties was largely responsible for their use. Ethnobotanical surveys list hundreds of traditional medicinal herbs with reported aphrodisiac properties [23, 111, 112]. Knowledge of herbal medicine is based on long-term historical uses of plants for various diseases contributing to our healthcare worldwide. Currently, modern evidence-based clinical research determines whether there is justification for such claims. In randomized, double-blind, placebo-controlled trials the herbs ashwagandha, fenugreek, maca, and tongkat ali show many and quite promising evidence-based clinical qualities in managing men's (sexual) health. A huge variety of herbal ingredients with possible bioactive potential have been identified; however, their contribution to beneficial effects thus showing significance is limited and the underlying mechanisms of action are still not clear. The dosage used for each herb is quite wide with the lowest dosage for efficacy reported for tongkat ali. Besides efficacy, safety aspects of daily herbal supplementation are of major concern. Only for tongkat ali has it been demonstrated, in addition to safety profiles, that the ratio T:E was not influenced during supplementation and was stable, falling within the normal range, indicating that this herb is good for physical performance without doping effects.

References

[1] Pan SY, Litscher G, Gao SH, Zhou SF, Yu ZL, Chen HQ, Zhang SF, Tang MK, Sun JN, Ko KM. Historical perspective of traditional indigenous medical practices: the current renaissance and conservation of herbal resources. Evid Based Complement Alternat Med 2014;2014, 525340.

[2] Lemonnier N, Zhou GB, Prasher B, Mukerji M, Chen Z, Brahmachari SK, Noble D, Auffray C, Sagner M. Traditional knowledge-based medicine: a review of history, principles, and relevance in the present context of P4 systems medicine. Prog Prev Med 2017;2(7):e0011.

[3] Wang G, Mao B, Xiong ZY, Fan T, Chen XD, Wang L, Liu GJ, Liu J, Guo J, Chang J, Wu TX. The quality of reporting of randomized controlled trials of traditional Chinese medicine: a survey of 13 randomly selected journals from mainland China. Clin Ther 2007;29:1456–67.

[4] Gwin P. How ancient remedies are changing modern medicine long overlooked by Western science, traditional Chinese treatments are yielding cutting-edge cures, https://www.nationalgeographic.com/magazine/2019/01/; 2019. [Accessed 2 February 2019].

[5] Subhose V, Srinivas P, Narayana A. Basic principles of pharmaceutical science in Ayurvĕda. Bull Indian Inst Hist Med 2005;35(2):83–92.

[6] Abdel-Azim NS, Shams KA, Shahat AA, El Missiry MM, Ismail SI, Hammouda FM. Egyptian herbal drug industry: challenges and future prospects. Res J Med Plants 2011;5(2):136–44. https://doi.org/10.3923/rjmp.2011.136.144.

[7] Zolla C. Traditional medicine in Latin America, with particular reference to Mexico. J Ethnopharmacol 1980;2(1):37–51.

[8] Euromonitor International. Herbal/traditional products-market size. Retrieved from http://www.euromonitor.com/herbal-traditional-products-in-Malaysia; 2016.

[9] Prnewswire. Herbal medicine market size, forecast and trend analysis, 2014–2024. Retrieved from https://www.prnewswire.com/news-releases/the-global-herbal-medicine-market-is-expected-to-reach-usd-117-02-billion-by-2024- -300726926.html; 2018.

[10] Simons J, Carey MP. Prevalence of sexual dysfunction: results from a decade of research. Arch Sex Behav 2001;30(2):177–219.

[11] Laumann EQ, Nicolosi A, Glasser DB, Paik A, Gingell C, Moreira E, Wang T. Sexual problems among women and men aged 40-80y: prevalence and correlates identified in the Global Study of Sexual Attitudes and Behaviors. Int J Impot Res 2005;17:39–57.

[12] Nicolosi A, Buvat J, Glasser JB, Hartmann U, Laumann EO, Gingell C. Sexual behavior, sexual dysfunctions and related help seeking patterns in middle-aged and elderly Europeans: the global study of sexual attitudes and behaviors. World J Urol 2006;24:423–8.

[13] Laumann EO, Glasser DB, Neves RCS, Moreira Jr ED. A population-based survey of sexual activity, sexual problems and associated help-seeking behavior pattern in mature adults in the United States of America. Int J Impot Res 2009;21:171–8.

[14] Nicolosi A, Glasser DB, Kim SC, Marumo K, Laumnn EO. Sexual behavior and dysfunction and help-seeking patterns in adults aged 40-80 years in the urban population of Asian countries. BJU Int 2005;95:609–14.

[15] Park K, Hwang EC, Kim S-O. Prevalence and medical management of erectile dysfunction in Asia. Asian J Androl 2011;13:543–9.

[16] Lewis RW. Epidemiology of sexual dysfunction in Asia compared to the rest of the world. Asian J Androl 2011;13:152–8.

[17] Ayta IA, McKinlay JB, Krane RJ. The likely worldwide increase in erectile dysfunction between 1995 and 2015 and some possible policy consequences. BJU Int 1999;84(1):50–6.

[18] Tharyan P, Gopalakrishanan G. Clinical evidence: erectile dysfunction. Men Health BMJ 2006;03:1803.

[19] Woolven L, Snider T. Herbs and erectile dysfunction: a review of traditional use and modern clinical evidence. American Botanical Council ABC HerbalGram 2013;99:35–45.

[20] Tan HM, Tong SF, Ho CCK. Men's health: sexual dysfunction, physical and psychological health—is there a link? J Sex Med 2012;9(3):663–71.

[21] Arasalingam S, Sidi H, Guan NC, Das S, Midin M, Musa R. Premature ejaculation in urban Malaysian population: the association between erectile dysfunction (ED), anxiety and depression. Int Med J Malaysia 2016;15(1):89–96.

[22] Tsertsvadze A, Fink HA, Yazdi F, MacDonald R, Bella AJ, et al. Clinical guidelines. Oral phosphodiesterase-5 inhibitors and hormonal treatment for erectile dysfunction: a systematic review and meta-analysis. Ann Intern Med 2009;15:650–61.

[23] MacKay D. Nutrients and botanicals for erectile dysfunction: examining the evidence. Altern Med Rev 2004;9(1):4–16.

[24] Malviya N, Jain S, Gupta VP, Vyas S. Recent studies on aphrodisiac herbs for the management of male sexual dysfunction—a review. Acta Pol Pharm Drug Res 2011;68(1):3–8.

[25] Lee JKC, Tan RBW, Chung E. Erectile dysfunction treatment and traditional medicine—can East and West medicine coexist? Transl Androl Urol 2017;6(1):91–100.

[26] Rao A, Steels E, Inder WJ, Abraham S, Vitetta L. Testofen, a specialized *Trigonella foenum-graecum* seed extract reduces age-related symptoms of androgen decrease, increases testosterone levels and improves sexual function in healthy aging males in a double-blind randomised clinical study. Aging Male 2016;19(2):134–42. Available at: www.ncbi.nlm.nih.gov/pubmed/26791805. [Accessed 5 June 2018].

[27] Steels E, Steele ML, Harold M, Coulson S. Efficacy of a proprietary *Trigonella foenum-graecum* L. de-husked seed extract in reducing menopausal symptoms in otherwise healthy women: a double-blind, randomized, placebo-controlled study. Phytother Res 2017;31(9):1316–22. Available at: www.ncbi.nlm.nih.gov/pubmed/28707431. [Accessed 5 July 2018].

[28] Maheshwari A, Verma N, Swaroop A, et al. Efficacy of Furosap, a novel *Trigonella foenum-graecum* seed extract, in enhancing testosterone level and improving sperm profile in male volunteers. Int J Med Sci 2017;14(1):58–66. Available at: www.ncbi.nlm.nih.gov/bmed/28138310. [Accessed 5 July 2018].

[29] Smith T, Kawa K, Eckl V, Morton C, Stredney R. Herbal supplement sales in US increase 8.5% in 2017, topping $8 billion. Strongest sales growth in more than 15 years bolstered by continued popularity of Ayurvedic herbs and new formulations of botanicals with general health and nutrition benefits. HerbalGram 2018;119:62–71.

[30] Wachtel-Galor S, Benzie IFF. Herbal medicine an introduction to its history, usage, regulation, current trends, and research needs. In: Herbal medicine: Biomolecular and clinical aspects. 2nd ed. Boca Raton, FL: CRC Press/Taylor & Francis; 2011 [chapter 1].

[31] Nocerino E, Amato M, Izzo AA. The aphrodisiac and adaptogenic properties of ginseng. Fitoterapia 2000;71(Suppl. 1):1–5.

[32] Talbott SM. Improving biochemical balance and energy, https://www.doctoroz.com/article/improving-biochemical-balance-and-energy; 2013.

[33] Biotropics Malaysia Berhad. Application for the approval of tongkat ali root extract as a novel food, https://ec.europa.eu/food/sites/food/files/safety/docs/novel-food_sum_ongoing-app_eurycoma-longifolia.pdf; 2016.

[34] George A, Udani J, Abidin NZ, Yusof A. Efficacy and safety of *Eurycoma longifolia* (Physta®) water extract plus multivitamins on quality of life, mood and stress: a randomized placebo-controlled and parallel study. Food Nutr Res 2018;62. https://doi.org/10.29219/fnr.v62.1374. Published 2018 Oct 16.

[35] Macpherson H, Rowsell R, Cox KH, Reddan J, Meyer D, Scholey A, Pipingas A. The effects of four-week multivitamin supplementation on mood in healthy older women: a randomized controlled trial. Evid Based Complement Alternat Med 2016;2016. https://doi.org/10.1155/2016/3092828. Published online 2016 Nov 15.

[36] Tyler VE. The honest herbal: a sensible guide to the use of herbs and related remedies. 3rd ed. New York, London Norwood: iPPP Pharmaceutical Products Press; 1993. 375 pp.[37]Hudson T. Fenugreek (*Trigonella foenum-graecum*): An overview of research and clinical indications. Retrieved from http://cdn.naturaldispensary.com/downloads/A_Research_Review_of_Fenugreek.pdf. [Accessed July 2016].Hudson T. Fenugreek (*Trigonella foenum-graecum*): An overview of research and clinical indications. Retrieved from http://cdn.naturaldispensary.com/downloads/A_Research_Review_of_Fenugreek.pdf. [Accessed July 2016].

[38] Aswar U, Bodhankar SL, Mohan V, Thakurdesai PA. Effect of furostanol glycosides from *Trigonella foenum-graecum* on the reproductive system of male albino rats. Phytother Res 2010;24:1482–8.

[39] *Foenugraeci* semen Fenugreek seed—Bockshornsamen. German Commission E; February 1, 1990. Bundesanzeiger.

[40] Community herbal monograph on *Trigonella foenum-graecum* L., semen. EMA; 27 January 2011. Retrieved from http://www.ema.europa.eu/docs/en_GB/document_library/Herbal_-_Community_herbal_monograph/2011/02/WC500102315.pdf.

[41] Semen *Trigonellae Foenugraeci*. In: WHO monographs on selected medicinal plants, Part 3; 2007. p. 338–48.

[42] *Trigonellae Foenugraeci* semen—Fenugreek. In: European Scientific Cooperative on Phytotherapy ESCOP monographs. 2nd ed; 2003. p. 511–20.

[43] Wani SA, Kumar P. Fenugreek: a review on its nutritional properties and utilization in various food products. J Saudi Soc Agric Sci 2016. http://www.sciencedirect.com/science/article/pii/S1658077X15301065.

[44] European Food Safety Authority EFSA. Conclusion on the peer review of the pesticide risk assessment of the active substance fenugreek seed powder (FEN560). EFSA J 2010;8(3):1448.

[45] Wankhede S, Mohan V, Thakurdesai P. Beneficial effects of fenugreek glycoside supplementation in male subjects during resistance training: a randomized controlled pilot study. J Sport Health Sci 2015;5(2):176–82.

[46] Poole C, Bushey B, Foster C, Campbell B, Willoughby D, et al. The effects of a commercially available botanical supplement on strength, body composition, power output, and hormonal profiles in resistance-trained males. JISSN 2010;7:34.

[47] Wilborn C, Taylor L, Poole C, Foster C, Willoughby D, et al. Effects of a purported aromatase and 5 α-reductase inhibitor on hormone profiles in college-age men. Int J Sport Nutr Exerc Metab 2010;20(6):457–65.

[48] Steels E, Rao A, Vitetta L. Physiological aspects of male libido by standardized *Trigonella foenum-graecum* extract and mineral formulation. Phytother Res 2011;25(9):1294–300.

[49] Park HJ, Lee KS, Lee EK, Park NC. Efficacy and safety of a mixed extract of *Trigonella foenum-graecum* seed and *Lespedeza cuneata* in the treatment of testosterone deficiency syndrome: a randomized, double-blind, placebo-controlled clinical trial. World J Mens Health 2018;36(3):230–8. Published online 2018 Mar 22 https://doi.org/10.5534/wjmh.170004.

[50] Engels G, Brinckmann J. Ashwagandha—*Withania somnifera* family: Solanaceae. American Botanical Council ABC HerbalGram 2013;99:1–7.

[51] *Withania somnifera*—monograph. Altern Med Rev 2004;9(2):211–4.

[52] Upton R, editor. Ashwagandha root. *Withania somnifera*. Analytical, quality control and therapeutic monograph. American Herbal Pharmacopoeia; 2000. 25 pp.

[53] Radix *Withaniae*. In: WHO monographs on selected medicinal plants, Part 4; 2009. p. 373–91.

[54] Kumar V, Dey A, Hadimani M, Marcovic T, Emerald M. Chemistry and pharmacology of *Withania somnifera*: an update. Review. Association of Humanitas Medicine, 2015;5(1). http://koreascience.or.kr/article/ArticleFullRecord.jsp?cn=TJHOBI_2015_v5n1_1.1.

[55] Ashwagandha. Health Canada; April 18 2007. p. 1–3.

[56] Singh N, Bhalla M, de Jager P, Gica M. An overview on ashwagandha: a rejuvenator of Ayurveda. Afr J Tradit Complement Altern Med 2011;8(S):208–13.

[57] Public statement on *Withania somnifera* (L) Dunal, radix. EMA HMCP; 9 July 2013.

[58] Committee on Herbal Medicinal Products (HMPC). Call for scientific data for use in HMPC assessment work on *Withania somnifera* (L.) Dunal, radix. London: European Medicines Agency (EMA); 2011. Available at: www.ema.europa.eu/docs/en_GB/document_library/Herbal__Call_for_data/2011/07/WC500109102.pdf. [Accessed 4 July 2013].

[59] Committee on Herbal Medicinal Products (HMPC). Public statement on *Withania somnifera* (L.) Dunal, radix. London: European Medicines Agency (EMA); 20 November 2012. Available at: www.ema.europa.eu/docs/en_GB/document_library/Public_statement/2012/12/WC500136129.pdf. [Accessed 4 July 2013].

[60] Andrade C, Aswath A, Chaturvedi SK, Srinivasa M, Raguram R. A double-blind, placebo-controlled evaluation of anxiolytic efficacy of an ethanolic extract of *Withania somnifera*. Indian J Psychiatry 2000;42(3):295–301.

[61] Auddy B, Hazra J, Mitra A, Abedon B, Ghosal S. A standardized *Withania somnifera* extract significantly reduces stress-related parameters in chronically stressed humans: a double-blind, randomized, placebo-controlled study. JANA 2008;11(1):50–6.

[62] Cooley K, Szczurko O, Perri D, Mills EJ, Bernhardt B, et al. Naturopathic care for anxiety: a randomized controlled trial ISRCTN78958974. PLoS One 2009;4(8):e6628.

[63] Chandrasekhar K, Kapoor J, Anishetty S. A prospective, randomized double-blind, placebo-controlled study of safety and efficacy of a high-concentration full-spectrum extract of ashwagandha root in reducing stress and anxiety in adults. Indian J Psychol Med 2012;34(3):255–62.

[64] Khyati S, Anup T. A randomized double-blind placebo-controlled study of ashwagandha on generalized anxiety disorders. IAMJ 2013;1(5):1–7.

[65] Choudhary D, Bhattacharyya S, Joshi K. Body weight management in adults under chronic stress through treatment with ashwagandha root extract: a double-blind, randomized, placebo-controlled trial. J Evid Based Complement Alternat Med 2016;1–11.

[66] Mamidi P, Thakar AB. Efficacy of ashwagandha (*Withania somnifera* Dunal Linn) in the management of psychogenic erectile dysfunction. AYU 2011;32(3):322–8.

[67] Ambiye VR, Langade D, Dongee S, Aptikar P, Kulkarni M, et al. Clinical evaluation of the spermatogenic activity of root extract of ashwagandha (*Withania somnifera*) in oligospermic males: a pilot study. Evid Based Complement Alternat Med 2013;, 571420.

[68] Gonzales GF. Ethnobiology and ethnopharmacology of *Lepidium meyenii* (Maca), a plant from the Peruvian highlands. Evid Based Complement Alternat Med 2012;, 193496. 1–10.

[69] Wankhede S, Langade D, Joshi K, Sinha SR, Bhattacharyya S. Examining the effect of *Withania somnifera* supplementation on muscle strength and recovery: a randomized controlled trial. J Int Soc Sports Nutr 2015;12:43.

[70] Ahmad MK, Mahdi AA, Shukla KK, Islam N, Rajender S, et al. *Withania somnifera* improves semen quality by regulating reproductive hormone levels and oxidative stress in seminal plasma of infertile males. Fertil Steril 2009;94:989–96.

[71] Mahdi AA, Shukla KK, Ahmad MK, Rajender S, Shankhwar SN, et al. *Withania somnifera* improves semen quality in stress-related male fertility. Evid Based Complement Alternat Med 2011;2011. https://doi:10.1093/ecam/nep138.

[72] Shukla KK, Mahdi AA, Mishra V, Rajender S, Sankhwar SN, et al. *Withania somnifera* improves semen quality by combating oxidative stress and cell death and improving essential metal concentrations. Reprod Biomed Online 2011;22:421–7.

[73] Smith E. Maca root: modern rediscovery of an ancient Andean fertility food. J Am Herbalists Guild 2004;1:1–3.

[74] Hudson T. Maca: new insights on an ancient plant. Integr Med 2008/2009;7(6):54–7.

[75] Rosales-Hartshorn M. Maca: botanical medicine from the Andes. Adv Food Technol Nutr Sci Open J 2015;1(2):e1–6. https://doi.org/10.17140/AFTNSOJ-1-e001.

[76] Maca—*Lepidium meyenii*. In: Health natural product monograph. Health Canada; March 6, 2013. p. 1–6.

[77] Maca. USP Safety Review. http://www.usp.org/sites/default/files/usp_pdf/EN/dietarySupp/dsc2012samplesafety_review.pdf.Maca. USP Safety Review. http://www.usp.org/sites/default/files/usp_pdf/EN/dietarySupp/dsc2012samplesafety_review.pdf.

[78] Biopirateria, https://biopirateria.org/peruvian-maca-exports-up-109-last-year/?lang=en; 2015.

[79] Smith T. Maca madness: Chinese herb smugglers create chaos in the Peruvian Andes—consequences for the market, consumers, and local farming communities. American Botanical Council ABC HerbalGram 2015;105:47–55. Also in HerbalEGram 2014;11 (12).

[80] Beharry S, Heinrich M. Is the hype around the reproductive health claims of maca (*Lepidium meyenii* Walp.) justified? J Ethnopharmacol 2018;211(30):126–70.

[81] Gonzales GF, Cordova A, Vega K, Chung A, Villena A, Góñez C, Castillo S. Effect of *Lepidium meyenii* (Maca) on sexual desire and its absent relationship with serum testosterone levels in adult healthy men. Andrologia 2002;34(6):367–72.

[82] Zenico T, Cicero AFG, Valmorri L, Mercuriali M, Bercovich E. Subjective effects of *Lepidium meyenii* (Maca) extract on well-being and sexual performance in patients with erectile dysfunction: a randomized, double-blind clinical trial. Andrologia 2009;41:95–9.

[83] Stone M, Ibarra A, Roller M, Zangara A, Stevenson E. A pilot investigation into the effect of maca supplementation on physical activities and sexual desire in sportsmen. J Ethnopharmacol 2009;126(3):574–6.

[84] Gonzales GF, Cordova A, Vega K, Chung A, Villena A, Góñez C. Effect of *Lepidium meyenii* (Maca), a root with aphrodisiac and fertility-enhancing properties, on serum reproductive hormone levels in adult healthy men. J Endocrinol 2003;176(1):163–8.

[85] Melnikovova I, Fait T, Kolarova M, Fernandez EC, Milella L. Effect of *Lepidium meyenii* Walp. on semen parameters and serum hormone levels in healthy adult men: a double-blind, randomized, placebo-controlled pilot study. Evid Based Complement Alternat Med 2015;324369. https://doi.org/10.1155/2015/324369.

[86] Shin BC, Lee MS, Yang EJ, Ernst E. Maca (*L. meyenii*) for improving sexual function: a systematic review. BMC Complement Altern Med 2010;10:44.

[87] Bhat R, Karim AA. Tongkat Ali (*Eurycoma longifolia* Jack): a review on its ethnobotany and pharmacological importance. Fitoterapia 2010;81:669–79.

[88] Rehman SU, Choe K, Yoo HH. Review on a traditional herbal medicine, *Eurycoma longifolia* Jack (Tongkat Ali): its traditional uses, chemistry, evidence-based pharmacology and toxicology. Molecules 2016;21:331.

[89] Ulbricht C, Conquer J, Flanagan K, Isaac R, Rusie E, et al. An evidence-based systematic review of Tongkat Ali (*Eurycoma longifolia*) by Natural Standard Research Collaboration. J Diet Suppl 2013;10(1):54–83.

[90] Ang HH, Lee EL, Cheang HS. Determination of mercury by cold vapor atomic absorption spectrophotometer in Tongkat Ali preparations obtained in Malaysia. Int J Toxicol 2004;23(1):65–71.

[91] Tongkat Ali gains approval. Natural Outlook; November 18, 2013.

[92] Patent *Eurycoma longifolia* extract LJ100®/Physta® (http://biotropicsmalaysia.com/manufacturing/; http://phytesbiotek.com.my/).Patent *Eurycoma longifolia* extract LJ100®/Physta® (http://biotropicsmalaysia.com/manufacturing/; http://phytesbiotek.com.my/).

[93] Tambi MI, Saad JM. Water-soluble extract of *Eurycoma longifolia* jack as a potential natural energizer for healthy aging in men. First Asian Andrology Forum in Shanghai China; 2002.

[94] Tambi MI, Imran MK. *Eurycoma longifolia* Jack in managing idiopathic male infertility. Asian J Androl 2010;12:376–80.

[95] Muhamad AS, Kiew CC, Kiew OF, Abdullah MR, Lam CK. Effects of *Eurycoma longifolia* Jack supplementation on recreational athletes' endurance running capacity and physiological responses in the heat. Int J Appl Sports Sci 2010;22(2):1–19.

[96] Ismail SB, Mohammad WMZW, George A, Hussain NHN, Kamal ZMM, Liske E. Randomized clinical trial on the use of Physta® freeze-dried water extract of *Eurycoma longifolia* for the improvement of quality of life and sexual well-being in men. Evid Based Complement Alternat Med 2012;2012. https://doi:10.1155/2012/429268.

[97] Talbott SM, Talbott JA, George A, Pugh M. Effect of Tongkat Ali on stress hormones and psychological mood state in moderately stressed subjects. J Int Soc Sports Nutr 2013;10(1):28.

[98] George A, Liske E, Chen CK, Ismail SB. The *Eurycoma longifolia* freeze-dried water extract-Physta® does not change normal ratios of testosterone to epitestosterone in healthy males. J Sports Med Doping Stud 2013;3:3. http://www.omicsonline.org/the-eurycoma-longifolia-freeze-dried-water-extract-physta-does-not-change-normal-ratios-of-testosterone-to-epitestosterone-in-healthy-males-2161-0673.1000127.php?aid=18813.

[99] Chen CK, Wan Mohamad WMZ, Ooi FK, Ismail SB, Abdullah MR, et al. Supplementation of *Eurycoma longifolia* Jack extract for 6 weeks does not affect urinary testosterone: epitestosterone ratio, liver and renal functions in male recreational athletes. Int J Prev Med 2014;5:728–33.

[100] Udani JK, George AA, Musthapa M, Pakdaman MN, Abas A. Effects of a proprietary freeze-dried water extract of *Eurycoma longifolia* (Physta®) and *Polygonum minus* on sexual performance and well-being in men: a randomized double-blind, placebo-controlled study. Evid Based Complement Alternat Med 2014;2014. https://doi:10.1155/2014/179529.

[101] Muhamad AS, Ooi FK, Chen CK. Effects of *Eurycoma longifolia* on natural killer cells and endurance running performance. Int J Sports Sci 2015;5(3):93–8.

[102] Ooi FK, Afifah MH, Chen CK, Asnizam AM. Combined effects of *Eurycoma longifolia* Jack supplementation and a circuit training programme on bone metabolism markers, muscular strength and power, and immune functions in adult men. IJERSS 2015;2(3):1–10.

[103] George A, Suzuki N, Abas AB, Mohri K, Utsuyama M, et al. Immunomodulation in middle-aged humans via the ingestion of Physta® standardized root water extract of *Eurycoma longifolia* Jack—a randomized, double-blind, placebo-controlled parallel study. Phytother Res 2016;30(4):627–35.

[104] Hamzah S, Yusof A. The ergogenic effects of Tongkat ali (*Eurycoma longifolia*): a pilot study. Br J Sports Med 2003;37:464–70.

[105] Talbott S, Talbott J, Negrete J, Jones M, Nichols M, Roza J. Effect of *Eurycoma longifolia* extract on anabolic balance during endurance exercise. J Int Soc Sports Nutr 2006;3(1):S32.

[106] Henkel RR, Wang R, Bassett SH, Chen T, Liu N, Zhu Y, Tambi MI. Tongkat Ali as a potential herbal supplementation for physically active male and female seniors—a pilot study. Phytother Res 2014;28:544–50.

[107] National Dope Testing Laboratory. Laboratory report of selected athletes for doping dated 13th May 2017; 2017. New Delhi, India.

[108] Tambi MI, Imran MK, Henkel RR. Standardised water-soluble extract of *Eurycoma longifolia*, Tongkat Ali, as testosterone booster for managing men with late-onset hypogonadism? Andrologia 2012;44:226–30.

[109] Thu HE, Mohamed IN, Hussain Z, Jayusman PA, Shuid AN. *Eurycoma longifolia* as a potential adoptogen of male sexual health: a systematic review on clinical studies. Chin J Nat Med 2017;15(1):71–80.

[110] European Food Safety Authority (EFSA). Tracing seeds, in particular fenugreek (*Trigonella foenum-graecum*) seeds, in relation to the Shiga toxin-producing *E. coli* (STEC) O104: H4 2011 Outbreaks in Germany and France. EFSA Support Publ 2011;8(7):176E.

[111] Singh B, Gupta V, Bansal P, Singh R, Kumar D. Pharmacological potential of plants used as aphrodisiacs. Int J Pharm Sci Rev Res 2010;5(1):104–13.

[112] Singh R, Singh S, Jeyabalan G, Ali A. An overview on traditional medicinal plants as aphrodisiac agents. J Pharmacogn Phytother 2012;1(4):43–56.

Chapter 10

The status of integration of herbal medicines into modern clinical practice and possible development of the market

Samuel Ayodele Egieyeh and Elizabeth Oyebola Egieyeh

School of Pharmacy, University of the Western Cape, Cape Town, South Africa

1 Introduction

Universal health coverage, an overarching goal of the World Health Organization (WHO), is intended to ensure that all people and communities get equitable access to needed health services [1]. These include good quality preventive, promotional, curative, rehabilitative, and palliative health services [1]. The integration of complementary and traditional medicine which includes herbal medicine (HM) with conventional medicine (modern clinical practice (MCP)) is one of the strategic objectives of the WHO's Traditional Medicine Strategy 2014–2023 to promote universal health coverage [2]. Integration of HM into MCP will be a significant driver of the universal health coverage.

HMs (also referred to as phytomedicine or phytotherapy) may be referred to as naturally occurring, raw, and minimally processed substances from one or more plants that have been used to treat illness within local or regional cultural healing practices and currently used for its therapeutic or other human health benefits [3–5]. The substances used in HM are not limited to whole, fragmented, or cut plants but may include algae, fungi, and lichen in dried or fresh form [2, 3]. These herbal substances may be processed by extraction, distillation, expression, fractionation, purification, concentration, and fermentation into herbal or botanical preparations like tinctures, aqueous or alcoholic extracts, essential oils, expressed juices, and exudates.

Modern pharmaceutical formulation strategies are being used to process herbal preparations into standardized pharmaceutical dosage forms like liquid extracts, granules, powders, capsules and tablets, syrups, ointments, emulsions, nanoparticles, etc., for the global market [6]. In the succeeding sections, we examine the current status and factors that affect the integration of HM with MCP. Specifically, we highlight the process and context of integration, global market of HM, instances of integration of HM into MCP, discuss factors affecting the integration of HM into MCP, and finally propose strategies to improve the integration of HM into MCP.

2 The process and context of integration of HM into/with MCP

Integration is the action or process of integrating, i.e., adding parts to find the whole (integer). In the context under discussion, it may be considered as a process to combine, amalgamate, incorporate, unify, merge, and concatenate two different medicine philosophies. The difference in the paradigm of HM and MCP is not trivial and may mar the approach of amalgamating modern medicine to traditional HM even in cases where potential integration may be visible.

For example, efficacy takes on different meanings in the practice of HM and MCP. While the efficacy of conventional drugs in MCP can be measured by using defined parameters or symptoms, e.g., reduction in inflammation, cancer shrinkage, etc., the efficacy of HM may only be obvious over a long term, with parameters such as better health, reduction in symptoms, and restoration of healthy functions. In addition, this divergent paradigm may lead to a situation where HM is taken out of context and adapted to resemble modern medicine during the integration process. For example, HM uses whole plants, usually as unpurified extract containing multiple phytochemicals (polypharmacy) to treat "underlying causes" of multiple ailments and support the body's physiological system to recover from such ailments. As such, they may be more suitable for diseases with multiple factors, such as diabetes, Alzheimer's

Herbal Medicine in Andrology. https://doi.org/10.1016/B978-0-12-815565-3.00010-2

disease, and chronic fatigue. On the other hand, MCP use of HM (Western herbalism) emphasizes the effects of herbs on distinctive body systems, e.g., herbs may be used for their supposed expectorant, immune-stimulatory, antiinflammatory, or antispasmodic properties.

This raises the question: should we pursue collaboration instead of integration of HM and MCP in light of the divergent philosophies? Studies suggest, "integration requires collaboration as a precondition" [7, 8]. Hence, the starting point for integration of HM and MCP is a collaborative practice of both medicine philosophies. This is evidenced by the progress made in this regard by China, Vietnam, Korea, and India. Integration of HM and MCP has been achieved via integrated medical education and parallel practice of HM and MCP under one national health-care system. For example, significant progress has been made in China with regard to the integration of traditional Chinese medicine (TCM) into MCP via parallel practice (integrative medicine) [9, 10]. Significant attempts at the integration of HM and MCP have also been made by Western countries, such as the United States, Australia, and the European Union by the inclusion of courses on HM in conventional medical schools [11–13]. The establishment of agencies such as the US National Center for Complementary and Integrative Health (NCCIH) that take the lead in scientific research on complementary medicine (including HM) [14] also attest to integration of HM and MCP.

3 Current status of integration of HM with MCP

3.1 Global market analysis of herbal medicinal products

The popular use of HM in the form of complementary and alternative medicine (CAM) or phytomedicine in the last two to three decades has led to a multinational, multibillion-dollar industry. The global market share of HM is likely to reach USD 111 billion by the end of 2023 [15]. Market analysis reports show that the hospital and retail pharmacies sectors were major (55.82%) outlets for HM in 2017 [15]. Within the global market, HM may be classified into four products: herbal pharmaceuticals, herbal dietary supplements, herbal functional foods, and herbal beauty products.

Herbal dietary supplements are herbal preparations that are intended to supplement the diet. In terms of regulatory control, herbal dietary supplement may only make claims that the product affect the body's function and structure, e.g., Cranberry (*Vaccinium macrocarpon*) marketed as a herbal supplement may make the claim "cranberry juice support the health of the urinary tract" as opposed to "cranberry juice may be used to prevent and treat urinary tract infections (UTI)." The herbal pharmaceuticals and preparations have shown evidence of pharmacological activity possibly by interaction of the phytochemicals with proteins within biological systems.

Manufacturers of herbal pharmaceuticals may make health claims that their products can treat, diagnose, prevent, or cure minor or major diseases depending on the level of regulatory requirements that such products meet. For example, *Pygeum africanum* (African cherry) has been shown to have growth factor inhibitory, antiinflammatory, and antiandrogenic actions. The herbal pharmaceuticals class accounted for USD 50,972.4 million of the HM market in 2017 [16]. The growth in the HM may be attributed to the reliance on HM by a greater proportion of the populace (70%–80% of people globally rely on herbal sources) [16], primarily for chronic noncommunicable diseases such as diabetes, arthritis, cancer, sleep disorders, and digestive problems especially within the increasing aging population [17]. In addition, a rekindled interest in "whole person care" or holistic health care [18], perception that HMs are safe and have fewer side effects [19, 20], and mounting evidence from preclinical and clinical studies on various herbs to validate reported medicinal properties drives the herbal medicinal product global market. Moreover, the rising prices of conventional drugs and the limited health budgets for the modern medicinal system drive the consumers toward the more economical and safer HM [21].

3.2 Instances of integration of HM into MCP

It is noteworthy to mention that the consumers/patients are somewhat charting the course for "integration" of HM into modern medicine by "complementary" use of herbal products with modern medicinal products. A number of studies show that patients attending health facilities for modern medicine also actively use HM with or without the knowledge of their health practitioners [22]. This has progressively led to changes in government policies concerning HM. For example, in Switzerland the government has given homeopathy and traditional Chinese medicine the same status as conventional medicine [23]. This is a case of the consumers' preference affecting the government policy. Table 1 presents the status of the integration of HM into MCP in Ghana (Africa), China (Asia), and India (Asia). A few of the herbal medicinal products that are relevant to sexual dysfunction in males are listed in Table 2.

TABLE 1 A summary of the current status of the integration of herbal medicine (HM) into modern clinical practice (MCP) in Ghana, China, and India.

Country	Instances and progress
Ghana [22]	• In 2001, Trained Herbal Medical practitioners are licensed to consult and prescribe therapy as well as cause many side effects or adverse events. • National Health Policy for the integration of herbal medicine into mainstream health care established in 2005 • Traditional Medicine Practice Council (TMPC) set up after release of the 2nd edition of the Ghana Herbal Pharmacopoeia (GHP) in 2007. • In 2012, HM practice was officially integrated into the clinical practice (using 18 government facilities nationwide).
China [2]	• In China, Chinese herbalism (an aspect of Traditional Chinese medicine (TCM)) and conventional medicine are practiced alongside each other at every level of the health-care service • Public and private insurance cover available for both Chinese herbalism and modern clinical practice (conventional medicine). • About 440–700 health-care institutions providing Chinese herbalism services • Chinese herbalism is available at all levels of general hospitals, clinics, and health stations in urban and rural areas. • About 90% of general hospitals include a Chinese herbalism department and provide Chinese herbalism services for both outpatients and inpatients. • Public or patients are free to choose Chinese herbalism or conventional medicine for health-care services, or their doctors can provide advice on which therapies may be better suited to their health problems.
India [2]	• Ayurveda, Yoga, Naturopathy, Unani Medicine, Siddha, and Homeopathy all have official recognition • There are institutionalized education systems for these traditional medicine practices. • India has 508 colleges with an annual admission capacity of 25,586 undergraduate students • 117 of these colleges also admitting 2493 postgraduate students • Colleges can only be established with the permission of central government and the prior approval of their infrastructure, syllabi and course curricula. • Annual and surprise inspections ensure that educational and infrastructural standards are met. • Central Government has the power to recognize or rescind any qualification and college.

Integration may be achieved by parallel practice of HM and MCP and official educational system for HM.

TABLE 2 A few herbal medicinal products that have been formulated for commercial sale in conditions related to sexual dysfunction in males.

Herb or herbal extract	Dosage form of commercial product	Potential mechanism of action
Angelica sinensis ("female ginseng") [24]	Capsules and oil	Enhances nitric oxide synthases activity
Tribulus terrestris (Devil's-thorn, Devil's-weed, Puncture vine) [25, 26]	Capsules	Increases testosterone level
Kaempferia parviflora (Thai ginseng) [27]	Powder	Reduces intracellular Ca^{2+} concentration in corpus cavernosum
Panax notoginseng (Chinese ginseng) [28]	Capsule and liquid	Reduces oxidative stress

4 Factors affecting the integration of HM into MCP

4.1 Quality of herbal medicinal products

The quality of herbal medicinal products is related to the effectiveness and safety of the products. According to ISO 8402-1986 standard *quality* may be defined as "the totality of features and characteristics of a product or service that bears its ability to satisfy stated or implied needs (including satisfying the stated claim of efficacy and safety)" [29]. The quality of herbal medicinal products is fundamental to the assurance of their efficacy and safety. Unlike conventional medicinal products that have well-defined and documented quality parameters in pharmacopeias, the qualities of most herbal medicinal products may vary widely (e.g., nonuniformity of chemical constituents and physical quality parameters).

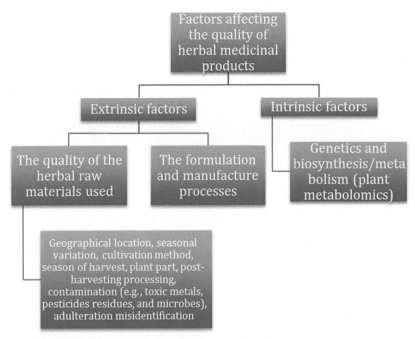

FIG. 1 Extrinsic and intrinsic factors that may affect the quality of herbal medicinal products.

A recent study on St. John's Wort (*Hypericum perforatum* L.) commercial products sold via the Internet, revealed significant compositional variation among the products [30]. This observation was attributed to adulteration with incorrect species (36%) and food dyes (19%). Another study showed that 33 out of 35 samples of *Ginkgo biloba* L. (Ginkgoaceae), an herbal product with a high economic value, contain elevated levels of rutin and quercetin, and low levels of Ginkgo metabolites [31]. These observations were attributed to poor extraction technique or deliberate adulteration (e.g., one product was adulterated with a 5-hydroxytryptophan derivative). Saffron (*Crocus sativus*), an expensive spice and medicinal plant, has also invited fraudulent behavior [32]. Aside deliberate or unintentional adulteration, the varying quality of herbal products may be due to a number of other extrinsic and intrinsic factors (see Fig. 1). In response to this challenge, the WHO has published various guidelines that address the issues regarding the herbal raw materials (WHO Guidelines on Good Agricultural and Collection Practices for medicinal plants) [5, 33] and herbal product manufacturing processes (WHO Guidelines on Good Manufacturing Practices (GMP) for Herbal Medicines) [34, 35].

In spite of the availability of these guidelines, some countries do not regulate herbal medicinal products at the same level as conventional drugs. For example, in the United States, most herbal medicinal products are marketed as dietary supplements under the jurisdiction of the Dietary Supplement Health and Education Act (DSHEA), thus preventing the US Food and Drug Administration from regulating them as strictly as conventional drugs with respect to their quality, efficacy, and safety. In contrast, HMs are regulated as conventional medicine and subject to required standards in Europe [36, 37]. Consequently, the quality of herbal medicinal product may vary within and among countries. The inconsistent quality of herbal medicinal products may discourage both practitioners and patients, thus limiting the effective integration of HM into MCP. Therefore, the regulatory agencies are saddled with the responsibility of assuring the consistency of the quality of herbal medicinal products, which can drive effective integration of HM into MCP.

4.2 Safety of herbal medicinal products

Efforts to integrate HMs into the MCP should take cognizance of the issues of adverse effects and drug-herb interactions because of their effect on human well-being and safety. HMs, in the public opinion, are generally perceived as safe (perhaps due to the venerable use by various cultures without reported adverse effects) though this may be a fallacy. Safety is a fundamental principle in the practice of HM and a critical component of its regulatory control. Adverse effects from HM may range from mild and frequent effects like gastrointestinal or dermatological reactions to severe and infrequent effects like kidney failure and liver damage (usually from contaminants like toxic chemicals or heavy metals, or harmful interactions with other drugs).

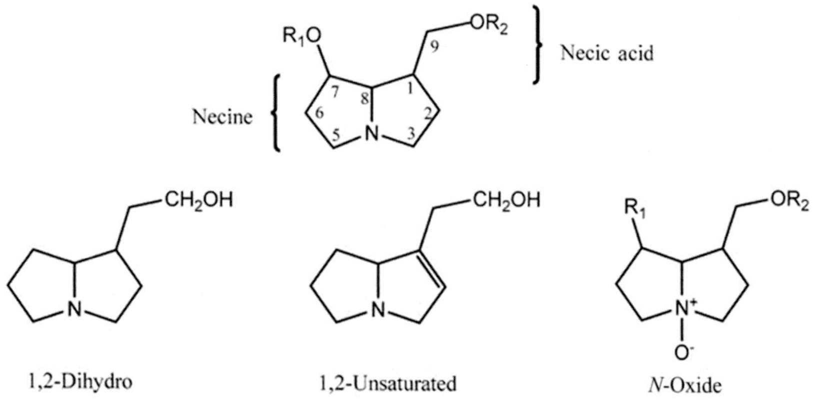

Necic acid

Necine

1,2-Dihydro   1,2-Unsaturated   N-Oxide

FIG. 2 Pyrrolizidine alkaloids with potential for hepatotoxicity (excluding the N-oxides and saturated pyrrolizidine alkaloids).

The regulatory body in Europe had drawn the attention of the public to the risk of hepatotoxicity from herbal medicinal products prepared from plants that contain pyrrolizidine alkaloids (Fig. 2) [38]. About half of the over 350 different pyrrolizidine alkaloids, excluding the N-oxides and saturated pyrrolizidine alkaloids, identified from over 300 plant species of up to 13 families, mainly in the families of Boraginaceae (all genera), Asteraceae (tribes Senecioneae and Eupatorieae) and Fabaceae (genus Crotalaria), are hepatotoxic [38–41].

Therefore, premarketing safety evaluation, including acute and chronic toxicity tests (e.g., immunotoxicity, genotoxicity, carcinogenicity, and reproductive toxicity), is required to assure the safety of herbal medicinal products. In addition, postmarketing surveillance that involves the inclusion of HMs in the pharmacovigilance system will significantly contribute to the identification of risks associated with the use of these products. Most important of which is the harmful HM-conventional medicine (drug) interactions that may lead to undesirable pharmacokinetic and pharmacodynamic effects [42, 43]. For example, concurrent use of herbal preparations containing *H. perforatum* (St. John's Wort) and digoxin, a drug used in cardiovascular conditions, has led to a significant reduction in effectiveness of digoxin [44, 45]. *H. perforatum* increases the metabolism of digoxin by inducing the metabolic enzymes, thus leading to a substantial reduction in the serum concentration of digoxin, often below the minimum effective concentration [44, 45]. A contrasting example was observed in the concomitant use of ginkgo (*G. biloba*) and the anticoagulant, warfarin, which leads to an enhancement in the anticoagulant effect of warfarin with an attendant increase risk of excessive bleeding [46].

Therefore, an unbiased attitude to increase knowledge in the safety profile of HM on the part of the conventional medicine practitioners and encouragement of disclosure of the use of HM by the patient to their health care providers will lead to safer clinical care for patients using both HM and conventional medicine. It should be noted that the current dearth of reported or documented adverse effects for these herbal medicinal products are not an absolute assurance of safety. Pharmacovigilance for herbal medicinal product is in its infancy and postmarket monitoring of these products presents unique challenges (depending on the prevailing regulatory system). National and international regulatory systems should enforce pre- and postmarket safety evaluation in order to promote a safe integration of efficacious HM into MCP.

4.3 Efficacy of herbal medicinal products

Efficacy may be referred to as a measure of the ability of an intervention (medicine) to produce the intended or claimed results (therapeutic effects). Most herbal medicinal products, especially those marketed as dietary supplements, health supplements, or food supplements, have little or no scientific documentation of their efficacy. Some have argued that for a valid scientific-based integration, it is important to demonstrate efficacy of HM (as it is done for conventional medicine) via pharmacological and clinical studies [47, 48]. The effectiveness of a number of HMs has been assessed (Table 3) using pharmacological and clinical studies.

Pharmacological and clinical evaluation approaches for the assessment of the efficacy of HM present a scientific justification for the integration of HM into MCP. The WHO has published guidelines for pharmacological and clinical evaluation of HM [5]. The reliability of the results from pharmacological and clinical evaluations depends on the quality of herbal medicinal products (in light of the various issues alluded to earlier) and the indicators used to assess the effectiveness of the HM (e.g., the choice of the pharmacological assays and clinical outcome parameters). The choice

TABLE 3 A few herbal medicines that have been investigated for specific indications.

Herbal medicine	Indications investigated	References
Garlic bulb (*Allium sativum* L.)	Antioxidant, antinematode, antimicrobial, antiproliferative	[49–51]
Horehound (*Marrubium vulgare*)	Antioxidant, antiinflammatory, antifungal	[52, 53]
Purple coneflower (*Echinacea purpurea*) root	For upper respiratory tract infection	[54–56]
Ginkgo leaf (*Ginkgo biloba*)	For dementia	[57, 58]
Ginseng root (*Panax ginseng*)	Antidiabetic	[59, 60]
Ginger (*Zingiber officinale*)	Antidysmenorrhea, antiemetic	[61, 62]

of the pharmacological assays (in vivo and/or in vitro studies), used prior to clinical studies, depends on the therapeutic claims of the herbal medicinal preparation available from the current practices by traditional health practitioners, from literature, or anecdotal evidences. Although it is important to establish a correlation of pharmacological activity with specific component(s) in the HM preparation (often referred to as active constituents), the synergistic effect among the components of such preparations to bring about the effect being assessed should not be overlooked.

Based on credible in vitro and/or in vivo pharmacological studies, herbal products may be evaluated with follow-up clinical studies (i.e., double blinded, placebo-controlled or multicenter clinical trials). Echoing this, the WHO has published a number of guidelines for clinical evaluation of the herbal products [5]. The robustness of the clinical outcome parameters measured in the clinical studies of herbal product is key to the deductions that may be drawn from such studies. Regardless of whether the clinical studies involve conventional medicine or HM, it is advocated that the Consolidated Standards of Reporting Trials (CONSORT) checklist [63, 64] including information on patient eligibility criteria, sample size calculation, objectives and hypotheses, statistical analysis, outcomes, etc., should be implemented. This will boost the acceptability of the conclusions from the clinical studies of herbal products by conventional medicine practitioners, because the efficacy measurements and outcomes used are objective, quantifiable, and based on conventional scientific principles, e.g., the reduction in a specific symptom(s) following the intervention of, usually, a single component conventional medicine. However, the foregoing did not take cognizance of the holistic concept and unique philosophy of HM.

In herbal medicinal practice, the patient is treated as an intact entity and given a product that is intended to support the natural innate ability of the body to heal and improve health over time. Hence, some subjective outcomes, including the percentage of patients with perceived benefits, patients "recovering" from the condition, and patients with improved quality of life are usually used as a measure of efficacy. Thus, assessment of efficacy using parameters that are based on conventional scientific principles put HM at an enormous disadvantage in comparison to conventional medicine during clinical studies.

Overall, it has been advocated that HMs should be subjected to the same evidence-based searchlight as conventional medicines with respect to safety, efficacy, and quality of the products [47, 48]. However, the disparity in the paradigm of HM and conventional medicine may make this a bigoted assessment of safety, efficacy, and quality. Therefore, expanding the knowledge base of herbal medicinal products, with due cognizance to the different cultures from which these products originated and evolved, will lead to design of relevant strategies to evaluate safety, efficacy, and quality of herbal medicinal products.

5 Conclusions

The 11th revision of the World Health Assembly Compendium, International Statistical Classification of Diseases and Related Health Problems (ICD-11), included the conditions related to traditional medicine in Chapter 26 [65, 66]. The inclusion of traditional medicine (including HM) in ICD-11 will further increase the accelerating proliferation of traditional medicine and related practices and eventually help them to integrate these practices into global modern health care [66]. WHO member states can follow-up this laudable development by implementing strategies that can drive integration of HM into MCP. Table 4 outlines a number of such strategies. However, the implementation of these strategies must not take HM out of context to resemble conventional/allopathic medicine.

TABLE 4 Proposed strategies that can drive integration of herbal medicine (HM) into modern clinical practice (MCP).

Strategies	Responsible persons or organizations
Develop a national policy and legislation for herbal medicine	Local and National Government, World Health Organization
Provide public funding for research on herbal medicine and health insurance for herbal medicine services	Local and National Government, Private sector
Develop and recognize a professional education for herbal medicine practitioners	Local and National Government
Encourage and recognize professional bodies or organizations for herbal medicine practitioners	Local and National Government
Improved regulation of herbal medicinal products and practices to assure safety and quality	Local and National Government, World Health Organization
Encourage the practice of herbal medicine by conventional medical practitioner	Local and National Government, World Health Organization

References

[1] Hogan DR, Stevens GA, Hosseinpoor AR, Boerma T. Monitoring universal health coverage within the Sustainable Development Goals: development and baseline data for an index of essential health services. Lancet Glob Health 2018;6(2):e152–68.

[2] Qi DZ. WHO traditional medicine strategy 2014-2023; 2015. p. 28.

[3] Alostad AH, Steinke DT, Schafheutle EI. International comparison of five herbal medicine registration systems to inform regulation development: United Kingdom, Germany, United States of America, United Arab Emirates and Kingdom of Bahrain. Pharm Med 2018;32(1):39–49.

[4] Ahmad Khan MS, Ahmad I. Herbal medicine: current trends and future prospects. In: Ahmad Khan MS, Ahmad I, Chattopadhyay D, editors. New look to phytomedicine. Academic Press; 2019. p. 3–13. [chapter 1, cited 2019 Jul 8] Available from: http://www.sciencedirect.com/science/article/pii/B978012814619400001X.

[5] Parveen A, Parveen B, Parveen R, Ahmad S. Challenges and guidelines for clinical trial of herbal drugs. J Pharm Bioallied Sci 2015;7(4):329–33.

[6] Byeon JC, Ahn JB, Jang WS, Lee S-E, Choi J-S, Park J-S. Recent formulation approaches to oral delivery of herbal medicines. J Pharm Investig 2019;49(1):17–26.

[7] Boon HS, Mior SA, Barnsley J, Ashbury FD, Haig R. The difference between integration and collaboration in patient care: results from key informant interviews working in multiprofessional health care teams. J Manipulative Physiol Ther 2009;32(9):715–22.

[8] Bångsbo A. Collaborative challenges in integrated care: Untangling the preconditions for collaboration and frail older people's participation. [cited 2019 Jul 8]. Available from: https://gupea.ub.gu.se/handle/2077/56888; 2018.

[9] Chen W, Li E, Zheng W. Policies on Chinese medicine in China may have enlightenments to complementary and alternative medicine in the world. Chin J Integr Med 2018;24(10):789–93.

[10] Griffiths S. Integrating traditional Chinese medicine: experiences from China. Australas Med J 2010;30:385–96.

[11] Chao MT, Adler SR. Integrative medicine and the imperative for health justice. J Altern Complement Med 2018;24(2):101–3.

[12] Micozzi MS. Fundamentals of complementary, alternative, and integrative medicine—E-book. Elsevier Health Sciences; 2018. 784 pp.

[13] Eckert M, Amarell C, Anheyer D, Cramer H, Dobos G. Integrative pediatrics: successful implementation of integrative medicine in a German hospital setting—concept and realization. Children 2018;5(9):122.

[14] NCCIH. NCCIH. [cited 2019 Jul 9]. Available from: https://nccih.nih.gov/.NCCIH. NCCIH. [cited 2019 Jul 9]. Available from: https://nccih.nih.gov/.

[15] Rickets Market Research Report—Forecast to 2023, MRFR. [cited 2019 Jul 9]. Available from: https://www.marketresearchfuture.com/sample_request/4671.Rickets Market Research Report—Forecast to 2023, MRFR. [cited 2019 Jul 9]. Available from: https://www.marketresearchfuture.com/sample_request/4671.

[16] Future trend of herbal medicine market 2018 scope—Reuters. [cited 2019 Jul 9]. Available from: https://www.reuters.com/brandfeatures/venture-capital/article?id=32992.Future trend of herbal medicine market 2018 scope—Reuters. [cited 2019 Jul 9]. Available from: https://www.reuters.com/brandfeatures/venture-capital/article?id=32992.

[17] Non communicable diseases. [cited 2019 Jul 9]. Available from: https://www.who.int/news-room/fact-sheets/detail/noncommunicable-diseases.Non communicable diseases. [cited 2019 Jul 9]. Available from: https://www.who.int/news-room/fact-sheets/detail/noncommunicable-diseases.

[18] Thomas H, Mitchell G, Rich J, Best M. Definition of whole person care in general practice in the English language literature: a systematic review. BMJ Open 2018. [cited 2019 Jul 9]. Available from: https://bmjopen.bmj.com/content/8/12/e023758.

[19] Msomi NZ, Simelane MBC. Herbal medicine. [cited 2019 Jul 9]. Available from: https://www.intechopen.com/books/herbal-medicine/herbal-medicine; 2018 Nov 5.

[20] Ekor M. The growing use of herbal medicines: issues relating to adverse reactions and challenges in monitoring safety. Front Pharmacol 2014;4. [cited 2019 Jul 9]. Available from: https://www.ncbi.nlm.nih.gov/pmc/articles/PMC3887317/.

[21] George A, Oluwatobi OS, Joseph B, Oluwatobi OS, Joseph B. Integrative pharmacology–Interconnecting the world of ayurveda (traditional Indian medicine–TIM), traditional Chinese medicine (TCM), and conventional medicine (CM). Holistic Healthcare; 2017. [cited 2019 Jul 10]. Available from: https://www.taylorfrancis.com/.

[22] Ameade EPK, Ibrahim M, Ibrahim HS, Habib RH, Gbedema SY. Concurrent use of herbal and orthodox medicines among residents of Tamale, Northern Ghana, who patronize hospitals and herbal clinics. Evid Based Complement Alternat Med 2018. [cited 2019 Jul 11]. Available from: https://www.hindawi.com/journals/ecam/2018/1289125/abs/.[23]Swiss to recognise homeopathy as legitimate medicine. SWI swissinfo.ch. [cited 2019 Jul 13]. Available from: https://www.swissinfo.ch/eng/society/complementary-therapies_swiss-to-recognise-homeopathy-as-legitimate-medicine/42053830.Swiss to recognise homeopathy as legitimate medicine. SWI swissinfo.ch. [cited 2019 Jul 13]. Available from: https://www.swissinfo.ch/eng/society/complementary-therapies_swiss-to-recognise-homeopathy-as-legitimate-medicine/42053830.

[24] Gong AGW, Lau KM, Zhang LML, Lin HQ, Dong TTX, Tsim KWK. Danggui Buxue tang, Chinese herbal decoction containing Astragali Radix and Angelicae Sinensis Radix, induces production of nitric oxide in endothelial cells: signaling mediated by phosphorylation of endothelial nitric oxide synthase. Planta Med 2016;82(5):418–23.

[25] Kamenov Z, Fileva S, Kalinov K, Jannini EA. Evaluation of the efficacy and safety of *Tribulus terrestris* in male sexual dysfunction—a prospective, randomized, double-blind, placebo-controlled clinical trial. Maturitas 2017;99:20–6.

[26] Roaiah MF, El Khayat YI, GamalEl Din SF, Abd El Salam MA. Pilot study on the effect of botanical medicine (*Tribulus terrestris*) on serum testosterone level and erectile function in aging males with partial androgen deficiency (PADAM). J Sex Marital Ther 2016;42(4). [cited 2019 Jul 13]. Available from: https://www.tandfonline.com/doi/abs/10.1080/0092623X.2015.1033579.

[27] Stein RA, Schmid K, Bolivar J, Swick AG, Joyal SV, Hirsh SP. *Kaempferia parviflora* ethanol extract improves self-assessed sexual health in men: a pilot study. J Integr Med 2018;16(4):249–54.

[28] Robinson TJ, Koontz BF. Role of oxidative stress in erectile dysfunction after prostate cancer therapy. In: Batinić-Haberle I, Rebouças JS, Spasojević I, editors. Redox-active therapeutics. Oxidative stress in applied basic research and clinical practice. Cham: Springer International Publishing; 2016. p. 499–508. doi:https://doi.org/10.1007/978-3-319-30705-3_21 [cited 2019 Jul 13].

[29] Hoyle D. ISO 9000 quality systems handbook-updated for the ISO 9001: 2015 standard: Increasing the quality of an organization's outputs. Routledge; 2017. [cited 2019 Jul 16]. Available from: https://www.taylorfrancis.com/books/9781315642192.

[30] Booker A, Agapouda A, Frommenwiler DA, Scotti F, Reich E, Heinrich M. St John's wort (*Hypericum perforatum*) products—an assessment of their authenticity and quality. Phytomedicine 2018;40:158–64.

[31] Booker A, Frommenwiler D, Reich E, Horsfield S, Heinrich M. Adulteration and poor quality of *Ginkgo biloba* supplements. J Herb Med 2016;6(2):79–87.

[32] Petrakis EA, Polissiou MG. Assessing saffron (*Crocus sativus* L.) adulteration with plant-derived adulterants by diffuse reflectance infrared Fourier transform spectroscopy coupled with chemometrics. Talanta 2017;162:558–66.[33]WHO guidelines on good agricultural and collection practices (GACP) for medicinal plants. 80.WHO guidelines on good agricultural and collection practices (GACP) for medicinal plants. 80.

[34] He T-T, Ung COL, Hu H, Wang Y-T. Good manufacturing practice (GMP) regulation of herbal medicine in comparative research: China GMP, cGMP, WHO-GMP, PIC/S and EU-GMP. Eur J Integr Med 2015;7(1):55–66.

[35] Ghosh D. Quality issues of herbal medicines: internal and external factors. Int J Complement Altern Med 2018;11(2). [cited 2019 Jul 16]. Available from: https://medcraveonline.com/IJCAM/IJCAM-11-00350.php.

[36] Santini A, Cammarata SM, Capone G, Ianaro A, Tenore GC, Pani L, et al. Nutraceuticals: opening the debate for a regulatory framework. Br J Clin Pharmacol 2018;84(4):659–72.

[37] Pereira C, Barros L, C. F.R. Ferreira I. Dietary supplements: foods, medicines, or both? A controversial designation with unspecific legislation. Curr Pharm Des 2017. [cited 2019 Jul 16]. Available from: https://www.ingentaconnect.com/contentone/ben/cpd/2017/00000023/00000019/art00003.

[38] Ma C, Liu Y, Zhu L, Ji H, Song X, Guo H, et al. Determination and regulation of hepatotoxic pyrrolizidine alkaloids in food: a critical review of recent research. Food Chem Toxicol 2018;119:50–60.

[39] Mulder PPJ, López P, Castelari M, Bodi D, Ronczka S, Preiss-Weigert A, et al. Occurrence of pyrrolizidine alkaloids in animal- and plant-derived food: results of a survey across Europe. Food Addit Contam A 2018;35(1):118–33.

[40] Tamariz J, Burgueño-Tapia E, Vázquez MA, Delgado F. Pyrrolizidine alkaloids. In: Knölker H-J, editor. The alkaloids: Chemistry and biology. Academic Press; 2018. p. 1–314. [chapter 1, cited 2019 Jul 16]. Available from: http://www.sciencedirect.com/science/article/pii/S1099483118300130.

[41] Letsyo E, Jerz G, Winterhalter P, Beuerle T. Toxic pyrrolizidine alkaloids in herbal medicines commonly used in Ghana. J Ethnopharmacol 2017;202:154–61.

[42] Gupta RC, Chang D, Nammi S, Bensoussan A, Bilinski K, Roufogalis BD. Interactions between antidiabetic drugs and herbs: an overview of mechanisms of action and clinical implications. Diabetol Metab Syndr 2017;9(1):59.

[43] Mehmood Z, Khan MS, Qais FA, Samreen, Ahmad I. Herb and modern drug interactions: efficacy, quality, and safety aspects. In: Ahmad Khan MS, Ahmad I, Chattopadhyay D, editors. New look to phytomedicine. Academic Press; 2019. p. 503–20. [chapter 18, cited 2019 Jul 16]. Available from: http://www.sciencedirect.com/science/article/pii/B9780128146194000197.

[44] Greener M. The hidden problem of herb-drug interactions. Prescriber 2016;27(9):22–7.

[45] Chrubasik-Hausmann S, Vlachojannis J, McLachlan AJ. Understanding drug interactions with St John's wort (*Hypericum perforatum* L.): impact of hyperforin content. J Pharm Pharmacol 2019. Wiley Online Library. [cited 2019 Jul 16]. Available from: https://onlinelibrary.wiley.com/doi/full/10.1111/jphp.12858.

[46] Choi S, Oh D-S, Jerng UM. A systematic review of the pharmacokinetic and pharmacodynamic interactions of herbal medicine with warfarin. PLoS ONE 2017;12(8):e0182794.

[47] Firenzuoli F, Gori L. Herbal medicine today: clinical and research issues. Evid Based Complement Alternat Med 2007;4(Suppl. 1):37–40.

[48] Mutua DN, Juma KK, Munene M, Njagi EN. Safety, efficacy, regulations and bioethics in herbal medicines research and practice. J Clin Res Bioeth 2016;7(3). [cited 2019 Jul 16]. Available from: https://www.omicsonline.org/open-access/safety-efficacy-regulations-and-bioethics-in-herbal-medicines-research-and-practice-2155-9627-1000270.php?aid=72665.

[49] Fratianni F, Ombra MN, Cozzolino A, Riccardi R, Spigno P, Tremonte P, et al. Phenolic constituents, antioxidant, antimicrobial and anti-proliferative activities of different endemic Italian varieties of garlic (*Allium sativum* L.). J Funct Foods 2016;21:240–8.

[50] Mohammadi KHH, Heidarpour M, Borji H. *Allium sativum* methanolic extract (garlic) improve therapeutic efficacy of albendazole against hydatid cyst: in vivo study. J Invest Surg 2018;32(8):1–8.

[51] Mahmoudvand H, Sepahvand P, Jahanbakhsh S, Azadpour M. Evaluation of the antileishmanial and cytotoxic effects of various extracts of garlic (*Allium sativum*) on *Leishmania tropica*. J Parasit Dis 2016;40(2):423–6.

[52] Namoune I, Khettal B, Assaf AM, Elhayek S, Arrar L. Antioxidant and anti-inflammatory activities of organic and aqueous extracts of northeast Algerian *Marrubium vulgare*. Phytothérapie 2018;16(S1):S119–29.

[53] Akbari Z, Dastan D, Maghsood AH, Fallah M, Matini M. Investigation of *in vitro* efficacy of *Marrubium vulgare* L. essential oil and extracts against *Trichomonas vaginalis*. Zahedan J Res Med Sci 2018;20(9). [cited 2019 Jul 16]. Available from: http://zjrms.com/en/articles/67003.html.

[54] Schapowal A, Klein P, Johnston SL. Echinacea reduces the risk of recurrent respiratory tract infections and complications: a meta-analysis of randomized controlled trials. Adv Ther 2015;32(3):187–200.

[55] Ross SM. *Echinacea purpurea*: a proprietary extract of *Echinacea purpurea* is shown to be safe and effective in the prevention of the common cold. Holist Nurs Pract 2016;30(1):54.

[56] Daneshmehr MA, Tafazoli A. Providing evidence for use of Echinacea supplements in Hajj pilgrims for management of respiratory tract infections. Complement Ther Clin Pract 2016;23:40–5.

[57] von Gunten A, Schlaefke S, Überla K. Efficacy of *Ginkgo biloba* extract EGb 761® in dementia with behavioural and psychological symptoms: a systematic review. World J Biol Psychiatry 2016;17(8):622–33.

[58] Yuan Q, Wang C, Shi J, Lin Z. Effects of *Ginkgo biloba* on dementia: an overview of systematic reviews. J Ethnopharmacol 2017;195:1–9.

[59] Choi HS, Kim S, Kim MJ, Kim M-S, Kim J, Park C-W, et al. Efficacy and safety of *Panax ginseng* berry extract on glycemic control: a 12-wk randomized, double-blind, and placebo-controlled clinical trial. J Ginseng Res 2018;42(1):90–7.[60]The efficacy of ginseng-related therapies in type 2 diabetes mellitus. [cited 2019 Jul 16]. Available from: https://www.ncbi.nlm.nih.gov/pmc/articles/PMC4753873/.The efficacy of ginseng-related therapies in type 2 diabetes mellitus. [cited 2019 Jul 16]. Available from: https://www.ncbi.nlm.nih.gov/pmc/articles/PMC4753873/.

[61] Chen CX, Barrett B, Kwekkeboom KL. Efficacy of oral ginger (*Zingiber officinale*) for dysmenorrhea: a systematic review and meta-analysis. Evid Based Complement Alternat Med 2016. [cited 2019 Jul 16]. Available from: https://www.hindawi.com/journals/ecam/2016/6295737/abs/.

[62] Soltani E, Jangjoo A, Afzal Aghaei M, Dalili A. Effects of preoperative administration of ginger (*Zingiber officinale* Roscoe) on postoperative nausea and vomiting after laparoscopic cholecystectomy. J Tradit Complement Med 2018;8(3):387–90.

[63] Schulz KF, Altman DG, Moher D, the CONSORT Group. CONSORT 2010 statement: updated guidelines for reporting parallel group randomised trials. BMC Med 2010. [cited 2019 Jul 16]. Available from: https://bmcmedicine.biomedcentral.com/articles/10.1186/1741-7015-8-18?report=reader.

[64] Pandis N, Chung B, Scherer RW, Elbourne D, Altman DG. CONSORT 2010 statement: extension checklist for reporting within person randomised trials. Br J Dermatol 2019. Wiley Online Library. [cited 2019 Jul 16]. Available from: https://onlinelibrary.wiley.com/doi/full/10.1111/bjd.17239.[65]ICD-11—Mortality and morbidity statistics. [cited 2019 Jul 17]. Available from: https://icd.who.int/browse11/l-m/en#/http%3a%2f%2fid.who.int%2ficd%2fentity%2f718687701.ICD-11—Mortality and morbidity statistics. [cited 2019 Jul 17]. Available from: https://icd.who.int/browse11/l-m/en#/http%3a%2f%2fid.who.int%2ficd%2fentity%2f718687701.

[66] Cyranoski D. Why Chinese medicine is heading for clinics around the world. Nature 2018;561:448.

Index

Note: Page numbers followed by *f* indicate figures and *t* indicate tables.

Printed in the United States
By Bookmasters